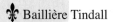 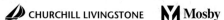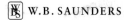

Electrotherapy: Evidence-Based Practice

For Churchill Livingstone:

Editorial Director, Health Professions: Mary Law
Project Development Manager: Mairi McCubbin
Project Manager: Alison Ashmore
Design Direction: George Ajayi/Judith Wright
Illustrator (new figures for 11e): Graeme Chambers

Electrotherapy: Evidence-Based Practice

Edited by

Sheila Kitchen MSc PhD DipTP MCSP
Head, Division of Physiotherapy,
King's College London, London, UK

In consultation with

Sarah Bazin MCSP
Director of Therapy Services, Department of Physiotherapy,
Solihull Hospital, Solihull, UK

ELEVENTH EDITION

(Previous edition entitled *Clayton's Electrotherapy*)

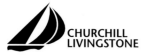

CHURCHILL
LIVINGSTONE

EDINBURGH LONDON NEW YORK PHILADELPHIA ST LOUIS SYDNEY TORONTO 2002

CHURCHILL LIVINGSTONE
An imprint of Harcourt Publishers Limited

First published 1948 as *Clayton's Electrotherapy and Actinotherapy*
Eighth edition 1981 as *Clayton's Electrotherapy*
Ninth edition 1985 as *Clayton's Electrotherapy*
Tenth edition 1996 as *Clayton's Electrotherapy*
Eleventh edition 2002

ISBN 0 443 07216 7

British Library Cataloguing in Publication Data
A catalogue record for this book is available from the British Library

Library of Congress Cataloging in Publication Data
A catalog record for this book is available from the Library of
Congress

Note
The publisher, the editors, The University of Melbourne as licensee
and the contributors to this work do not assume any responsibility for
any injury and/or damage to persons or property arising out of or
related to any use of the material contained in the book and CD-ROM.
It is the responsibility of the student or the practitioner to determine
the best treatment and method of application for the patient. Medical
knowledge is constantly changing. The editors, contributors, The
University of Melbourne as licensee and publishers have taken care to
ensure that the information given in this text and CD-ROM is accurate
and up-to-date. However, readers are strongly advised to confirm that
the information, especially with regard to drug usage and the use of
equipment, complies with the latest legislation and standards of practice as well as with the recommendations of the manufacturers of any
equipment involved.

The
publisher's
policy is to use
**paper manufactured
from sustainable forests**

Printed in China by RDC Group Limited

Contents

The CD-ROM accompanying this text includes simulations that may assist readers in understanding concepts presented in the text. These are indicated in the text by the following symbol ⊙.
The CD-ROM is designed to be used in conjunction with the text and not as a stand-alone teaching aid.

Contributors

Kate Ballard BSc(Hons) RGN
Clinical Nurse Specialist, Tissue Viability Unit,
Guy's Nuffield House, London, UK

Sarah Bazin MCSP
Director of Therapy Services, Department of
Physiotherapy, Solihull Hospital, Solihull, UK

David Baxter TD BSc(Hons) DPhil MCSP
Head of School of Rehabilitation Sciences,
University of Ulster, Jordanstown, UK

Sara Carroll BAppSc MSc
Senior Lecturer, Director of Research, School of
Physiotherapy, Curtin University of Technology,
Perth, Australia

Robert A. Charman DipTP MCSP FCSP
Lecturer in Physiotherapy, Department of
Physiotherapy Education, University of Wales
College of Medicine, Cardiff, UK

Brian Diffey BSc AKC PhD DSc FInstP FIPEM
Head of Regional Medical Physics Department,
Professor of Medical Physics, Professor of
Photobiology, Newcastle General Hospital,
Newcastle upon Tyne, UK

Mary Dyson BSc PhD LHD(Hon) FCSP(Hon)
Director of Dyderm Ltd; Executive
Vice-President of Longport Inc.; Emeritus
Reader in the Biology of Tissue Repair at King's
College London, London, UK; Visiting Professor,
University of Kansas, Kansas City, USA

Peter Farr MD FRCP
Consultant Dermatologist, Department of
Dermatology, Royal Victoria Infirmary,
Newcastle upon Tyne, UK

Tracey Howe MSc PhD GradDipPhys CertEd MCSP
Director, Postgraduate Institute for Health,
School of Health, University of Teesside,
Teesside, UK

Mark Johnson BSc(Hons) PhD
Principal Lecturer in Human Physiology,
Leeds Metropolitan University, Leeds, UK

Sheila Kitchen MSc PhD DipTP MCSP
Head, Division of Physiotherapy,
King's College London, London, UK

Denis Martin BSc(Hons) MSc DPhil
Assistant Director, Scottish Network for
Chronic Pain Research, Department of
Physiotherapy, Queen Margaret University
College, Edinburgh, UK

Stephen Martin BAppSc
Research Fellow in Online Learning, Deputy
Director of the Technology Unit, School of
Physiotherapy, Faculty of Medicine, Dentistry
and Health Sciences, University of Melbourne,
Parkville, Australia

Suzanne McDonough BPhysio(Hons) PhD
Lecturer in Rehabilitation Sciences, School of
Rehabilitation Sciences, University of Ulster,
Newtownabbey, UK

Joan McMeeken BSc(Hons) MSc DipPhysio MAPA
Professor and Head of School of Physiotherapy,
Faculty of Medicine, Dentistry and Health
Sciences, University of Melbourne, Parkville,
Australia

Shea Palmer BSc(Hons)
Lecturer in Physiotherapy, Department of
Physiotherapy, Queen Margaret University
College, Edinburgh, UK

Oona Scott PhD MCSP
Reader, Department of Rehabilitation
Sciences, University of East London,
London, UK

Shona Scott MSc MCSP
Lecturer, School of Life Sciences, Napier
University, Edinburgh, UK

Barry Stillman PhD DipPhysio MAPA MCSP FACP
School of Physiotherapy, Faculty of Medicine,
Dentistry and Health Sciences, University of
Melbourne, Parkville, Australia

Gail ter Haar MSc DSc PhD
Head of Therapeutic Ultrasound, Royal
Marsden Hospital, Sutton, UK

Margaret Trevor BSc(Hons) MSc CEng MIEE MIPEM
ILTM
Senior Lecturer in Medical Imaging, School of
Health, University of Teesside, Teesside, UK

Tim Watson BSc(Hons) PhD MCSP
Head of Department of Physiotherapy,
University of Hertfordshire, Hatfield, UK

Leslie Wood BSc PhD
Senior Lecturer in Physiology, School of
Biological and Biomedical Sciences, Glasgow
Caledonian University, Glasgow, UK

Steve Young PhD
Director, Tissue Viability Unit, Guy's Nuffield
House, London, UK

Preface

Electrotherapy has been one of the key skills of the physiotherapy profession from its earliest inception, with the use of heat, cold and electrical stimulation having a long history in clinical practice. Recent years have seen the addition of a number of other treatment agents to the repertoire. Despite this history, and its continued wide usage, both the physical and physiological principles underlying its use are still often misunderstood and the evidence for its efficacy—or otherwise—often not taken into account in daily practice.

This text, which has been revised and extended by a large number of experts in the field, is designed to provide the reader with up-to-date knowledge of the most commonly used agents. It has been expanded to take into account recent developments in research, and to enhance certain aspects which had limited coverage in the last edition of *Clayton's Electrotherapy*. It simultaneously provides the student with information about the safe and appropriate application of treatments, whilst avoiding the 'cookbook' approach, which inhibits informed clinical decision making. In a new venture, a CD-ROM is provided with this text with a number of interactive tasks related to the use of many of the agents. It is hoped that this will be both useful and fun for those reading the book!

The change in title for this text—*Electrotherapy: Evidence-Based Practice*—is designed to reflect the strong emphasis placed on the need to practise therapeutic techniques in the light of a solid and informed knowledge base. Watson (2000) draws attention to the importance of the role of knowledge and evidence in clinical decision making. He notes that both the quantity and quality of that evidence are steadily improving and provides a useful model for decision making in electrotherapy. It is essential that we learn from the underlying theory (both physical and physiological) and research evidence, as well as reflecting on our experience in clinical practice. This material may then be used to select suitable treatment for individuals for whom we have identified clear therapeutic aims. The decision-making model illustrated (Fig. 1) shows the interrelationship between theory, learning, clinical decision making and clinical effects, and has been developed by Watson (2000).

The editor wishes to thank all the contributors, who come from a wide variety of specialist fields and are experts in their areas, for their work and their determination to deliver accessible and well-informed information.

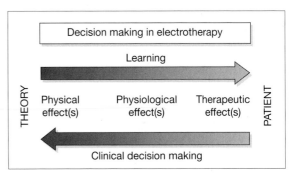

Figure 1 A bidirectional model of electrotherapy (Watson, 2000).

Credit should also go to Kenneth Collins, for his work in the last edition, in Chapter 6. Thanks are also expressed to the producers and editors of the interactive material, and to the publishers, who have provided continued support throughout the project.

REFERENCE

Watson, T (2000) The role of physiotherapy in contemporary physiotherapy practice. *Manual Therapy* **5**(3): 132–141.

Scientific background

1

Electrophysical and thermal principles

Gail ter Haar

INTRODUCTION

Electrophysical agents are used by physiotherapists to treat a wide variety of conditions. These agents include both electromagnetic and sound waves, in addition to muscle- and nerve-stimulating currents. In part, these techniques are used to induce tissue heating. This chapter contains, in simple terms, an introduction to the effects of heat on tissue and the basic physics necessary for the understanding of the remainder of the book. The electrical properties of cells and the implications for electrotherapy are described in Chapter 2.

For centuries, early philosophers have speculated on the nature of heat and cold. Opinions have been divided as to whether heat was a substance or an effect of the motion of particles, but in the eighteenth century, physicists and physical chemists came to the conclusion that what gave our senses the impression of heat or cold was the speed of motion of the constituent molecules within the body or object. The accurate investigation of the relationship between the work done in driving an apparatus designed to churn water, and the heat developed while doing so, was taken up by Dr JP Joule of Manchester in the year 1840. He showed quite clearly that the amount of heat produced by friction depended on the amount of work done. Subsequently, his work also contributed to the theory of the correlation of forces, and in 1847 he stated the law of the conservation of energy (the basis of the first law of thermodynamics).

It became the accepted view that heat can be regarded as a form of energy, which is interchangeable with other forms such as electrical or mechanical energy. The theory supposed that, when a body is heated, the rise in temperature is due to the increased energy of motion of molecules in that body. The theory went further, and explained the transmission of radiant energy from one body to another, as from the sun to an individual on earth. Evidence was found in favour of the supposition that light is an electromagnetic wave, and exactly the same evidence was adduced with regard to radiant energy. Apart from the fact that radiant heat waves (e.g. infrared radiations) have a longer wavelength than light waves, their physical characteristics are the same. It was therefore suggested that molecules of a hot body are in a state of rapid vibration, or are the centre of rapid periodic disturbances, producing electromagnetic waves, and that these waves travel between the hot body and the receiving body causing a similar motion in the molecules. The sense of heat may thus be excited in an organism by waves of radiant heat energy which start from a hot object, just as the sense of sight is excited by waves of light which start from a luminous object.

An understanding of wave motion is central to getting to grips with the physics of any form of therapy that uses either electrical or mechanical energy. A general description of wave motion therefore precedes more detailed treatment of electricity and magnetism, and of ultrasound.

WAVE MOTION

Wave motion transfers energy from one place to another. Think of a cork floating in a pond into which a stone is dropped. Ripples move out from where the stone enters the water, and some of the stone's energy is transferred to the pond's edge. The cork bobs up and down, but does not move within the pond.

An easy way to demonstrate wave motion is to use a Slinky spring toy. Two types of wave exist: *transverse waves*, which can be mimicked by raising and lowering one end of the spring rapidly, as shown in Figure 1.1, and *longitudinal*

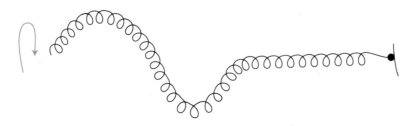

Transverse wave

Figure 1.1 If a spring that is attached at one end is flicked up and down, a transverse wave is produced.

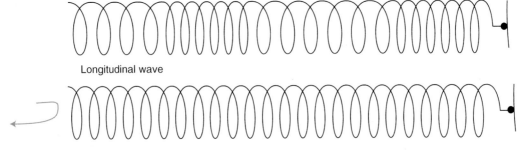

Longitudinal wave

Unstretched spring

Figure 1.2 Extending a spring along its length and letting it go again produces a longitudinal wave.

waves, which can be demonstrated by extending the spring along its length and then letting it go (Fig. 1.2). Water waves, the motion of a violin string, and electromagnetic waves, as used in short-wave diathermy, infrared and interferential current therapy, are examples of transverse waves. Sound, as used in ultrasound therapy, propagates mainly as longitudinal waves.

It is much more difficult to picture a longitudinal wave than a transverse wave. If the spring with the wave travelling down it (Fig. 1.2) is compared with an unstretched spring, some regions can be seen where the coils are closer together, and other regions where the coils are further apart. The part of the spring where the coils are closely spaced is called a region of *compression*, and the region where they are separated further apart, is termed a region of *rarefaction*.

Waves on the sea are generally described in terms of peaks and troughs. The movement up to a wave crest, down to a trough, and back up to the crest again is known as a *cycle of oscillation*. A cork floating in the sea bobs up and down as the waves go past. The difference in height of the cork between a crest and a trough is twice the *amplitude*. Perhaps a simpler way of visualising the amplitude is as the difference in water height above the seabed between a flat, calm sea and the crest of the wave. The number of wave crests passing the cork in a second is the wave *frequency* (*f*). Frequency is measured in *hertz* (Hz), where 1 Hz is 1 cycle/second. The time that elapses between two adjacent wave crests passing the cork is the *period* (*τ*) of the oscillation. This has units of time; if each cycle takes *τ* seconds, there must be $1/\tau$ cycles in each second. The number of cycles that occur in a second has already been defined as the frequency, and so can be written as follows:

$$f = 1/\tau, \quad \text{or} \qquad [1]$$
$$\tau = 1/f. \qquad [2]$$

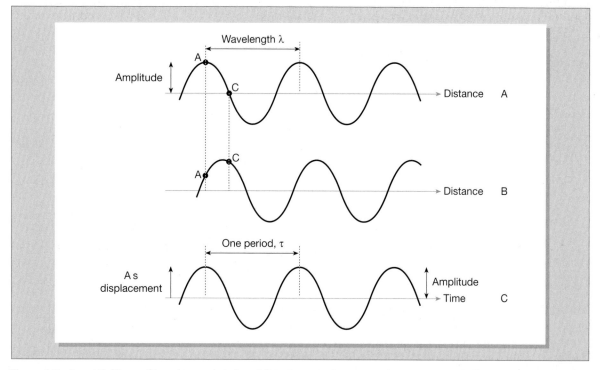

Figure 1.3 A and B: The position of two points A and C in the path of a wave as it passes through. The displacements shown are frozen at two different times, between which the wave has moved on a fraction of a wavelength. C: The displacement of the point during two cycles.

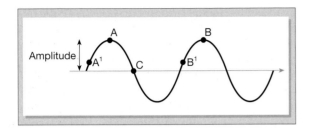

Figure 1.4 Points A and B, and also A¹ and B¹, are always in the same relative position in the wave. They are in phase. Points A and C are out of phase.

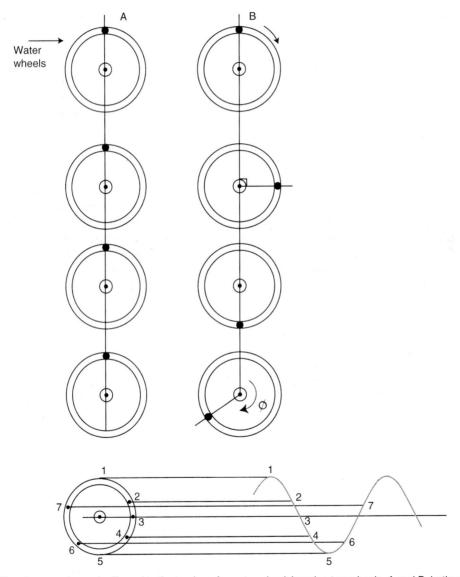

Figure 1.5 The phase angle can be likened to the turning of a water wheel. Imagine two wheels, A and B, both with a mark on their rim. A does not move, but B turns, and as it does the rim mark executes the circles, each complete turn representing one *cycle*. The angle through which the mark turns in one cycle is 360° (2π radians). Thus, for example, compared with A, when the mark on B's rim has moved around a quarter of a turn (cycle), the angle between the two marks is a quarter of 360° (90° or π/2 radians); after half a turn the angle between the two marks is 180° or π radians. This angle between the two marks is analagous to the *phase difference*. As B rotates, the height of the mark above the wheel's hub varies. If the wheel turns at a constant speed, then the mark's height traces out a *sine wave* when plotted against time.

The distance between two adjacent wave crests is the *wavelength* (λ).

Figure 1.3A and B shows a wave frozen at two moments, a short time apart. It can be seen that the different points on the wave have changed position relative to the central line, but have not moved in space. In fact, if you tracked the motion of point A over several periods, the movement up and down would look like the picture shown in Figure 1.3C. The speed at which the wave crests move is known as the wave *speed*. Since the wave moves a wavelength (λ) in one cycle, and one cycle takes a time equal to the period τ, then the wave speed (c) is given by the equation:

$$c = \lambda / t. \qquad [3]$$

It is known that $1/t$ is the same as the frequency f, and so

$$c = f\lambda. \qquad [4]$$

In Figure 1.4, points A and B on the wave (or A^1 and B^1) are moving in the same way and will reach the crest (or trough) together. These points are said to be in *phase* with each other. The movement from A to B (or A^1 to B^1) represents one cycle of the wave motion. A and C are not in phase; C is a quarter of a cycle ahead of A and they are said to have a *phase difference* (ϕ) of a quarter cycle. Phase is usually expressed as an angle, where a complete cycle is 2π radians (or 360°). A quarter cycle therefore represents a phase difference of $\pi/2$ radians (90°). This is illustrated in Figure 1.5.

Reflection and refraction of waves

When waves travelling through a medium arrive at the surface of a second medium some of the energy is reflected back into the first medium, and some of the energy is transmitted through into the second medium. The proportion of the total energy that is reflected is determined by the properties of the two media involved. Figure 1.6 shows what happens when waves are reflected by a flat (plane) surface. An imaginary line that is perpendicular to the surface is called the *normal*. The *law of reflection* states that the angle between the incident (incoming) wave and the normal is always equal to the angle between the reflected wave and the normal. If the incident wave is at normal incidence, the wave is reflected back along its path.

The waves that are transmitted into the second medium may also undergo *refraction*. This is the bending of light towards the normal when it travels from one medium into one in which the wave speed is lower, or away from the normal when the wave speed in the second medium is higher. This is shown in Figure 1.7. For example, light bends towards the normal as it enters water from air since it travels more slowly in water than in air, and so a swimming pool may appear shallower than it really is.

As has been discussed earlier, waves carry energy. There are conditions, however, under which the transport of energy can be stopped, and the energy can be localised. This happens in a *standing (stationary) wave*. A standing wave is produced when an incident wave meets a

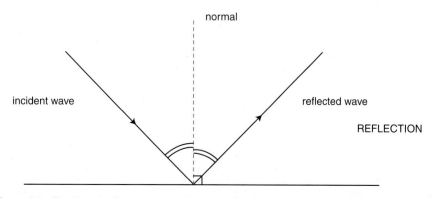

Figure 1.6 The law of reflection states that the angle of incidence equals the angle of reflection.

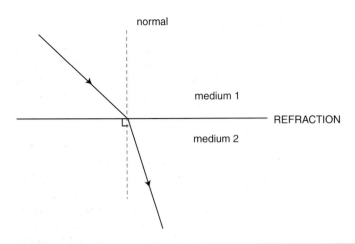

Figure 1.7 When a beam passes from one medium to another, it may be refracted (i.e. it changes its direction).

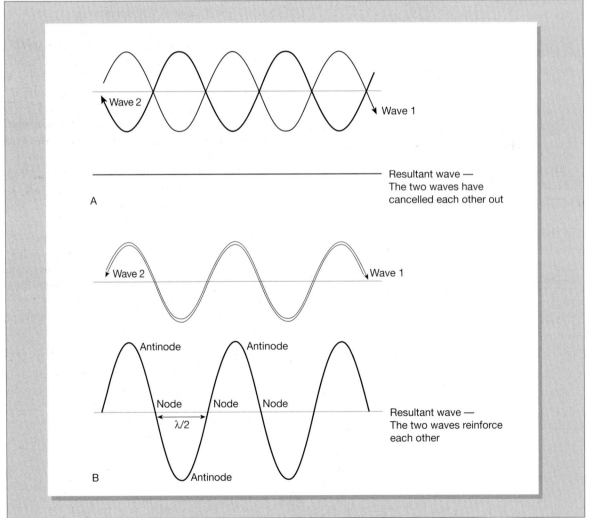

Figure 1.8 A standing wave is formed when two waves of equal amplitude travelling in opposite directions meet. A: The two waves cancel each other out. B: The two waves add to reinforce each other.

returning reflected wave with the same amplitude. When the two waves meet, the total amplitude is the sum of the two individual amplitudes. Thus, as can be seen in Figure 1.8A, if the trough of one wave coincides with the crest of the other, the two waves cancel each other out. If, however, the crest of one meets the crest of the other, the wave motion is reinforced (Fig. 1.8B) and the total amplitude doubles. In the reinforced standing wave there are points that always have zero amplitude; these are called *nodes*. Similarly, there are points that always have the greatest amplitude, and these are called *antinodes*. Nodes and antinodes are shown in Figure 1.8B. The distance between adjacent nodes, or adjacent antinodes, is one-half of the wavelength.

Polarisation

In flicking the Slinky spring up and down to produce a transverse wave, one has an infinite number of choices as to which direction to move it, so long as the motion is at right angles to the line of the spring. If the spring is always moved in a fixed direction, the wave is said to be *polarised*—the waves are in that plane only. However, if the waves (or directions in which the spring is moved) are in a number of different directions, the waves are *unpolarised*. It is possible to polarise the waves by passing them through a filter that allows only waves that are in one plane to pass through. This can be visualised by envisaging a piece of card with a long narrow slit in it. This will allow the waves formed in the plane of the slit to go through, but no others—the card therefore acts as a polarising filter.

ELECTRICITY AND MAGNETISM

All are familiar with effects of electrical charges even if all are not aware of their causes. The 'static' experienced when brushing newly-washed hair or undressing and the electrical discharge obvious in lightning are examples of the effects of charges.

Electricity

Matter is made up of atoms, an atom being the smallest particle of an element that can be identified as being from that element. The atom is made up of a positively charged central nucleus (made up of positively charged *protons* and uncharged *neutrons*), with negatively charged particles (*electrons*) orbiting around it, resembling a miniature solar system. An atom contains as many protons as there are electrons, and so has no net charge. If this balance is destroyed, the atom has a non-zero net charge and is called an *ion*. If an electron is removed from the atom it becomes a *positive ion*, and if an electron is added the atom becomes a *negative ion*.

Two particles of opposite charge attract each other, and two particles of the same charge repel each other (push each other away). Hence, an electron and a proton are attracted to each other, whereas two electrons repel each other.

The unit of charge is a *coulomb* (C). An electron has a charge of 1.6×10^{-19} C, so it takes a very large number (6.2×10^{18}) of electrons to make up one coulomb.

The force between two particles of charge q_1 and q_2 is proportional to the product of q_1 and q_2 ($q_1 \times q_2$), and inversely proportional to the distance between them (d) squared (Fig. 1.9). Thus, the force is proportional to $q_1 q_2 / d^2$. The constant of proportionality (i.e. the invariant number) necessary to allow one to calculate the force between two charges is $1/4\pi\varepsilon$, where ε is the *permittivity* of the medium containing the two charges:

$$F = q_1 q_2 / 4\pi\varepsilon d^2 \qquad [5]$$

If one of the charges is negative, then the force is attractive. If the particles are in a vacuum, the permittivity used is ε_0; this is known as the *permittivity of free space*. For a medium other than a vacuum, the permittivity is often quoted as a multiple of ε_0, where the multiplying factor, κ,

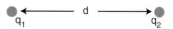

Figure 1.9 Two particles of charge q_1 and q_2 a distance of d apart experience a force between them that is proportional to $q_1 q_2 / d^2$.

is known as the *relative permittivity* or *dielectric constant*. So:

$$\varepsilon = \kappa \varepsilon_0, \quad \text{or} \quad [6a]$$

$$\kappa = \varepsilon/\varepsilon_0. \quad [6b]$$

Electric fields

An *electric field* exists around any charged particle. If a smaller charge that is free to move is placed in the field, the paths it will move along are called *lines of force* (or *field lines*). Examples of fields and their patterns are shown in Figure 1.10.

The *electric field strength, E,* is defined as the force per unit charge on a particle placed in the field. A little thought shows that $E = F/q$, where F is the force and q is the particle's charge. The units used to describe E are newtons/coulomb (N/C).

If E is the same throughout a field, it is said to be uniform. In this case, the field lines are parallel to each other as shown in Figure 1.10D. If a charged particle is moved in this field, work is done on it, unless it moves perpendicular to the field lines. This is somewhat analogous to moving a ball around on Earth. If the ball is always kept at the same height, and moved

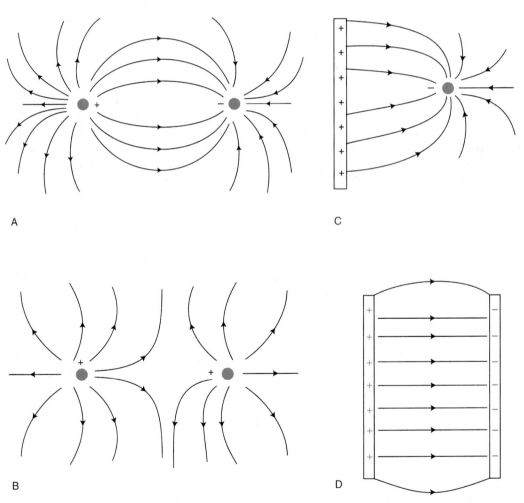

Figure 1.10 Examples of electric fields near charged particles and plates. A: Field between two particles of equal and opposite charges. B: Field between two positively charged particles. C: Field between a charged particle and an oppositely charged plate. D: Field between two oppositely charged plates.

horizontally, its potential energy remains constant. If the ball is raised or lowered, its potential energy is changed. The ball has no potential energy when it lies on the ground. In a non-uniform field where the lines are not parallel, moving a charged particle always results in a change of potential energy. The *electric potential*, V, is defined as the potential energy per unit charge of a positively charged particle placed at that point. Electric potential is measured in units of *volts*. Since the position at which the electric potential energy is zero is taken as infinity, another way of thinking of the electrical potential at a point is as the work done in moving the charge to that point from infinity. In practice it is easier to compare the electrical potential at two points in the field than to consider infinity. The difference in the work required to move a charge from infinity to a point, A, and that required to move it to another point, B, is called the *potential difference* (p.d.) between the two points; this is also measured in *volts*. The p.d. is best thought of as a kind of pressure difference. Between the two points there will be a gradient in potential (just as there is a pressure gradient between the top and bottom of a waterfall). This gradient is described in units of volts/metre. In a uniform field between parallel plates with potential difference V, and separation d, the potential gradient is given by V/d. If a particle of charge q is moved from one plate to another, the work done is qV. Work is force × distance, and so the force, F, is given by:

$$F = qV/d.\qquad [7]$$

Since the electric field strength, E, is given by:

$$E = F/q,\qquad [8]$$

it follows that:

$$E = V/d.\qquad [9]$$

Remember that V/d is the potential gradient. From this equation we can see that the electric field strength can be increased by bringing the two plates closer together. Although the derivation is more complicated, the electric field strength at any point in a non-uniform field can

also be shown to be the same as the potential gradient at that point.

Any electric circuit needs a supply of power to drive the electrons around the conductors. A power source has one positive and one negative terminal, and the source forces the electrons out from its negative terminal. Electrical energy can be produced within the source by a number of means. Dynamos convert mechanical energy into electrical energy, solar cells convert the sun's energy into electrical energy, and batteries convert chemical energy into electrical energy. The force acting on the electrons is called the *electromotive force* (e.m.f.). This is defined as the electrical energy produced per unit charge inside the source. The unit in which e.m.f. is measured is the volt, because 1 volt is 1 joule/coulomb.

Electric current

An *electric current* is the flow of electric charge (usually electrons). In some materials (e.g. metals) where the atoms are bound into a lattice structure, the charge is carried by electrons. In materials in which the atoms are free to move, the charge is carried by ions. A liquid in which the ions are the charge carriers is called an *electrolyte*. An *insulator* is a material that has no free charge carriers, and so is unable to carry an electric current. Current is measured using an ammeter, and the unit in which it is given is the *ampere*. An ampere represents 1 coulomb of charge flowing through a point in 1 second.

There are two types of electric current. A *direct current* (DC) is one in which the flow of electrons is in one direction only, and an *alternating current* (AC) is one in which the current flows first one way and then another. In considering electric circuits, it is easiest to think first of direct currents. A later section points to the differences between AC and DC circuits.

Resistance and Ohm's law

The flow of electric charge through a conductor is analogous to the flow of water through pipes. If water is pumped round the system, narrow pipes put up more resistance to flow than wide ones. Electrical conductors also put up a *resistance* to the flow of charge. As the charged particles move through a conductor they collide with other charge carriers and with the resident atoms; the constituents of the conductor thus impede the current flow.

Georg Ohm was able to demonstrate that the current flowing in a circuit is proportional to the potential difference across it. His law (*Ohm's law*), formally stated, is:

The current flowing through a metallic conductor is proportional to the potential difference that exists across it, provided that all physical conditions remain constant.

So, $I \propto V$; this can also be written as $V \propto I$, where the constant of proportionality is the *resistance*. The equation resulting from Ohm's law is therefore:

$$V = IR. \tag{10}$$

R is measured in ohms (Ω). The ohm is defined as the resistance of a body such that a 1 volt potential difference across the body results in a current of 1 ampere through it.

The resistance of a piece of wire increases with its length, and decreases as its cross-sectional area increases. A property called *resistivity* is defined which is a property of the material only, and not of the material's shape. The resistance R of a piece of wire with resistivity ρ, length L and area A is given by:

$$R = \rho L / A. \tag{11}$$

When electrons flow through a conductor, they collide with the atoms in the conductor material and impart energy to those atoms. This leads to heating of the conductor. The unit used for measuring energy is the *joule*. It has been seen earlier (see equation 7) that the potential difference measured in volts is the work done in moving a unit charge between two points. So it follows from this that since the potential difference is the work done per unit charge:

$$\text{volt} = \text{joule/coulomb}, \tag{12a}$$

and so:

$$\text{joule} = \text{volt coulomb}. \tag{12b}$$

The unit of power measurement is the *watt*. Power is the rate of doing work, so a watt is a joule/second. It follows from the equation above that:

$$1 \text{ watt} = 1 \text{ joule/second} \tag{13a}$$

$$= 1 \text{ volt coulomb/second}. \tag{13b}$$

From the definition given it is known that a coulomb/second is an ampere. So, therefore:

$$1 \text{ watt} = 1 \text{ volt.ampere}. \tag{14}$$

In other words, the electrical power developed in a circuit is given by:

$$\text{power} = VI, \tag{15}$$

where V is in volts, I is in amperes, and the power is in watts.

From Ohm's law substitutions can be made in this equation to express power in terms of different combinations of V, I and R. So:

$$W = VI, \tag{16a}$$

$$W = I^2 R, \tag{16b}$$

$$W = V^2 / R, \tag{16c}$$

are equivalent equations, where W is in watts, V is in volts and R is in ohms.

Capacitance

Any passive device capable of storing electric charge is called a *capacitor*. This is the electrical equivalent of a compressed spring, which stores energy until it is allowed to expand. A capacitor stores charge until it can release it by becoming part of a completed electrical circuit. If you apply an electric potential, V, between two plates of a capacitor, one plate becomes positively charged and the other becomes charged with an equal but opposite negative charge. If an insulating material known as a *dielectric* is placed between the plates, the capacity to store charge is increased. The *relative permittivity*, or *dielectric constant* mentioned earlier has another definition: it is also the ratio of the charge that can be stored between two plates with a dielectric material between them, to that which can be stored without the dielectric.

A capacitor is drawn in a circuit diagram as a pair of vertical parallel lines. Its *capacitance, C*, is defined as the charge (Q) stored per unit potential difference across its plates.

$$C = Q/V. \qquad [17]$$

Since Q is measured in coulombs, and V is measured in volts, the unit for capacitance is the coulomb/volt, known as the *farad*. Commonly, the capacitance of a capacitor found in an electric circuit is a few micro- (10^{-6}) or pico- (10^{-12}) farads.

A capacitor is *charged* by applying a potential difference across its plates. It is *discharged* (i.e. the charge is allowed to flow away from the plates) by providing an electrical connection between the plates.

Electric circuits

The symbols used to denote different components used in electrical circuits are shown in Figure 1.11.

Two electrical components are said to be in *series* if they carry the same current. The potential difference across a series of components is the sum of the potential differences across each one. The components are in *parallel* if they have the same potential difference across them. The current is then the sum of the currents flowing through them.

Resistors in series. If several resistors are joined in series with each other, the same current flows through them all since electrons cannot be lost on the way through. From Ohm's law, the potential, V_i, across each resistance in Figure 1.12A, is given by:

$$V_i = IR_i. \qquad [18]$$

If the total potential across the whole string is V, then:

$$V = V_1 + V_2 + V_3 + \cdots + V_i. \qquad [19]$$

So:

$$V = IR_1 + IR_2 + IR_3 + \cdots + IR_i$$
$$= I[R_1 + R_2 + R_3 + \cdots + R_i]. \qquad [20]$$

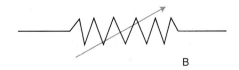

A

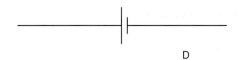

B

C

D

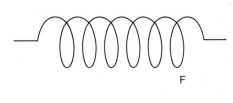

E

F

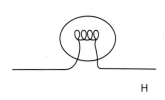

G

H

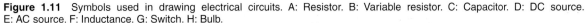

Figure 1.11   Symbols used in drawing electrical circuits. A: Resistor. B: Variable resistor. C: Capacitor. D: DC source. E: AC source. F: Inductance. G: Switch. H: Bulb.

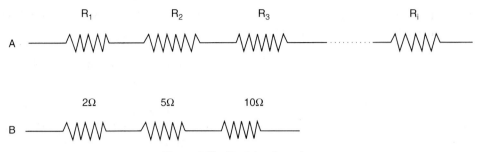

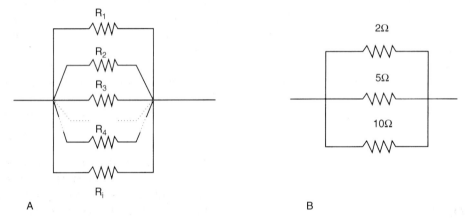

Figure 1.12 Resistors in series.

Figure 1.13 Resistors in parallel.

Thus the single resistance needed to have the same effect as the string of resistors, R_{total}, is the sum of all the resistances:

$$R_{total} = R_1 + R_2 + R_3 + \cdots + R_i. \qquad [21]$$

For example, in the string shown in Figure 1.12B, the total resistance R_{total}, is $2+5+10\,\Omega = 17\,\Omega$.

Resistors in parallel. Resistors may also be wired up in parallel, as shown in Figure 1.13A. The electron flow splits up at A, electrons taking different routes to B where they join up again. The total flow of current through all resistors, I, is the same as the sum of the currents through each resistor:

$$I = I_1 + I_2 + I_3 + \cdots + I_i. \qquad [22]$$

The potential difference across each resistor is identical. Using Ohm's law in the above equation, we can write:

$$I = V/R_1 + V/R_2 + V/R_3 + \cdots + V/R_i$$
$$= V[1/R_1 + 1/R_2 + 1/R_3 + \cdots + 1/R_i]. \qquad [23]$$

Therefore the single resistance that could replace these parallel resistors has a value:

$$1/R_{total} = 1/R_1 + 1/R_2 + 1/R_3 + \cdots + 1/R_i. \qquad [24]$$

For example, if three resistors of 2, 5 and $10\,\Omega$ are in parallel, as shown in Figure 1.13B, the equivalent resistor to replace these is $1/(1/2+1/5+1/10)$, which is $1/(0.5+0.2+0.1)= 1/0.8 = 1.25\,\Omega$.

Capacitors in series. A voltage applied across four capacitors in series induces charges of $+Q$ and $-Q$ on the plates of each (Fig. 1.14). Using equation 17 we know that:

$$1/C = V/Q.$$

The potential difference across the series row is the sum of the potentials across each capacitor,

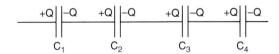

Figure 1.14 Capacitors in series.

and so the single capacitance, C, equivalent to the four capacitors C_1, C_2, C_3 and C_4 is given by:

$$1/C = [V_1+V_2+V_3+V_4]/Q \qquad [25]$$
$$= V_1/Q+V_2/Q+V_3/Q+V_4/Q$$
$$= 1/C_1+1/C_2+1/C_3+1/C_4. \qquad [26]$$

If the capacitances are 2, 1, 5 and $10\,\mu\text{F}$, then $C = 0.56\,\mu\text{F}$.

Capacitors in parallel. If capacitors are connected in parallel as shown in Figure 1.15, the total charge developed on them is the sum of the charges on each of them. The current is never negative. The potential difference is the same across all the capacitors.

The effective capacitance of all the capacitors put together is given by the expression:

$$C = Q/V,$$

where:

$$Q = Q_1+Q_2+Q_3+Q_4,$$

and so:

$$C = Q_1/V+Q_2/V+Q_3/V+Q_4/V \qquad [27]$$
$$= C_1+C_2+C_3+C_4. \qquad [28]$$

If the capacitances are 1, 2, 5 and $10\,\mu\text{F}$, then C is $18\,\mu\text{F}$.

Direct and alternating current. As discussed earlier, two types of electric current exist: direct current (DC) and alternating current (AC). The most common type of alternating current has a sinusoidal waveform, such as that found in the electricity mains. For sinusoidal AC, the relationships between frequency and period, etc., defined in the first section hold true. The variation of

current can be described by the relationship:

$$I = I_0 \sin [2\pi ft], \qquad [29]$$

and, similarly, the voltage is described by:

$$V = V_0 \sin [2\pi ft], \qquad [30]$$

where $\sin [2\pi ft]$ is the expression which tells you that the wave form is a sine wave of frequency f, and I_0 and V_0 are the maximum values of current and voltage (the amplitude of the oscillation). Clearly, the average current over one cycle in Figure 1.16 is zero—the current is positive as much as it is negative—and the same applies to the voltage.

In some instances, an alternating current may be *rectified*, as shown in Figure 1.16B and C. Here, the average current is clearly not zero. For *half-wave rectification*, the average current is $0.318I_0$, and for *full-wave rectification* the average current is $0.636I_0$.

If an alternating current flows through a resistor the average current is zero, but the heating effect is not. On each pass through the resistor, the electrons heat it slightly, whatever the direction of flow. Clearly, despite the zero net current, some energy is expended in the circuit, and an *effective current* is defined to account for this. The effective current (also known as the *root mean square (RMS) current*, I_{RMS}), is the value of the constant current that if allowed to flow for the same length of time would expend the same amount of electrical energy for a fixed voltage as the alternating current. An *effective voltage (root mean square (RMS) voltage*, V_{RMS}) is defined in a similar way as the constant voltage that, if present for the same length of time, would expend the same amount of electrical energy for a fixed voltage as the alternating voltage.

From equation 16 the power, W, in DC circuits is given by:

$$W = VI,$$

where W is in watts, V is in volts, and I is in amperes. Similarly, in an AC circuit:

$$W = V_{RMS}I_{RMS} \qquad [31]$$

Ohm's law can be used if the effective currents and voltages are used. Thus the power may also

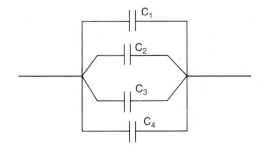

Figure 1.15 Capacitors in parallel.

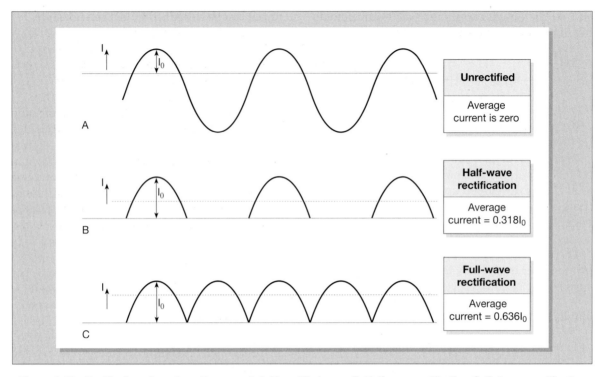

Figure 1.16 Rectification of an alternating current. A: Unrectified wave. B: Half-wave rectification. C: Full-wave rectification.

be written:

$$W = I_{eff}^2 R,$$ [32]

or

$$W = V_{eff}^2 / R.$$ [33]

It can be shown that $I_{eff} = I_0/\sqrt{2} = 0.707I_0$ and that $V_{eff} = V_0/\sqrt{2} = 0.707V_0$.

Capacitors allow alternating currents to flow. The resistance across capacitor plates is known as *impedance* (Z). This is defined as the ratio of the amplitudes of the voltage and current in the same way as resistance is given by V/R for direct current. It can be shown that:

$$Z = 1/\omega C,$$ [34]

where C is the capacitance and ω (the *angular frequency*) $= 2\pi f$.

Magnetism

Most of us have used a compass, and know that the needle swings around to point North–South.

The compass is a permanent bar magnet that aligns itself with the earth's magnetic field.

There are two magnetic poles: the North and the South pole. In many ways, the two poles of a magnet act in the same way as opposite electric charges. Like magnetic poles repel each other, and unlike poles attract. There is a force between two magnets a distance d apart from each other, and the equation describing this force is very similar to that in equation 5:

$$F = m_1 m_2 / 4\pi\mu d^2.$$ [35]

Here, μ is the *permeability* of the medium, μ_0 (the permeability of free space) is used when the magnets lie in a vacuum. The strength of a magnet is measured in units of *webers* (Wb). The unit of permeability is the *henry/metre* (H/m). *Relative permeability*, μ_r, is defined by the relationship:

$$\mu_r = \mu/\mu_0.$$ [36]

A *magnetic field* exists at a point if a small magnet put there experiences a force. It will line up along the *magnetic field lines*. The fields around some permanent magnets are shown in Figure 1.17.

The number of magnetic lines of force passing through an area, *A*, is known as the *magnetic flux* (*N*). The magnetic flux going through a unit area that is aligned perpendicular to the field is the *magnetic flux density* (*B*). Magnetic flux density is measured in units of *teslas* (T); 1 tesla = 1 Wb/m^2.

Electromagnetism

Wires carrying an electric current produce magnetic fields around them. The magnetic field around a long straight wire forms a series of concentric circles with the wire at their centre. A solenoid (i.e. a coil of wire) creates a field somewhat similar to that produced by a permanent bar magnet, the main difference being that there is a uniform field inside it. This uniformity of field is used to advantage in short-wave diathermy applications. Figure 1.18 illustrates these fields.

Electromagnetic spectrum. Light is a form of electromagnetic radiation. It can be split up into its different component parts using a prism, with each colour of the 'rainbow' having a different wavelength. Electromagnetic waves are

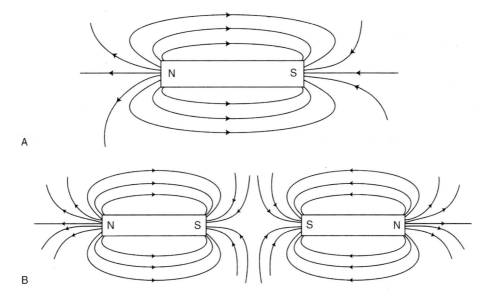

Figure 1.17 A: Magnetic field around a single permanent bar magnet. B: Magnetic field around two bar magnets.

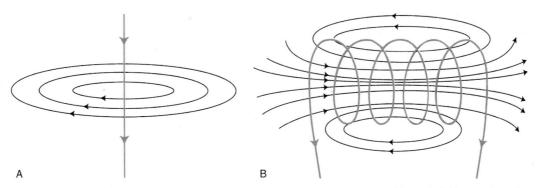

Figure 1.18 A: Magnetic field around a long straight wire carrying an electric current. B: Magnetic field around a coil carrying an electric current.

electrical and magnetic fields that travel together through space without the need for a carrier medium (Fig. 1.19). They travel at a speed of 3×10^8 m/s in a vacuum. There is a whole spectrum of such waves of which light is only a small part. Other radiations in the electromagnetic spectrum include radio waves, microwaves and X-rays; the spectrum is shown in Figure 1.20. The behaviour of electromagnetic radiation can be usefully described, not only in terms of wave motion, but also in terms of 'particles'. It can be thought of as discrete 'packets' of energy and momentum, sometimes referred to as *quanta*. The energy in joules of a quantum of radiation is determined by its frequency, and is given by the equation:

$$E = h\nu, \qquad [37]$$

where ν is the frequency, and h is *Planck's constant* ($h = 6.62 \times 10^{-34}$ Js). It is more usual to quote electromagnetic energies in *electron-volts* (eV); $1\,\text{eV} = 1.6 \times 1.10^{-13}$ J. It can be seen from Figure 1.20 that energies in the long-wavelength end of the spectrum are very small. It is generally thought that energies in excess of 30 eV are required to ionise atoms, and so this allows the spectrum to be classified into two bands: ionising and non-ionising radiation.

The wavelength of the radiation determines the size of objects with which it will interact. A wave with a wavelength of 100 m (a radio wave) will not 'see' something of the size of an atom and will pass by undisturbed. However, a wave with a wavelength of 10^{-12} m (a gamma ray) will interact with the atomic nucleus, with which it has a comparable size. Infrared radiation has a wavelength comparable to the size of atoms or molecules and so can interact with them, imparting kinetic energy (heat).

Electromagnetic induction. The dynamo on a bicycle wheel that is used to power the bicycle's lights makes use of electromagnetic induction. Electromagnetic induction is in many ways the reverse of electromagnetism. When a magnet and a conducting wire move relative to one another, a current is induced in the wire. In the bicycle wheel, a magnet is made to rotate near a fixed coil of wire which forms part of a circuit that includes the lamp bulb. Current is induced in the wire, and the lamp is lit.

The electrons in the wire approaching (or being approached by) a magnetic field experience a force as they enter the field. All of the electrons are displaced towards one end of the wire, so that end becomes negatively charged. Conversely, the other end takes up a positive charge. Therefore an electromotive force is induced between the two ends, and, if the circuit is completed, a current will flow. If the wire is coiled, the induced current is increased. A coil of conducting wire used in this way is called an *inductor*. The e.m.f. induced in the conductor

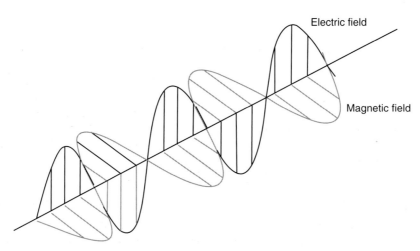

Figure 1.19 An electromagnetic wave; the electric and magnetic fields travel together.

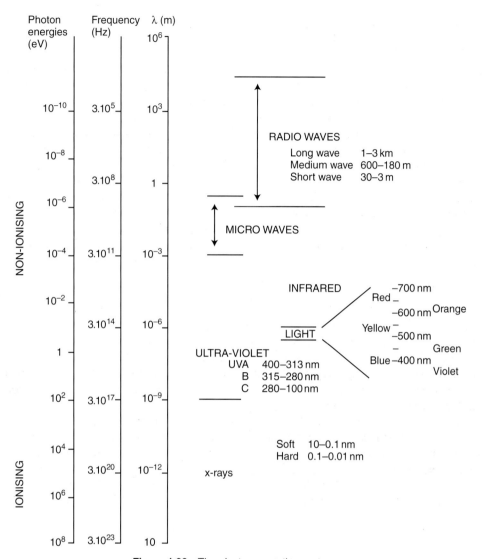

Figure 1.20 The electromagnetic spectrum.

equals the rate of change of flux linkage—this is *Faraday's law* of electromagnetic induction. The direction of the induced current is always such that it opposes the change which caused it—*Lenz's law*. In this sense, inductors act as resistances in circuits; they are often used to block changing voltages while allowing steady (DC) voltages through.

An inductor (L) and capacitor (C) are sometimes used in series or parallel to produce *LC-tuned circuits* (Fig. 1.21). It can be shown that these circuits have a resonant frequency, *f*, such that,

series LC-tuned circuits offer a very low impedance to waves of that frequency, but an extremely high impedance to everything else, whereas parallel LC-tuned circuits offer a very high resistance to waves of frequency *f* and allow other frequencies through. They therefore act as filters. The resonant frequency is given by the equation:

$$f = 1/2\pi r(LC).$$ [38]

Mutual induction. A changing magnetic field from a current-carrying conductor can induce an e.m.f. and current in a second conductor nearby.

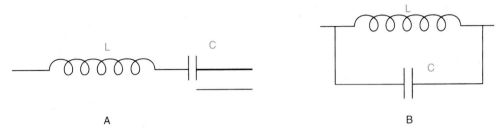

Figure 1.21 LC-tuned circuits. A: Series LC circuit. B: Parallel LC circuit.

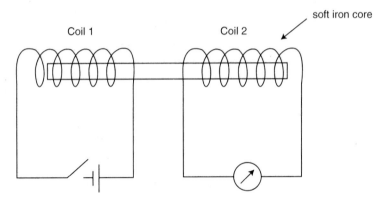

Figure 1.22 Mutual induction. The changing magnetic field in one coil can induce a current in a second coil. The magnetic field thus created will create a current in the first coil. A soft iron core enhances this effect.

This current will vary, and in its turn can produce its own varying magnetic field that induces an e.m.f. and current in the first conductor. Each conductor therefore induces a current in the other (Fig. 1.22). This is called *mutual inductance*. The mutual inductance is 1 henry if 1 volt is induced in one conductor by a current change of 1 ampere per second in the other. An AC transformer makes use of mutual inductance.

Self-inductance. When a current is switched on in a coil, the growing current in the coil causes a change in magnetic flux in the coil. This, in turn, causes an e.m.f. that opposes the e.m.f. of the battery. This is called a *back e.m.f.* This effect is increased if there is a soft iron core in the coil.

A conductor has a self-inductance of 1 henry if a back e.m.f. of 1 volt is induced by a changing current of 1 ampere/second.

MECHANICAL WAVES

The most important mechanical wave used in physiotherapy is ultrasound. Sound waves differ from electromagnetic waves in one major way: the waves are a form of *mechanical energy*, and as such cannot propagate through a vacuum. This is because energy passes through a medium by the movement of molecules, which transfer their momentum in the direction of the wave. Sound is produced by a moving surface; this may be a diaphragm in a loudspeaker, for example, or a transducer front face in medical ultrasound. As the surface moves forward, it *compresses* the molecules immediately in front. These molecules in turn push forward against their neighbours in an attempt to restore their former arrangement, and these in turn push their neighbours. The compression therefore moves away from its source. If the surface now moves in the opposite direction, the density of the molecules is reduced next to it (a region of *rarefaction* is created), and so molecules move in to fill the space. This in turn leaves a low-density region which is immediately filled by more molecules, and so the rarefaction moves away from the source. This has been illustrated in Figure 1.23.

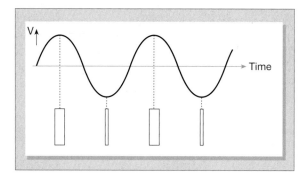

Figure 1.23 The piezoelectric effect. The crystal gets fatter and thinner, depending on the polarity of the voltage.

This type of wave is called a *longitudinal wave* because the displacement of the molecules is along the direction in which the wave moves.

Ultrasound

The velocity of sound in air is 330 m/s. The human ear can hear frequencies up to about 18 000 Hz (18 kHz). The wavelength of audible sound (calculated using equation 4) where the ear is most sensitive (about 1.6 kHz) is about 20 cm. At ultrasonic frequencies (above 18 kHz), the wavelength becomes so short that the sound does not travel far through air. (At 1.5 MHz, the wavelength is about 0.2 mm.) However, ultrasound will travel through water, a medium for which the sound velocity is 1500 m/s. At 1.5 MHz the wavelength in water is 1 mm. This fact is used in medicine since most body tissues are comprised mainly of water, and the millimetre wavelengths at the low megahertz frequencies used (0.75–10 MHz) are comparable with the size of the tissue structures with which interaction is required.

Ultrasound is generated from a *transducer.* A transducer is a device that transforms one form of energy into another. The transducer most commonly used in ultrasound changes electrical energy into mechanical energy using the *piezoelectric effect.* A piezoelectric crystal has the property that if a voltage is applied across it, it will change its thickness, and alternatively if the crystal thickness is changed then a voltage develops across the crystal (this is the

inverse piezoelectric effect). Thus, if an oscillating voltage is applied across the crystal it will alternately get thicker and thinner than its resting thickness, following the polarity of the voltage (Fig. 1.23). As the front face of the transducer moves backwards and forwards, regions of compression and rarefaction move out from it, forming an ultrasonic wave. The piezoelectric material most commonly used for physiotherapy transducers is lead zirconate titanate (PZT).

The voltage across the ultrasound transducer may either be applied continuously over the whole treatment time (*continuous wave*, CW), or may be applied in bursts—on for a time, off for a time, and so on; this is known as *pulsed mode.* The wave trains for a continuous wave and a pulsed mode are shown in Figure 1.24.

In the pulsed mode, the pulsing regimen may be described in one of three ways (Fig. 1.24B):

1. x seconds on; y seconds off
2. $m : s$, where m represents the 'mark' and s represents the 'space', where the ratio represents that of the on time to the off time; this is called the *mark : space ratio.* So, if x is twice y, $m : s$ is $2 : 1$. In order to discover the true pulsing regime, it is also necessary to know the pulse length
3. the *duty cycle*: this is the pulse length as a percentage of the total on and off time, so it is given by $x/(x + y) \times 100\%$.

Take, for example, a common pulsing regimen as shown in Figure 1.25. This may be described as 2 ms on : 8 ms off, as 1 : 4 mark : space ratio, pulse length 2 ms, or as a 20% ($2/10 \times 100\%$) duty cycle. It is worth noting that, at 1 MHz, a pulse of length 2 ms contains 2000 cycles.

Intensity

The energy in an ultrasound wave is characterised by *intensity.* This is the energy crossing a unit area perpendicular to the wave in unit time; the units used are *watts/m²*. However, for clinical applications, the square metre is an inappropriately large area in terms of regions of the human

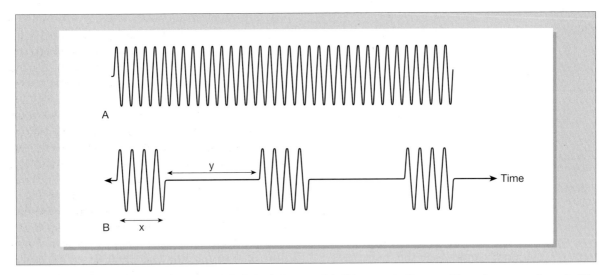

Figure 1.24 A: Continuous wave ultrasound. B: Pulsed ultrasound. In this example, the sound is on for *x* seconds, and off for *y* seconds.

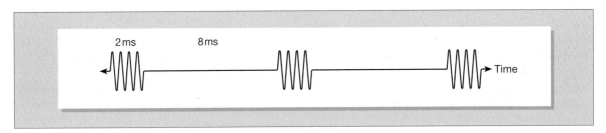

Figure 1.25 A typical physiotherapy pulsing regimen.

body to be treated, and so the unit used in medical ultrasound is watts/cm².

Several types of intensity are used to describe ultrasound exposures. The field from a circular piezoelectric disc is complex. Near the transducer there are many peaks and troughs, but as the beam moves further from the transducer the field pattern becomes more uniform. The region near the transducer is known as the *near field* or *Fresnel zone*; the region beyond that is called the *far field* or *Fraunhoffer zone*. The boundary between the two zones is at a distance given by r^2/λ where r is the transducer radius and λ is the wavelength of the ultrasound. This is the position of the peak of intensity on the beam axis that is furthest from the transducer. Physiotherapy ultrasound commonly operates at 0.75, 1.0, 1.5 or 3 MHz. The extent of the near field is

shown in Table 1.1 for a number of frequencies and transducer sizes. This demonstrates that most physiotherapy ultrasound exposures are carried out in the near field, which has many peaks of intensity. It also indicates that a number of intensities need to be identified.

The transverse field profiles shown in Figure 1.26 illustrate the problem. Both profiles have the same peak intensity I_0, but the levels are rather different if they are averaged over the whole beam. Peak levels are the most significant parameter if the beam is held stationary over one tissue volume for a long time, but if the transducer is kept in continuous motion the average value becomes more important as this is what the tissue will experience. In a continuous wave field, therefore, two intensities are defined, the *spatial peak intensity* (I_{SP}) and the *spatial average intensity* (I_{SA}).

Table 1.1 Extent of near field for different ultrasound transducers

Frequency MHz	r cm	r^2/λ cm
0.75	0.5	1.25
	1.0	5
	1.5	11.25
1.0	0.5	0.6
	1.0	6.7
	1.5	15
1.5	0.5	2.5
	1.0	10
	1.5	22.5
3.0	0.5	5
	1.0	20
	1.5	45

r is the transducer radius; λ is the ultrasonic wavelength.

Things become more complicated in a pulsed field. Here, the analogy is of a boy standing up to his ankles in the sea. As the waves come in, the water rises up his legs, and drops again as the wave moves past, only to come up again on the next wave. There is a high-water mark on the boy's legs, representing the highest point reached by the wave while he was standing there (the *temporal peak*) and there is an average

water level experienced during the paddle (the *temporal average*). In the same way, a *temporal peak intensity* and a *temporal average intensity* can be identified as the highest intensity experienced at a point in tissue over a period of time, and the average intensity experienced at that point over a time, where the averaging is done over both on-times and off-times. If these temporal intensities are measured at the point in tissue where the spatial peak intensity is found, then a *spatial peak temporal peak intensity* (I_{SPTP}) and a *spatial peak temporal average intensity* (I_{SPTA}) can be determined. If these temporal intensities are combined with spatial averaging, the *spatial average temporal average* (I_{SATA}) and *spatial average temporal peak intensities* (I_{SATP}) can also be defined. These are demonstrated in Figures 1.27 and 1.28.

For example, take a beam with $I_{SP} = 3\,W/cm^2$ and $I_{SA} = 2\,W/cm^2$ while the sound is on, pulsed 2 ms on, 8 ms off. Whatever the temporal peak, the temporal average will be 20% of this since the sound is on for only a fifth of the time. Thus, $I_{SPTP} = 3\,W/cm^2$, $I_{SPTA} = 0.6\,W/cm^2$, $I_{SATP} = 2\,W/cm^2$, $I_{SATA} = 0.4\,W/cm^2$.

The ultrasound field can also be described in terms of the pressures involved. It can

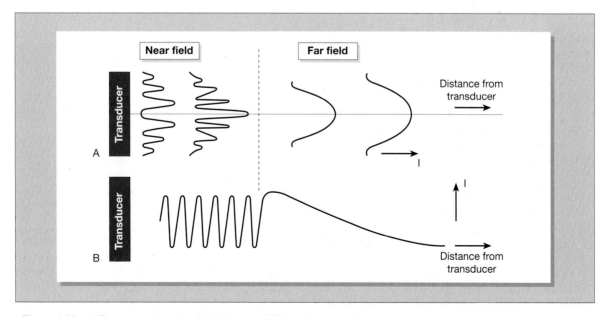

Figure 1.26 A: Transverse intensity distributions at different distances from the transducer. B: Intensity distribution on axis.

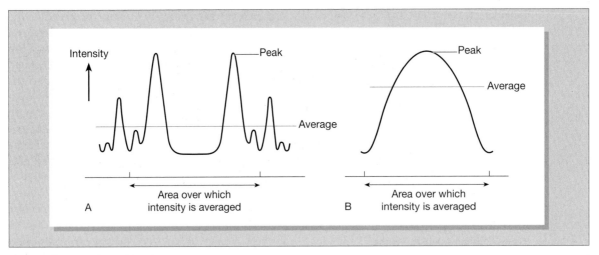

Figure 1.27 A: Example of a transverse beam profile in the near field. B: Transverse beam profile in the far field. This has the same peak intensity as the profile in A.

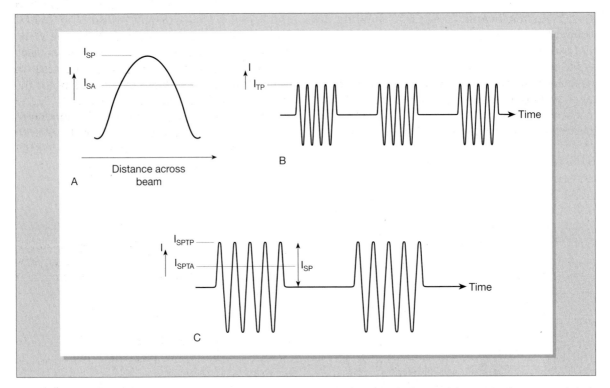

Figure 1.28 Diagram to illustrate the different types of intensity. I_{SP}: spatial peak; I_{SA}: spatial average; I_{TP}: temporal peak; I_{SPTP}: spatial peak–temporal peak; I_{SPTA}: spatial peak–temporal average.

be seen from Figure 1.29 that the pressure oscillates around the ambient level of the medium through which it passes. The field can therefore also be characterised in terms of *pressure amplitude* (usually the *peak positive pressure amplitude*, p_+, and the *peak negative pressure amplitude*, p_-) found anywhere in the field.

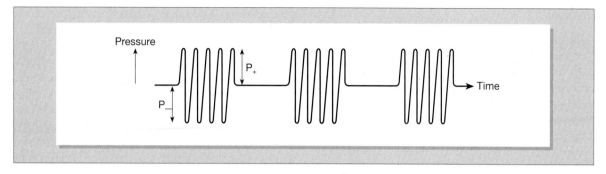

Figure 1.29 An ultrasound exposure can be described in terms of pressure. The peak positive pressure amplitude, p_+, and the peak negative pressure amplitude, p_-, is shown.

Intensity and pressure are related by the expression:

$$I = p^2/2\rho c, \qquad [39]$$

where ρ is the density and c is the speed of sound in the medium.

Ultrasound interacts with tissue in several ways. The two mechanisms thought to be most important are heat and cavitation. Cavitation is the activity of bubbles in an ultrasonic field. The oscillating pressure can cause bubbles to grow, and to oscillate. An oscillating bubble causes the liquids around it to stream, and considerable shear stresses may occur. In some instances they may become *resonant*, in which case they start to oscillate unstably and may undergo violent collapse, causing tissue damage in their vicinity. When the amount of tissue heating is being considered, spatially-averaged intensities are the most relevant parameters. However, when cavitation is considered, it is the peak negative pressure that is the most relevant parameter.

Calibration

Ultrasound fields can be calibrated using a number of methods, depending on the information required. The pressure distribution can be mapped using a pressure-sensitive PVDF (polyvinylidene–difluoride) membrane hydrophone which makes use of the inverse piezoelectric effect. Field plotting is a lengthy and detailed process usually undertaken by manufacturers or medical physics departments. It is always advisable to have transducers calibrated in this way before use, and again when a fault is suspected. It provides an easy way of identifying damaged crystals. The calibration method of choice within a physiotherapy department should be a radiation pressure balance. When ultrasound hits a target in water, it exerts a force on the target (radiation pressure) and tries to move it. If this is suitably counterbalanced, the radiation force can be calculated. This device averages over the target area, and allows a rapid assessment of reproducibility of output from day to day. This is an important check that should be incorporated into any treatment routine.

Reflection of ultrasound waves

Tissue offers resistance to the passage of ultrasound. This resistance is called the *acoustic impedance*, Z, and may be calculated from the expression:

$$Z = \rho c, \qquad [40]$$

where ρ is the density and c is the velocity of sound. The unit in which Z is measured is the *rayl*.

The amount of sound reflected from a plane surface between two materials of impedance Z_1 and Z_2 is $(Z_2 - Z_1)/(Z_2 + Z_1)$, and the amount of sound transmitted is $2Z_2/(Z_2 + Z_1)$. Water has an impedance of 1.5×10^6 rayl, fat has an impedance of 1.4×10^6 rayl, muscle of 1.7×10^6 rayl and bone of 7×10^6 rayl.

Attenuation

As ultrasound passes through tissue, some of the energy is reflected by the structures in the path (*scattering*), and some of the energy is absorbed by the medium itself, leading to local heating (*absorption*). *Attenuation* (the loss of energy from the beam) is due to these two mechanisms, with absorption accounting for 60–80% of the energy loss. If the intensity incident on tissue is I_0, and the intensity after travelling through x cm of tissue of attenuation coefficient α, is I, these are related by the expression:

$$I = I_0\, e^{-\alpha x}. \qquad [41]$$

The way in which the intensity drops as it goes through tissue is shown in Figure 1.30; this is known as *exponential decay*.

Attenuation coefficient values are often quoted in dB/cm/MHz or nepers/cm/MHz (1 dB/cm = 4.34 nepers/cm). The decibel (dB) represents a ratio of intensity levels such that the intensity level quoted in decibels is $10\log_{10} I_0/I$. It can be shown that when the intensity level is 3 dB the ratio of intensities is 2. The attenuation coefficient is quoted as a function of frequency, since they are approximately linearly related.

Table 1.2 shows relative attenuation coefficients for different biological tissues. Also shown are half-value thicknesses. This is the thickness of tissue needed to reduce the intensity by a factor two. It can be seen that bone and lung attenuate the sound very rapidly and very little energy gets into them. They are therefore not suited to physiotherapy ultrasound treatments. In fact, care should be taken when treating over such regions because the lost energy goes into heating the tissue locally. It can also be seen that the half-thickness layer decreases with increasing frequency and so, where deep treatments are required, low frequencies should be used.

Coupling agents. It can be seen from Table 1.2 that megahertz frequency sound does not travel through air. Therefore, when a patient is being treated, it is essential for an effective treatment that no air comes between the transducer and the skin. There are a number of methods by which ultrasound is applied. The most common method is to use a 'contact' application, where a thin layer of oil or gel is applied to the skin prior

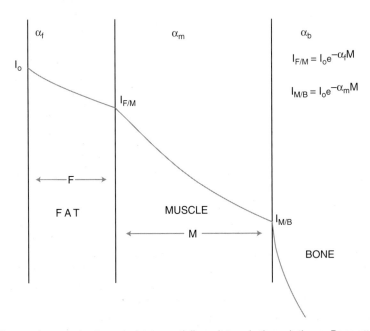

Figure 1.30 Ultrasound energy is attenuated exponentially as it travels through tissue. Bone attenuates most strongly.

Table 1.2 Tissue ultrasound attenuation coefficients and half-value layers

Tissue	Attenuation dB/cm/MHz	Half-value layer at 1 MHz	Half-value layer at 3 MHz
Blood	0.2	15 cm	5 cm
Fat	0.6	5 cm	1.6 cm
Liver	1.0	3 cm	1 cm
Muscle	1.3–3.3	1–2 cm	3–6 mm
Bone	20	1.5 mm	0.5 mm
Lung	41	0.7 mm	0.2 mm
Air	342 [1 MHz]	0.02 mm	
Water	0.002	1500 cm	500 cm

to treatment. The requirement for the coupling medium is that it has a similar acoustic impedance to skin. Mineral oils and water-based gels are most commonly used. Awkward geometries can most readily be treated in a water bath, with both the limb to be treated and the transducer being immersed.

HEAT AND TEMPERATURE

The fact that when various forms of energy are converted into heat there is always a constant ratio between the amount of energy that disappears and the amount of heat produced, suggests that in all these processes energy is neither created nor destroyed. This principle is a partial expression of the *first law of thermodynamics*: 'in all processes occurring in an isolated system, the energy of the system remains constant'. Electrical, chemical, magnetic and other forms of energy can be converted into heat energy with 100% efficiency, but it is not possible to achieve the reverse and transform all heat energy stored in the microstructure of matter to some other energy form. Again, if one form of energy is converted to another (e.g. chemical to mechanical) the process is not 100% efficient and some of the energy is always converted to heat. The tendency eventually to randomise molecular motion into heat energy suggests that heat is a primordial component in the structure of matter.

The concepts of *heat* and *temperature* are rigorously differentiated in physics and the distinction needs to be similarly maintained in the theory of electrotherapy. Supposing that the same quantity of heat (Q) is distributed over a large or a small volume of the same material, the larger volume will have a lower temperature (T_1) than the smaller volume (T_2). Thus, while the quantity of heat is a form of energy, the temperature of an object is a measure of the *average kinetic energy* of the constituent molecules. Because it is related to the 'average' movement of molecules, the concept of temperature can be applied only to bodies consisting of a large number of molecules.

The only term for temperature that allows consistent expression of all states of matter, solid, liquid and gas in accord with the laws of thermodynamics is the thermodynamic temperature, the base unit of which is the *kelvin* (K). In this system, introduced by Lord Kelvin in 1848, the linear scale starts at the absolute zero of temperature (0 K). The thermodynamic *Celsius* scale is subdivided into the same intervals as the Kelvin scale but has a zero point displaced by 273.15. The Celsius scale is divided into 100 unit intervals between two fixed points: the condensing point of steam (100°C = 373.15 K) and the melting point of ice (0°C = 273.15 K). Absolute zero on the Celsius scale is −273.15°C. The *Fahrenheit* (F) scale does not conform to the International System (SI) of units but continues to be used in many regions of the world particularly in meteorological data; 0°C is 32°F, 100°C is 212°F so 1° on the Celsius scale is equivalent to 1.8° on the Fahrenheit scale.

Heat units

Energy, work and the *amount of heat* are physical quantities with the same dimensions and ideally should be measured by a common unit. Traditional units such as the calorie are deeply rooted in technical as well as in dietary usage, but in accordance with SI strategy, the calorie is a 'non-coherent' unit. To conform with the SI, a quantity of heat should be expressed in *joules* (J). Heat exchanges are usually considered in terms of *power* (energy per unit time), for example joules per second (= 1 watt or W). The watt is probably more familiar in everyday use as a measure of power consumption of electrical appliances, for instance in kilowatt hours (kW h), which is actually energy per unit time × time. Table 1.3 derives the relationship between the physical expressions of *force, energy* and *power*.

The amount of heat energy required to raise a unit mass of material by 1°C is known as the *specific heat* of the material. The specific heat of water is 4.185 J/g per °C. Far less heat is needed to raise the temperature of a gas (e.g. the specific heat of air = 1.01 J/g per °C). The human body comprises approximately 60% water and not surprisingly has a relatively high specific heat (3.56 J/g per °C). The specific heats of skin, muscle, fat and bone are respectively 3.77, 3.75, 2.3 and 1.59 J/g per °C. It is thus readily calculated that if the mean body temperature of a 65 kg person is increased by 1°C over a period of 1 h then an extra 231 kJ of heat has been stored in the body.

Physical effects of heat

When heat is added to matter, a number of physical phenomena result from increasing the kinetic energy of its microstructure. These may be summarised as follows:

1. **Rise in temperature.** The average kinetic energy of constituent molecules increases.

2. **Expansion of the material.** Increased kinetic energy produces a greater vibration of molecules, which move further apart and expand the material. Gases will expand more than liquids and liquids more than solids. If, for example, a gas is enclosed so that expansion cannot take place, a rise in gas pressure will occur instead.

3. **Change in physical state.** Changing a substance from one physical state (phase) to another requires a specific amount of heat energy (i.e. latent heat). The latent heat of fusion is the energy required for, or released by, 1 gram of ice at 0°C in order to convert it to 1 gram of water at 0°C (336 joules), and the latent heat of vaporisation is the energy needed to convert 1 gram of water at 100°C to 1 gram of steam at 100°C (2268 joules).

4. **Acceleration of chemical reactions.** Van't Hoff's law states that 'any chemical reaction capable of being accelerated, is accelerated by a rise in temperature; the ratio of the reaction rate constants for a reaction occurring at two temperatures 10°C apart is the Q_{10} of the reaction'.

5. **Production of an electrical potential difference.** If the junction of two dissimilar metals (e.g. copper and antimony) is heated, an e.m.f. (electromotive force or electrical potential difference) is produced between their free ends (the Seebeck or thermocouple effect). Conversely, an e.m.f. applied to the junction of two metals can cause a rise in temperature at the junction (Peltier effect).

6. **Production of electromagnetic waves.** When energy is added to an atom (e.g. by heating) an electron may move out into a higher-energy electron shell. When the electron returns to its normal level, energy is released as a pulse of electromagnetic energy (a photon).

7. **Thermionic emission.** Heating of some materials (e.g. tungsten) may cause such molecular agitation that some electrons leave their atoms and may break free of the metal. This

Table 1.3 Derivation of coherent heat units

Physical quantity	Definition	SI unit	Dimension
Force	mass × acceleration	newton (N) (kg × metre s^{-2})	$M\,L\,T^{-2}$
Energy	force × distance	joule (J) (newton × metre)	$M\,L^2\,T^{-2}$
Power	energy/unit time	watt (W) (joule s^{-1})	$M\,L^2 T^{-3}$

M = mass; L = distance; T = time.
Non-coherent units:
1 calorie = 4.185 joules; 1 kcal/hour = 1.16 watts.

leaves a positive charge which tends to attract electrons back. A point is reached where the rate of loss of electrons equals the rate of return, and a cloud of electrons then exists as a space charge around the metal. This process is known as thermionic emission.

8. **Reduction in viscosity of fluids.** Dynamic viscosity is the property of a fluid (liquid or gas) of offering resistance (internal friction) to the non-accelerated displacement of two adjacent layers. The molecules in a viscous fluid are quite strongly attracted to one another. Heating increases the kinetic movement of these molecules, reducing their cohesive mutual attraction and making the fluid less viscous.

Heat transfer

The laws of thermodynamics govern processes involving the movement of heat energy from one point to another. Previously, mention has been made of the first law, which deals with the conservation and interchange of different forms of energy. The *second law of thermodynamics* states that 'heat cannot by itself, i.e. without performance of work by some external agency, pass from a colder to a warmer body'. These general laws establish the principles that govern heat exchanges (gain or loss) within the body and between the body and its environment. In electrotherapy we are concerned with the transfer of heat energy between the external environment and the body surface, and between the component tissues and fluids of the body itself as well as with the therapeutic effects of heat.

Conduction

Conduction is the mechanism of energy exchange between regions of different temperature, from hotter to colder regions, which is accomplished by direct molecular collision. The energy thus transferred causes an increased vibration of molecules, which is transmitted to adjacent molecules. A simple example of this process is the metal bar heated at one end which, by heat conduction, eventually becomes hot at its other end. The application of a cold pack to the skin surface induces skin cooling by heat conduction from the warm skin, and vice versa for a hot pack. The rate of heat transfer depends on the difference in temperature between the regions in contact, the surface area of contact at the boundary and the thermal conductivity of the materials in contact. Thermal conductivity is a specific property of the material itself; for example metals are better conductors than wood, water a better conductor than air.

Convection

Convection is the heat transfer mechanism that occurs in a fluid due to gross movements of molecules within the mass of fluid. If a part of a fluid is heated, the kinetic energy of the molecules in that part is increased, the molecules move further apart and the fluid becomes less dense. In consequence, that part of the fluid rises and displaces the more dense fluid above, which in turn descends to take its place. The immediate process of energy transfer from one fluid particle to another remains one of conduction, but the energy is transported from one point in space to another primarily by convective displacement of the fluid itself. Pure conduction is rarely observed in a fluid, owing to the ease with which even small temperature differences initiate free convection currents.

Thermal radiation

Heat may be transmitted by electromagnetic radiation emitted from the surface of a body whose surface temperature is above absolute zero. The heating of certain atoms causes an electron to move to a higher-energy electron shell; as it returns to its normal shell, this energy is released as a pulse of electromagnetic energy. This radiation occurs primarily in the infrared band, from wavelengths of about 10^{-5} cm to 10^{-2} cm (0.1–100 μm, or 10^{3}–10^{6} Å). A thermal radiation incident upon a surface can be:

1. reflected back from that surface
2. transmitted through it
3. absorbed.

In many everyday circumstances, objects are radiating and absorbing the same amount of infrared energy, thus maintaining a constant temperature. The amount of radiation from an object is proportional to the fourth power of the temperature (in kelvins). The rate of emission from a surface also depends on the nature of the surface, being greatest for a black body. A perfect black body absorbs all the radiation, whereas other surfaces absorb some and reflect the remainder.

Evaporation

Thermal energy is required to transform a liquid into vapour; the rate at which this proceeds is determined by the rate at which the vapour diffuses away from the surface. The rate depends on the power supplied and the vapour pressure of the air above the liquid. Evaporation follows laws very similar to those governing convection. When water vaporises from the body surface (e.g. during sweating) the latent heat required is extracted from the surface tissue, thereby cooling it. The converse process, condensation, entails latent heat gain at the surface as vapour is changed into liquid.

Body heat transfer

In thermoregulation, heat is exchanged by conductive, convective, radiative and evaporative transfer processes between the body surface and the environment so that the body's core temperature remains constant and equilibrium is maintained between internal (metabolic) heat production and heat loss (or gain) from the skin's surface.

Heat transfer within tissues takes place primarily by *conduction* and *convection*. The temperature distribution will depend on the amount of energy converted into heat at a given tissue depth and the thermal properties of the tissue (e.g. specific heat, thermal conductivity). Physiological factors are important in determining tissue temperature; for example when a raised tissue temperature produces an increased local blood flow, cooler blood reperfusing the heated tissue will selectively tend to cool the tissue by conduction. The technique of application of a treatment modality will also clearly modify the tissue temperature through variations in time and intensity, etc. When deep treatment is applied (e.g. short-wave diathermy, microwave, or ultrasound) conversion of the energy into heat occurs as it penetrates into the tissues. Heating modalities may be subdivided according to their primary mode of heat transfer during selective heating of superficial or deep tissues (Table 1.4).

In thermotherapy, the important properties concerned with heat conduction in tissues are thermal conductivity, tissue density and specific heat. Convection involves these properties also but, in addition, fluid viscosity becomes important. Understanding of the interaction of electromagnetic waves within biological media requires knowledge of the dielectric properties of tissues with different water contents.

Table 1.4 Heating modalities and their primary mode of heat transfer. (After Lehmann JF (1990) *Therapeutic Heat and Cold*, 4th edn. Baltimore, MD, Williams & Wilkins.)

Primary method of heat transfer	Modality
Conduction	Hot packs
	Paraffin wax baths
Convection	Hydrotherapy
	Fluidotherapy
	Moist air
'Conversion'	Radiant heat
	Laser
	Short-wave
	Ultrasound
	Microwave

2

Electrical properties of cells and tissues

Robert A. Charman

INTRODUCTION

Chapter 1 has introduced the basic concepts, units and laws of electrical theory and electromagnetism and explained how the construction and properties of common components of electrical and electronic circuitry, such as conductors, insulators, switches, semiconductors, resistors and capacitors, are designed and connected in accordance with the appropriate theory.

Biological tissues seem so different in their wet and salty nature compared, for example, with the metallic wiring of a television set, that they would appear to have nothing in common. Yet the astonishing fact is that living cells are dependent upon electrical activity for their very existence and the tissues that they make, such as bone and fascia, exhibit a wide range of electrical properties. The same theory applies to their use of electrical components; they obey the same laws and use the same units of, for example, voltage, capacitance, current flow and resistance.

As will be seen, the main difference between electricity in biological tissues and electricity in equipment is that cells and tissues use charged atoms, or ions, for the movement of charge whereas electrical and electronic systems use electrons. (See Charman, 1990a–e, 1991a–d for a detailed discussion.)

With this relationship between biological tissues and electrical circuitry in mind the rest of this chapter will be devoted to biological electricity, or *bioelectricity*.

CELLS AS ELECTRICAL SYSTEMS

Living cells employ many of the properties of electrical systems. For example, they generate electromotive force (e.m.f.), maintain a required difference in potential (p.d.), increase or decrease that p.d. as necessary, use varying resistances in series and in parallel, switch current on and off, control current flow, rectify current flow, possess impedance and, of crucial importance, store charge (capacitance).

Cells achieve their electrical purposes by using circuit components that are very different in their nature and construction to those used in ordinary electrical apparatus, but the principles, such as separation of charge to create an e.m.f., remain the same.

The average body cell, with all of its ordered complexity and function (Fig. 2.1), is between 10 and 50 micrometres (μm) in diameter ($1\,\mu$m = 1 millionth, or 10^{-6} of a metre). This means that it is some 5 to 20 times smaller than the smallest particle that the eye can see—a scale of miniaturisation approached only by very advanced microchip construction.

In electrical terms, cells have the great advantage of being very compact, with extremely short conducting pathways of about 10–20 nanometers ($1\,$nm = 10^{-9}m), but, against that, they work under some major disadvantages compared with ordinary electrical and electronic circuitry.

Cells are *wet circuits* that operate in a salty, conductive medium. They must *continually*

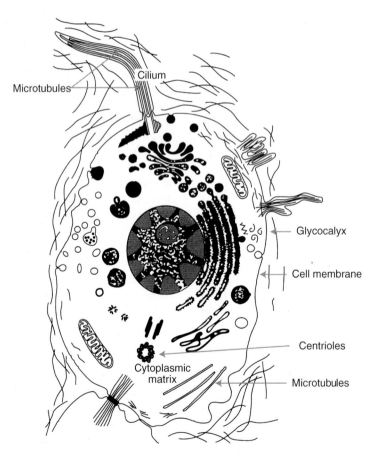

Figure 2.1 Composite diagram of main cell structures, which will vary according to cell type. Named structures are discussed in the text. (After *Gray's Anatomy*, with permission of Harcourt Health Sciences.)

make the replace all of their electrical components, *continuously* work to generate and maintain regions of differing electrical components, *continuously* work to generate and maintain regions of differing electrical properties against *continuous* leakage of charge, *continually* control rates of desired current flow against possible shorting of current, and *continually* work to prevent unwanted current flow when a pathway is switched off. The ceaseless work involved in achieving and maintaining these essential electrical ends consumes some 50–60% of the metabolic activity of a cell (Alberts *et al.*, 1989).

In marked contrast, ordinary circuits are *dry circuits* whose components need only occasional replacement. Because they are dry there is a clear distinction between conducting and non-conducting components. They possess the enormous advantage that they can store and move charge without leakage, and energy is required only when the circuit is in use. No work, for example, is required to resist an externally applied e.m.f. such as the 230 volts of the mains, when the circuit is switched off because the e.m.f. is passively resisted by the non-conducting properties of the 'off' switch insulator, whereas cells have to use active electrical pumps against the e.m.f. generated by capacitance charge separation to maintain that e.m.f. and prevent current leakage.

Another major difference lies in the type of charge used. Ordinary circuit use electrons, which have negligible mass, are highly mobile and have a diameter some 100 thousand times smaller than an atom (10^{-15} m compared with 10^{-10} m). Cells use atoms that have become charged as a result of gaining, or losing, valency shell electrons. Compared with electrons, charged atoms, or *ions*, are very 'heavy' by virtue of their nuclear mass of protons and neutrons. For example, the single proton nucleus of the hydrogen ion (H^+), atomic mass unit (μ) of 1μ, has about 2000 times the mass of an electron, and the two main ions used by cells to store charge and generate e.m.f., namely sodium ions (Na^+) of 23μ and potassium ions (K^+) of 39μ, are some 46 000 times and 78 000 times respectively, more massive than an electron, yet they possess only the same, univalent, strength of charge of a single electron as they have each lost only one electron from their outer electron shell.

Another disadvantage for the cell is that all ions in solution are *hydrated* ions. This means that each ion is surrounded by polar water molecules (H_2O) that are attracted to the ion by their own, very weak, negative/positive end polarity. In the case of cations, such as Na^+ and K^+, the water molecules orientate themselves so that the weak negativity of the oxygen atom is closest to the positive ion, and in the case of anions the weak negativity of the hydrogen atoms lie closest to the negative ion. Thus every hydrated ion, whether positive (cation), or negative (anion), is closely surrounded by a cluster of water molecules. When ions pass through the very narrow ion channels in the membrane, whether by diffusion along electrochemical gradients or by active transport, the weak hydration bonds of the water cluster are broken as the H_2O molecules are 'scraped off' the ion as it moves through the membrane channel (Alberts *et al.*, 1989).

Because of their relatively unwieldy mass, ions require far more energy to control their movement, and accelerate much more slowly along a given p.d. gradient, in comparison to electrons. This is one reason why cellular ionic changes tend to have submillisecond to millisecond (10^{-3} s) response times compared with the nanosecond (10^{-9} s) to attosecond (10^{-18} s) response times achievable in electronic circuitry.

Cellular circuit components

The main components used by the cell are *membranes, ion pumps* and *ion diffusion channels.*

Membranes as capacitor plates

Cell membranes are 5–7.5 nm thick, and are composed of a highly mobile but closely packed array of proteolipid molecules arranged as a bilayer, with their lipid tails forming a central zone (Fig. 2.2) that is resistant to the passage of electricity and can act as an insulator. The *plasma membrane* forms the surface boundary of the cell, and the intracellular membranes enclose each of

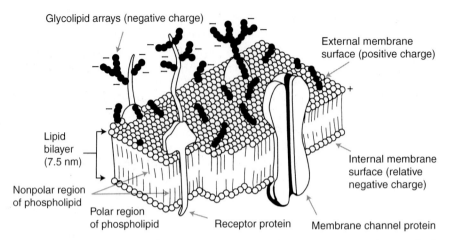

Figure 2.2 Fluid mosaic model of cell membrane. Note the transmembrane receptor protein, attached to the branched glycolipid array, and the charged surface.

the cell's organelles, with a double membrane around the nucleus. By means of selective permeability to ions, cell membranes being relatively impermeable to Na^+ ions and more permeable to K^+ ions, separate the two ions into different charge concentrations so that the outer membrane surface, as in the plasma membrane, is relatively more positive than the inner surface because the density, or number, of Na^+ ions and other cations per unit area is greater on the outside surface than the density of K^+ ions lining the inner surface. This charge separation results in an average 80 millivolt (mV) p.d. across the membrane, with the inner surface being relatively negative compared with the outer surface. Figure 2.3 illustrates the relative difference in cation concentration on either side of the cell membrane that creates the relative positive/negative (outside/inside) difference in charge concentration resulting in the 80 mV e.m.f. gradient across the membrane as shown by the arrow. In practical terms the inside of the cell is *negatively* charged to a difference of 80 mV compared with the outside. In cells, the gradient difference is created by separating cations into different concentration strengths either side of a membrane. This separation is also backed up by differences in negatively charged ions inside and outside of the cell.

Ion pumps and ion diffusion channels

Because fluid-filled ion channels are relatively leaky, ion separation across a membrane is controlled by directional ion pumps, such as the Na^+/K^+ pumps, which eject two Na^+ ions out of the cell for every Ka^+ ion into the cell to maintain the charge separation across the diameter of the membrane. Another vitally important ion pump is the Ca^{2+} ion pump, which keeps Ca^{2+} ions outside the cell at a concentration some 10 000 greater than inside the cell. Passive ion diffusion channels are controlled by varying the diameter and lining charge of the ion channel as necessary. Figure 2.4 summarises the activity of these ion channels and pumps; it is best read by starting at 'A' on the left-hand side of the diagram, where potassium ions are moving down an electrical gradient into the cell, and moving clockwise through the alphabet to 'K', where representative passive ion channels are shown. The transmembrane 75 mV p.d. shown here is the resulting average e.m.f. generated by these ionic movements and acts, in effect, as a capacitor store of charge that is available to do work. The 'bound cations' in the cell form a thin layer of potassium cations that are held to the boundary surface of the negatively charged cytosol by mutual attraction, and do not play any part in membrane ion pump exchange.

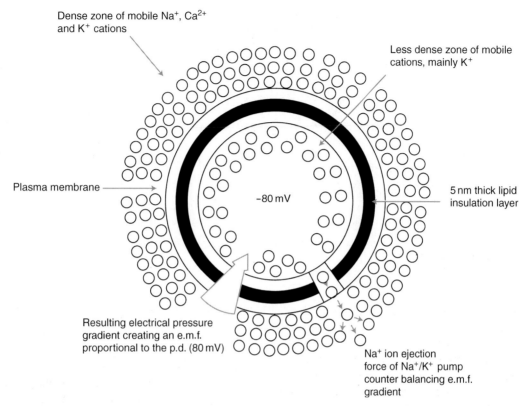

Figure 2.3 Schematic diagram illustrating the relative negativity of the cations inside the plasma membrane compared with those on the outside, the resulting transmembrane e.m.f. at a given p.d. in millivolts, and the resistance offered by the central lipid layer acting as an insulator and the Na^+ force of the Na^+/K^+ pump.

In summary, cell membranes act as capacitor plates when they hold a difference in ion charge concentration across their diameter. The charge is held on the continuous insulator surface of plasma membranes between the pores of the ion pump channels that help to maintain it. Cell membrane charge is measured in picofarad $(1\,pF = 10^{-12}\,F)$ and/or pico-coulombs (pC).

A quantity of 1 pF is 6×10^6 univalent charges, and cells operate in quantities of a few pC of ions stored upon their membranes, and around 0.01 to 0.001 pC flowing through individual ion channels. The rate of ion flow (amperage) through individual ion channels is measured in nanoamperes (nA), and the sum rates of ion channel flow across all the membranes of a cell at any given moment, acting as resistances in parallel, are measured in microamperes (μA).

Cell membrane p.d.

Charge separation creates a p.d., and a resulting e.m.f., between the two areas of charge on either side of the plasma membrane. As this cannot discharge through the middle lipid layer of the membrane it can be used to create a controlled driving force of ionic flow through the ionic channels. This force can be used as a transport system, and Na^+ ion exclusion from the cell helps to control cytoplasm osmolarity and cell volume. In neurons, the voltage-gated Na^+ pumps are used to transmit impulses. Depending upon the type of cell, membrane p.d.s range between 10 and 200 mV across their diameter. These are incredibly high voltages to sustain across a vanishingly thin membrane of some 7.5 nm diameter without breakdown when the membrane consists only of freely mobile lipid molecules at 37°C

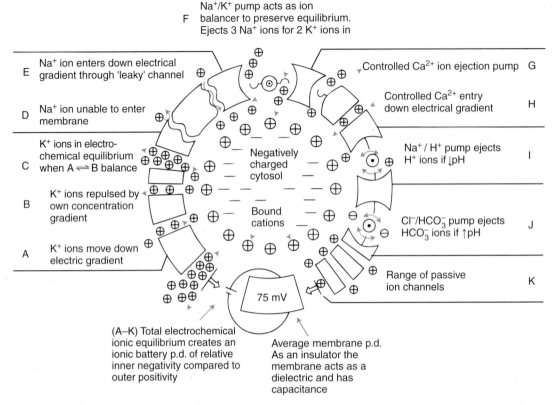

F Na+/K+ pump acts as ion balancer to preserve equilibrium. Ejects 3 Na+ ions for 2 K+ ions in

E Na+ ion enters down electrical gradient through 'leaky' channel

D Na+ ion unable to enter membrane

C K+ ions in electro-chemical equilibrium when A ⇌ B balance

B K+ ions repulsed by own concentration gradient

A K+ ions move down electric gradient

Negatively charged cytosol

Bound cations

75 mV

Controlled Ca2+ ion ejection pump G

Controlled Ca2+ entry down electrical gradient H

Na+ / H+ pump ejects H+ ions if ↓pH I

Cl−/HCO3− pump ejects HCO3− ions if ↑pH J

Range of passive ion channels K

(A–K) Total electrochemical ionic equilibrium creates an ionic battery p.d. of relative inner negativity compared to outer positivity

Average membrane p.d. As an insulator the membrane acts as a dielectric and has capacitance

Figure 2.4 Diagram summarising plasma membrane K+ leak channels, ion pumps and ion channels. Total electrochemical equilibrium acts as an ion battery creating a resting potential across the membrane, which is internally negative.

thermal agitation. Scaled up into round figures by assuming a central lipid diameter of 5 nm, and an average membrane p.d. of 100 mV, this is the equivalent of an e.m.f. of 2×10^4 V/mm.

THE CELL AS AN ELECTRIFIED SYSTEM

This sounds very similar to discussing cells as electrical systems, and the phenomenon is partly based upon active charge separation as discussed in the previous section. But it carries a more extended meaning and involves additional components of charge.

To consider the cell as an *electrified system* means considering it as an electrified, or charged, body with a surrounding electrical field that can influence other charged bodies, or objects. It also means looking at cell structure to see whether

different components of the cell act as collective wholes that create clearly defined subzones of particular charge, or sign.

Every cell is an electrified resultant of two types of electrical phenomena. One has already been discussed, and this is the active creation by the cell of charged capacitor membrane surfaces through selective ion channel diffusion and ion pump maintenance. The second type concerns electrostatics. Cell membranes can be considered in terms of electrostatics as their stored charge of inorganic ions creates an electrical field, consisting of an electric flux, or 'lines of force', radiating outwards from their surfaces. To this actively maintained surface charge must be added any organic molecules and compounds, such as proteins, amino acids, polysaccharides and simple sugars in the cytoplasm of the cell, that carry an overall charge and collectively act as an ionic mass. Some organic ions carry a positive charge but the majority are negative (Alberts *et al.*, 1989). To these must be added those compound molecules that are electrically neutral but carry charges of opposite sign at their ends. These are *dipoles*. They tend to rotate about their centre in response to an alternating field, and orientate themselves perpendicularly to a site of opposite charge, as if pointing at it like a stick.

When the cell is considered in these terms it is found to possess an external charge relative to other charged bodies, and is cross-sectionally divided into four charged zones, two of relatively steady charge strength, and two that vary about a mean value. Figure 2.5 shows the cell as an electrified system and should be referred to when reading the following description as it is a rather unusual way of looking at the cell. From the central zone outwards these four electrified zones are as follows:

• **Central negative zone (steady charge).** This zone is the negatively charged mass of cytoplasm that includes negatively charged proteins, amino acids and other organic molecules, and maintains a steady bulk negativity.

• **Inner positive zone (variable charge).** This consists of a thin zone of cations, mainly K^+ ions, that both 'coats' the outer surface of the central negative zone with a thin layer of cations (bound cations), and clusters along the inner surface of the plasma membrane as freely mobile cations that are available for transport in and out of the cell as required.

• **Outer positive zone (variable charge).** This consists of a more extended, and more dense, zone of mobile cations, mainly Na^+ ions and Ca^{2+} ions, with some K^+ ions, that cluster along the outer surface of the plasma membrane and are therefore extracellular.

• **Outermost negative calyx zone (steady charge).** This outermost zone of steady negativity is separated from the outer positive zone of the plasma membrane by a distance of some $20\,\mu m$. It is created by negatively charged sialic acid molecules that tip many of the glycolipid arrays that project outwards from the surface of the cell like cactus branches.

Many of these glycolipid structures are attached through the plasma membrane to the cell's microtubular framework (Fig. 2.6). *Microtubules* are

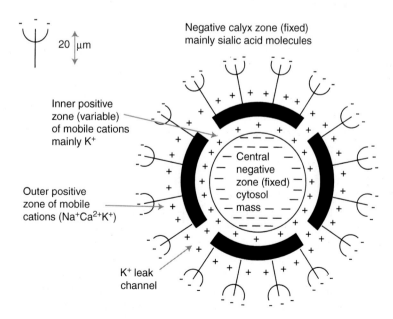

Figure 2.5 Schematic diagram of electrical zones of a cell. The membrane is relatively impermeable to Na^+ and Ca^{2+} ions, so the membrane p.d. is relatively internally negative.

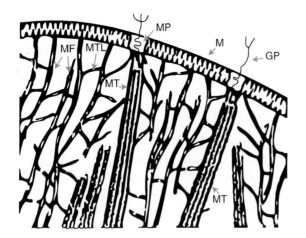

Figure 2.6 Schematic diagram of a cellular cytoplasmic membrane. M = cell membrane potential; GP = glycoprotein extending into extracellular space; MT = microtubule; MF = microfilaments (actin filaments or intermediate filaments); MTL = microtrabecular lattice. Cytoskeletal proteins that connect MT and membrane proteins include spectrin, fodrin and anhydrin. (From Hameroff, 1987, with permission from Elsevier Science.)

flexible hollow tubes, built from dipole-charged protein blocks like chimney bricks, that have an overall opposite sign charge at each end and are therefore bipolar, or dipoles. They radiate outwards from their centriole base near the central nucleus to the plasma membrane, and sometimes beyond. They help to give the cell shape, provide sites for enzymes, support the membrane, and act as active transport systems throughout the cytoplasm. In neurons they are the channels for axoplasmic flow.

It is this outermost calyx zone of steady negativity that makes each cell act as a negatively charged body. This means that every cell creates a negatively charged field around itself that influences any other charged body close to it. This electrostatic field has important consequences. Although the field is very weak, cell calyx fields mutually repulse each other, thus tending to maintain a 40 μm space between cells, except where there is actual junctional contact. All cellular tissue surfaces, such as the endothelial lining of the vascular system for example, carry a steady negative charge on their surfaces. In this example the endothelial surface charge repulses the negatively charged blood cells,

platelets and plasma proteins so that they are separated from the endothelium by a thin zone of pure plasma fluid. If the endothelium is damaged the damaged area loses its negativity, allowing the platelets to adhere with consequent risk of thrombus formation (Marino, 1988).

In addition to these four zones it should be noted that the immediate inner surface of the plasma membrane carries an overall negative charge that holds an important enzyme, protein kinase C, against its surface until it is activated and released by an influx of Ca^{2+} ions to initiate cascade reactions within the cell.

THE ELECTRICAL PROPERTIES OF TISSUES

All soft tissues include long-chain protein molecules such as collagen, elastin and keratin in their structure. These molecules have a regular, repeating subunit structure. Connective tissues, such as capsules, ligaments, fascia and tendon, consist of dense sheets of these molecules, especially collagen. Cartilage consists of collagen and proteoglycans, and bone is a calcified collagenous structure. All such tissue proteins possess one electrical feature in common: when they are mechanically distorted (strained) by an applied mechanical stress they develop *piezoelectric*-type p.d.s upon their external and internal surfaces (Becker and Marino, 1982; Black, 1986). Bone can be taken as a typical example of a tissue developing piezoelectric-like potentials when it is deformed, as shown in Figure 2.7. Surface voltages range from 10 to 150 mV and are proportional to the degree of strain deformation resulting from a given stress force acting upon the tissue.

Piezoelectric-type tissue surface potentials

These surface p.d.s may either be termed *stress-* or *strain-related potentials* (SRPs), or *stress-* or *strain-generated potentials* (SGPs). The terms employed are usually defined in the particular text. Some authorities consider that the applied *stress* force should be considered as the primary cause of

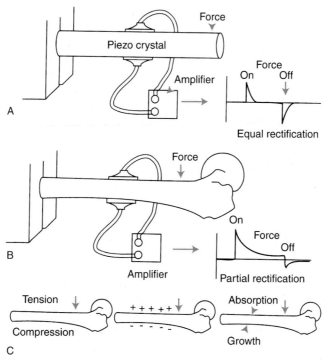

Figure 2.7   Apparent piezoelectricity in bone. A: Typical piezocrystal response to momentary deformation. B: Similar transducing response in bone. C: Tension/compression surface potentials of opposite sign to resulting bone cell response. (After Becker and Selden, 1985, with permission of HarperCollins Publishers, Inc.)

these surface p.d.s; others consider that the resulting *strain distortion* is the direct cause. Whichever definition is followed the p.d. is proportional to the stress or strain within the maximum that can be generated by the tissue. Each distorted protein molecule develops a p.d. and the surface tissue p.d. is the sum resultant (Black, 1986).

Each time a bone, such as the femur, takes a weight-bearing load it bends slightly. The compressed concave surface generates a *negative* p.d., and the stretched convex surface generates a *positive* p.d. The point charges are measured in picocoulombs, as shown in Figure 2.8. A similar effect occurs within fluid-filled channels, such as the Haversian canals, where the surface p.d. is termed a *streaming potential*, as it is the p.d. between the generated charge on the tissue surface and the ionised fluid that is flowing past it. A very thin, electrically neutral, interface develops between the two p.d.s, which is called the *slip plane*. In tendons, the tensile stress exerted

by muscle contraction against the external load carried by the tendon between the muscle and its skeletal or fascial insertion generates parallel planes of p.d. charge along its stretched length, and the same applies to all connective tissue.

DISCUSSION

This chapter shows how basic electrical theory can be applied to cell structure and function by considering the living cell as an electrical system and as an electrified system, respectively. It helps to provide a framework for understanding how the physical effects of various forms of applied electrical, magnetic, electromagnetic and ultrasonic energy may be converted to physiological effects when absorbed by cells. It is particularly relevant to those modalities that evoke a variety of *non-heating* (athermal) cellular responses, such as low-frequency stimulation, and to those modalities that are claimed to possess, and may indeed

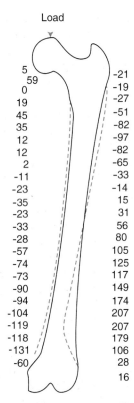

Load

5	-21
59	-19
0	-27
19	-51
45	-82
35	-97
12	-82
12	-65
2	-33
-11	-14
-23	15
-35	31
-23	56
-33	80
-28	105
-57	125
-74	117
-73	149
-90	174
-94	207
-104	207
-119	179
-118	106
-131	28
-60	16

Figure 2.8 Charge distribution (pC/cm^2) along femoral surfaces on loading. Hatched outline is theoretical profile change of growth and resorption proportional to charge strength. (After Becker and Marino, 1982, with permission of the State University of New York Press.) (See p. 39.)

possess, *non-thermal* (athermal) effects in addition to any physiological effects resulting from tissue temperature rise following energy absorption from them—for example pulsed and continuous high-frequency fields.

What must always be borne in mind is that cells are functional wholes. To discuss them only in electrical terms is to abstract one aspect of their function, and any consequences arising from such electrical activity must be considered in their physiological context of change in metabolism and function.

The known electrical properties of bone and soft tissues, as distinct from the living cells that manufacture them, is far less familiar. The probable reason for this is that the biological function and significance of these electrical effects are not known for certain, and many claims are hotly

disputed. This uncertainty centres upon highly contentious issues concerning cellular responses to the various forms of energy discussed in the text.

Leaving aside the *known* and undisputed cellular and body system responses to electrotherapy modalities as a consequence of, for example, heating, cooling, depolarisation, mechanical vibration and photochemical reactions, the unresolved question is whether cells can receive, decode and act upon specific frequencies, intensities and waveforms in the same way that they respond to, for example, the arrival of hormone molecules.

To put the question another way, can cells act as electrical receivers? Do they, like radio circuits, have 'frequency windows' that change according to their metabolic needs during normal function, or when traumatised? Can they, in effect, scan incoming frequencies and tune their circuitry to resonate at particular frequencies? Can they distinguish between signals that convey *meaning* upon reception and random noise? If so, can they distinguish, amplify and use very weak signals, perhaps a hundred to a thousand times weaker than normal membrane p.d.s, and measured in microvolts rather than the millivolts of membrane p.d.s, which may be emitted by very active nearby cells in the form of *biophotons* (Kert and Rose, 1989)? Or those oscillatory electrical and/or magnetic fields that are emitted from environmental sources, such as mains cables, high-tension cables and electronic equipment, and permeate the body by night and day?

If the answer to these questions is 'yes', then it means that particular forms of electrical and/or magnetic energy can act as incoming *first messengers*, like chemical molecules, and the cell will respond to them in a reasonably consistent way, as it does to, say, insulin or growth hormone. If this could be demonstrated beyond reasonable doubt then *electromagnetic medicine*, as electrotherapy would become, would develop as a recognised specialty. It would be able to deliver measured doses of electrotherapy appropriate to the diagnosis of a wide range of disorders, as, for example, it does now when specific J/cm^2 dosages of UVA radiation are applied to psoriatic skin in conjunction with psoralen drug therapy (PUVA).

A 'yes' answer also has deep implications concerning the possible role of naturally produced (endogenous) electricity. The piezoelectric-type tissue p.d. response to mechanical deformation offers an interesting, and unresolved, test case for discussion.

To those who consider that the evidence supports a working hypothesis that cells can interpret and respond to fluctuating patterns of external e.m.f. impinging upon their charged surfaces, these tissue p.d.s resulting from mechanical deformation are seen as a self-regulatory command system that instructs tissue cells what to do (Bassett, 1982; Becker and Marino, 1982; Becker and Selden, 1985; Becker, 1991; Black, 1986; Frochlich, 1988; Nordenstrom, 1983). According to this view, mechanical stress and the resulting strain distortion is transduced (i.e. energy transformation) into patterns and intensities of surface p.d.s proportional to localised strain deformation. These p.d.s act as a signaling system upon adjacent cells, such as fibrocytes in tendons, chondrocytes in cartilage, and osteoblasts and osteoclasts in bone, *instructing* them to increase or decrease tissue formation, or increase/ decrease tissue absorption, as a response to the imposed mechanical stress. Thus bone and tendon become proportionally thicker with increased load-bearing stress through exercise because the cells have 'read' the proportional intensity and frequency of tissue-generated surface p.d.s. Bone, for example, can undergo extensive remodelling in response to sustained changes in load. Figure 2.9 provides a diagrammatic summary of this hypothesis; it should be read clockwise, starting from the initiating agent of mechanical stress.

Conversely, the osteoporosis and connective tissue thinning associated with disuse is interpreted from this viewpoint as a lack of stress-induced p.d. stimulus to the cells with consequent loss of rate of tissue replacement compared with rate of absorption. The late stage of postfracture remodelling, in this view, is programmed by the intensity distribution of fracture site p.d.s as shown in Figure 2.10. The important point here is that the remodelling in this case *straightens* the femoral shaft against the compressional forces of weight bearing that should, by mechanical loading, *increase* the deformity of the malleable bone. The argument of those who consider that the tissue p.d.s act as an important information and control system is that the cells, as in this example, are responding to the p.d. intensity gradient created by the stress force and not to the stress force in itself, which would obviously crush the cells if they received it directly.

Suggested mechanisms whereby tissue p.d.s may act as first messengers are that they may activate ion channels, such as Ca^{2+}, which is an important second messenger that can initiate, through protein kinase C, specific enzyme cascades within the cell, or be picked up by the charged glycolipid strands that project outwards from the cell and conveyed into the cell via

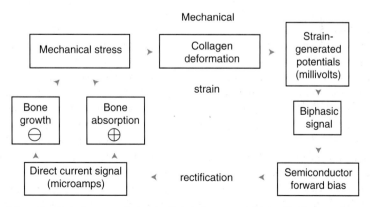

Figure 2.9 Summary of the role of strain-generated potentials in bone and, by implication, cartilage and connective tissue in adaptation to mechanical stress—Wolff's law control system. (After Becker and Marino, 1982, with permission of the State University of New York Press.)

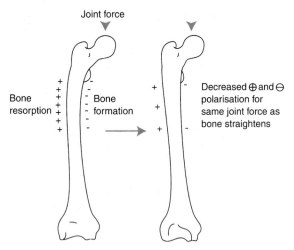

Figure 2.10 Adaptive remodelling of fracturing malunion under control of stress-generated potential polarity; concave surface negativity stimulates new bone, and convex surface positivity stimulates bone resorption (postulated feedback control system). (After Black, 1986, with permission of Greenwood Publishing Group, Inc., Westport, CT.)

connecting microtubule dipoles and 'read off' by enzyme systems attached to the microtubules, as shown in Figure 2.6.

A recent theory concerning the possibility that very weak signals, such as electromagnetic fields or cellular emission of biophotons, can be detected by cells is that the intrinsic random 'noise' energy created by the ceaseless activity of membrane ion channels may be *entrained* by very weak, incoming oscillatory signals to create strong signals at the same frequency (Wiesenfeld and Moss, 1995). In effect, the random fluctuations of membrane noise energy are converted to strong, regular oscillations that can modify cell behaviour. This conversion of random noise to controlled signal is known as *stochastic* (random noise) *resonance* (oscillatory frequency), or SR, and its magnitude can be expressed as a signal strength to noise ratio, or SNR. If, for example, these were shown to be at the same resonant frequency as the mechanical, electroconformational changes of transmembrane proteins that control the movement of charge across the membrane, then they could act as first messengers.

Another contentious example is the undoubted evidence that a wide range of microampere currents ebb and flow through the body along tissue channels connecting areas of differing metabolic activity (Becker, 1991; Borgens *et al.*, 1989; Nordenstrom, 1983). Areas of raised metabolic activity are negative relative to areas of low metabolic activity, and currents flow through, and around, localised areas of tissue trauma and healing. Most standard authorities see these currents, if they recognise their existence at all, as by-products of little significance. Others, as cited above, see them as an essential guiding, and regulatory, component of body function that works in synergy with the nervous system, vascular system and hormonal system. Nordenstrom (1983), for example, refers to them as a circulatory system that is additional to the former systems. He has modelled the body as an electrical circuit system in which sheets of connective tissue, as in organ capsules, fascial planes and the vascular system, act as relative insulators, and ionic tissue fluids act as ionic currents that can convey charged substances such as nutrients and waste products to and fro and alter tissue osmotic pressures. Nordenstrom considers the enclosed blood circulatory system as at zero electrical potential, analogous to 'earth' in electrical systems, and all other tissues as at a relative positive, or negative, p.d. to it according to their level of metabolism. The capillaries are the variable resistance points through which ionic currents between tissues and blood plasma can flow according to their relative difference in potential. There is considerable evidence (Borgens *et al.*, 1989; O'Connor, Bentall and Monahan, 1990) to show that electrical tissue gradients during embryonic development act as directional growth markers, that injured tissues generate so-called 'injury currents' which stimulate repair processes and that wound healing in skin, as a particular example, is more efficient if the area is kept moist so that micro-ampere currents, driven by e.m.f.s generated by the epidermal layers, can flow across it.

Chen (1996) and Tsui (1996) have demonstrated that the acupoint and meridian system has its own electrical properties and directional conductivity. Popp (1986) has found that the weak, low-frequency biophoton emission from cells is coherent (as in lasers), implying that the 'solid-state circuitry' of cells is the source, and that emission and reception of biophotons between cells, especially during embryonic development, is an important intercellular signalling system. New research into the bioelectrical properties of connective tissue has shown that its regular, repeating array of triple helix collagen molecules, encased by lattice sheaths of bound water molecules, has 'liquid crystalline' properties for very fast proton current conduction (Ho and Knight, 1998). This new research, and its associated concept that there is a fast-conducting body tissue communication system running alongside the nervous system, is summarised and explored by Ho (1998) and Oschman (2000). The latter, in particular, discusses the implications of these ideas for physical therapy procedures. For example, given the same voltage of application, low-frequency electrical currents meet a reduced ohmic resistance when applied longitudinally along fascial and ligamentous

planes of some one hundred times less compared with cross-fibre conduction. Barnes (2000) relates these new concepts of bodywide bioinformational systems to myofascial release techniques.

All electrotherapeutic modalities must interact with the ongoing bioelectrical activity already present. This activity, in turn, must reflect changes in tissue activity related to injury, disease, healing and health. Scott-Mumby (1999), for example, has taken this bioresonance approach by modelling body organs and tissues as interacting frequency systems. Equipment has been developed to detect bioelectrical anomalies in frequency and amplitude profiles emitted by the body as related to pathological processes and, in return, feed back the frequencies considered necessary to aid healing and restore normality. Assuming that further research confirms these claims, the future of electrotherapy as electromedicine may well develop along these lines.

REFERENCES

Alberts, B, Bray, D, Lewis, J, Raff, M, Roberts, K, Watson, D (1989) *Molecular Biology of the Cell*, 2nd edn. Galtand Publishing, New York.

Barnes, MF (2000) Myofascial release—morphological changes in connective tissue. In Charman RA (ed) *Complementary Therapies for Physical Therapists*. pp 171–185.

Bassett, CAL (1982) Publishing electromagnetic fields: a new method to modify cell behaviour in calcified and non calcified tissues. *Calcified Tissue International* **34**: 1–8.

Becker, RO (1991) *Cross Currents*. Bloomsbury, London.

Becker, RO, Marino, AA (1982) *Electromagnetism and Life*. State University of New York Press, USA.

Becker, RO, Selden, G (1985) *The Body Electric: Electromagnetism and the Foundation of Life*. W Morrow and Co, New York.

Black, J (1986) *Electrical Stimulation: Its Role in Growth, Repair and Remodelling of the Musculoskeletal System*. Praeger, New York.

Borgens, RB, Robinson, KR, Vanable, JW, McGinnis, ME (1989) *Electrical Fields in Vertebrate Repair*. Alan R Liss, New York.

Charman, RA (1990a) Introduction. Part 1. The electric cell. *Physiotherapy* **76**(9): 502–508.

Charman, RA (1990b) Part 2. Cellular reception and emission of electromagnetic signals. *Physiotherapy* **76**(9): 509–516.

Charman, RA (1990c) Part 3. Bioelectrical potentials and tissue currents. *Physiotherapy* **76**(10): 643–654.

Charman, RA (1990d) Part 4. Strain generated potentials in bone and connective tissue. *Physiotherapy* **76**(11): 725–730.

Charman, RA (1990e) Part 5. Exogenous currents and fields—experimental and clinical applications. *Physiotherapy* **76**(12): 743–750.

Charman, RA (1991a) Part 6. Environmental currents and fields—the natural background. *Physiotherapy* **77**(1): 8–14.

Charman, RA (1991b) Part 7. Environmental currents and fields—man made. *Physiotherapy* **77**(2): 129–140.

Charman, RA (1991c) Part 8. Grounds for a new paradigm? *Physiotherapy* **77**(3): 211–216.

Charman, RA (1991d) Bioelectromagnetics bookshelf. *Physiotherapy* **77**(3): 217–221.

Chen, KG (1996) Electrical properties of meridian. Pt 2. *IEEE Engineering in Medicine and Biology*. May/June: 58–63, 66.

Frochlich, H (ed) (1988) *Biological Coherence and Response to External Stimuli*. Springer-Verlag, Heidelberg.

Hameroff, SR (1997) *Ultimate Computing: Biomolecular Consciousness and Nanotechnology*. Elsevier-North, Amsterdam, Holland.

Ho, MW (1998) *The Rainbow and the Worm: The Physics of Organisms*, 2nd edn. World Scientific, Singapore.

Ho, MW, Knight, D (1998) The acupuncture system and the liquid crystalline collagen fibres of the connective tissues. *American Journal of Chinese Medicine* **26**(3–4): 1–15.

Kert, J, Rose, L (1989) *Clinical Laser Therapy: Low Level Laser Therapy*. Scandinavian Medical Laser Technology, Copenhagen.

Marino, AA (1988) *Modern Bioelectricity*. Marcel Dekker, New York.

Nordenstrom, BEW (1983) *Biologically Closed Circuits: Clinical, Experimental and Theoretical Evidence for an Additional Circulation*. Nordic Medical, Stockholm.

O'Connor, ME, Bentall, RHC, Monahan, JC (eds) (1990) *Emerging Electromagnetic Medicine*. Springer-Verlag, New York.

Oschman, JL (2000) *Energy Medicine: The Scientific Basis*. Churchill Livingstone, New York.

Popp, FA (1986) On the coherence of ultraweak photoemission from living tissues. In: Kilmister CW (ed) *Disequilibrium and Self Organisation*. pp 207–230.

Scott-Mumby, K (1999) *Virtual Medicine*. Thorsons, London.

Thibodeau, GA (1987). *Anatomy and Physiology*. Times Mirror/Mosby College Publishing, St Louis, MO.

Tsui, JJ (1996) The science of acupuncture—theory and practice. Pt 1. *IEEE Engineering in Medicine and Biology* May/June: 52–57.

Wiesenfeld, K, Moss, F (1995) Stochastic resonance and the benefits of noise: from ice ages to crayfish and SQUIBS. *Nature* **373**: 33–36.

3

Tissue repair

Sheila Kitchen
Steve Young

INTRODUCTION

Physiotherapists treat both acute and chronic inflammatory lesions, open and closed wounds, and problems associated with the healing process, such as oedema and haematomas. Use is made of a wide variety of electrophysical agents to initiate or enhance the repair process, including ultrasound, the diathermies, lasers, and low-frequency stimulating currents. In order to understand how electrophysical agents may affect the healing of tissues and the rationale underlying their selection and application, it is essential that the processes underlying healing be considered.

Healing is a complex but essential process without which the body would be unlikely to survive. It involves the integrated actions of cells, matrix and chemical messengers and aims to restore the integrity of the tissue as rapidly as possible. It is a homeostatic mechanism to restore physiological equilibrium, and may be initiated as a result of loss of communication between adjacent cells, between cells and their support, or by cell death. Healing can be described in terms of chemokinesis, cell multiplication and differentiation. A complex series of events occurs, involving the migration of cells of vascular and connective tissue origin to the site of injury. This process is governed by chemotactic substances liberated in situ. The healing process, which is common to all body tissue types, may be divided into three overlapping phases:

1. inflammation
2. proliferation
3. remodelling.

Healing of all tissue is based upon these phases and normally results in the formation of scar tissue. Limited regeneration of certain tissues such as the epidermis, skeletal muscle and adipose tissue may also occur. The basic principles that underlie repair which lead to scar formation will first be described; subsequently, a brief summary of the regenerative healing of epidermal and muscular tissue is provided.

THE PRINCIPLES OF TISSUE HEALING

Inflammatory phase

Inflammation is the immediate response to injury. The cardinal signs of inflammation are redness, swelling, heat and pain. The acute, or early, phase of inflammatory response lasts between 24 and 48 hours and is followed by a subacute, or late, phase which lasts between 10 and 14 days. The subacute phase can be extended if there is a continuing source of trauma or if some form of irritation, such as a foreign body or infection, is present.

Tissue injury causes both cell death and blood vessel disruption. The primary purpose of the inflammatory phase of healing is to rid the area of debris and dead tissue and to destroy any invading infection prior to the repair. This phase may be described in terms of vascular and cellular changes which are mediated through the actions of chemical agents.

Vasoregulation and blood clotting

The initial vascular reaction involves haemorrhage and fluid loss due to destruction of vessels; vasoconstriction, vessel plugging, and blood coagulation follow, to prevent further blood loss.

These processes lead to the activation of the repair process. Blood loss into the tissues initiates platelet activity and blood coagulation directly, both of which then result in the production of chemical factors which initiate and control the healing process. In addition, the blood clot provides a provisional matrix which facilitates the migration of cells into the wound (Clark, 1991).

Primary vessel constriction occurs, and is due to the release of noradrenaline (norepinephrine); this reaction lasts only for a few seconds to a few minutes. During vasoconstriction the opposing cell walls are brought into contact, and adhesion between the surfaces results. Secondary vessel vasoconstriction may follow, due to the action of serotonin, adenosine diphosphate, calcium and thrombin.

Both lymphatics and blood vessels are plugged in order to limit fluid loss. Initial platelet adhesion and aggregation is stimulated by the presence of thrombin (Terkeltaub and Ginsberg, 1988). The platelets adhere to one another, to the vessel walls and to the interstitial extracellular matrix, leading to the build-up of relatively unstable platelet plugs (Clark, 1991). The process is continued and consolidated by the release of adhesive proteins such as fibrinogen, fibronectin, thrombospondin and von Willebrand factor by the platelets (Ginsberg, Loftus and Plow, 1988).

Coagulation of extravascular blood is thought to be due to the action of platelets and intrinsic and extrinsic clotting mechanisms. Prothrombin is converted to thrombin and thus fibrinogen to fibrin, providing an early wound matrix.

Blood coagulation not only aids haemostasis through clot formation, but adds to the early wound matrix and results in the generation of chemical mediators such as bradykinin (Proud and Kaplan, 1988). These substances affect the local circulation, stimulate the production of further chemical mediators and act as attractants to cells such as neutrophils and monocytes (Clark, 1990a).

Following this period of vasoconstriction, secondary vasodilation and increased permeability of venules occur owing to the effects of histamine, prostaglandins and hydrogen peroxide production (Issekutz, 1981; Williams, 1988). Subsequently, both bradykinin and the anaphylatoxins initiate mechanisms which increase the permeability of undamaged vessels, leading to the release of plasma proteins which contribute to the generation of the extravascular clot.

Cell migration and action

Neutrophils and monocytes are the earliest cells to reach the site of injury. They migrate in response to a wide variety of chemical and mechanical stimuli, including the products of the clotting mechanism, the presence of bacteria and cell-derived factors.

The neutrophils' primary action is phagocytosis, and their task is to rid the site of bacteria and of dead and dying materials. Neutrophilic margination within the vascular structures leads to the passage on neutrophils through vessel walls by amoeboid action, enabling them to reach damaged extravascular tissues. Phagocytosis is achieved by neutrophilic lysis. This results in the release of protease and collagenase, which begin the lysis of necrotic protein and collagen respectively, as shown in Figure 3.1. Infiltration of the neutrophils into the extravascular tissue ends after a couple of days, marking the end of the early phase of inflammation.

Macrophages are essential to the healing process and can perform the normal function of neutrophils in addition to their other tasks. Monocytes migrate from the vasculature into the tissue space and rapidly differentiate into macrophages; the factors responsible for this change have not been fully identified, but may include the presence of insoluble fibronectin (Hosein, Mosessen and Bianco, 1985), low oxygen tension (Hunt, 1987), chemotactic agents (Ho, Lee and Snyderman, 1987) and bacterial lipopolysaccharides and interferons (Riches, 1988). Macrophages phagocytose pathogenic organisms, tissue debris and dying cells (including neutrophils), and release collagenase and proteoglycan, both of which are degrading enzymes the lyse necrotic material (Leibovich and Ross, 1975; Tsukamoto, Helsel and Wahl, 1981).

Chemical factors

Many factors that influence and control the initial inflammatory process and trigger further

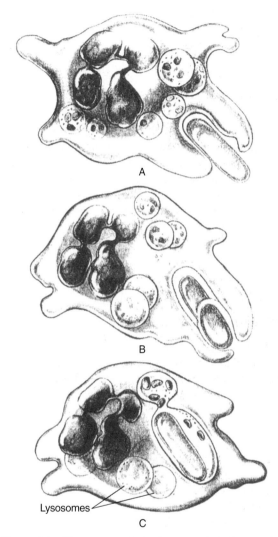

Figure 3.1 Phagocytosis. A: In phagocytosis, cells such as neutrophils and macrophages ingest large solid particles such as bacteria and dead and dying material. B: Folds of the plasma membrane surround the particle to be ingested, forming a small vacuole around it, which then pinches off inside the cell. C: Lysosomes may fuse with the vacuole and pour their digestive enzymes (such as protease and collagenase) on to the digested/ingested material.

developments in the proliferative phase are released by cells during the stage of inflammation. Macrophages release factors which attract fibroblasts to the area (Tsukamoto, Helsel and Wahl, 1981) and enhance collagen deposition (Clark, 1985; Weeks, 1972). Platelets release growth factors which contribute to the control of fibrin deposition, fibroplasia and angiogenesis through their action on a variety of cells (Clark, 1991). Platelets also release fibronectin, fibrinogen, thrombospondin and von Willebrand factor (Ginsberg, Loftus and Plow, 1988); these are necessary for the aggregation of platelets and for their binding to tissue structure. In addition, serotonin, adenosine diphosphate, calcium and thromboxin are released; these are necessary for blood vessel constriction to prevent haemorrhage (Clark, 1991).

Dead and dying cells release substances which influence the development of the neomatrix; these include a variety of tissue factors, lactic acid, lactate dehydrogenase, calcium, lysosomal enzymes and fibroblast growth factor (Clark, 1990a). In addition, prostaglandins (PG) are produced by almost all cells of the body following damage, due to alterations in the phospholipid content of the cell walls (Janssen, Rooman and Robertson, 1991); some types of PG are pro-inflammatory, increasing vascular permeability, sensitising pain receptors and attracting leucocytes to the area. Other classes of PG may be anti-inflammatory. Both may be involved in early stages of repair.

Proliferative phase

Granulation tissue is formed during the proliferative phase. This is a temporary structure that evolves after a period of a couple of days and comprises neomatrix, neovasculature, macrophages and fibroblasts. Granulation tissue precedes the development of mature scar tissue. 'Fibroplasia' is a term that encompasses the processes of fibroblast proliferation and migration, and the development of the collagenous and non-collagenous matrices.

Fibroplasia

Fibroblasts produce and organise the major extracellular components of the granulation tissue. They appear to originate from resting fibrocytes situated in the wound margins, and migrate into the wound in response to both chemical and physical attractants (Repesh, Fitzgerald and

Furcht, 1982; McCarthy, Sas and Furcht, 1988; Clark, 1990b).

The fibroblast is primarily responsible for the deposition of the new matrix. Once present within the wound, fibroblasts synthesise hyaluronic acid, fibronectin and types I and III collagen—these form the early extracellular matrix. As the matrix matures, certain changes take place: the presence of hyaluronic acid and fibrinogen is gradually reduced, type I collagen becomes the predominant component, and proteoglycans are deposited.

Hyaluronic acid, present only in early wound healing, appears to facilitate cell motility and may be important in fibroblast proliferation (Lark, Laterra and Culp, 1985; Toole, 1981). Fibronectin has many functions within a wound; these include action as a chemoattractant to cells such as fibroblasts and endothelial cells, augmentation of the attachment of fibroblasts to fibrin, facilitation of the migration of fibroblasts, and possibly provision of a template for collagen deposition (Clark, 1988). Proteoglycans contribute to tissue resilience and help to regulate cell motility and growth, and the deposition of collagen.

Collagen is a generic term covering a number of different types of glycoprotein found in the extracellular matrix. Collagen provides a rigid network which facilitates further healing. The types of collagen within a wound and their quantities are gradually modified with time. Type III (embryonic collagen) is gradually absorbed and replaced by type I collagen, which is mature fibrillar collagen. Type IV collagen may be produced as a part of the basement membrane when skin damage occurs, and type V collagen is deposited around cells, forming a structural support.

Two primary factors affect collagen metabolism and, therefore, production. The first is the effect of the cytokines; Table 3.1 lists some of the cytokines believed to affect collagen metabolism. There appears to be a balance between the stimulatory and inhibitory effects of these substances, leading to optimal healing with neither over- nor underproduction of collagen.

The second factor influencing collagen metabolism is the nature of the extracellular matrix

Table 3.1 Cytokines controlling collagen production

TGF-β	induces collagen synthesis	(Ignotz and Massague, 1986)
IL-1	induces collagen synthesis	(Prostlethwaite et al., 1988)
TNF	induces collagen synthesis	(Duncan and Berman, 1989)
IFN (α, β, γ)	decreases collagen synthesis	(Czaja et al., 1987)
TNF-α	decreases collagen synthesis	(Scharffetter et al., 1989)
PGE₂	decreases collagen synthesis	(Nicholas et al., 1991)

Key: TGF-β, transforming growth factor β; IL-1, intereukin 1; TNF, tumour necrosis factor; IFN, interferons; PGE_2, prostaglandin E_2.

(Kulozik et al., 1991; Mauch and Krieg, 1990). The extracellular matrix provides both a structural scaffold for the tissue and signalling for the cells. Reduced collagen synthesis results from cell contact with mature, type I collagen, upon which the production of collagenase is activated.

Angiogenesis

An extensive vascular system is required to provide for the needs of the proliferative phase. Angiogenesis is thought to be initiated by the presence of multiple stimuli. The process initially involves capillary budding, which involves the disruption of the basement membrane of the venule at a point adjacent to the angiogenic stimulus. Endothelial cells migrate towards the stimulus as a cord of cells surrounded by a provisional matrix (Ausprunk, Boudreau and Nelson, 1981; Clark et al., 1982a). Individual sprouts link to form capillary loops, which may in turn develop further sprouts. Lumina appear within the arched cords and blood flow is gradually established, initially in immature, permeable vessels, and later in more mature capillary beds having developed basement membrane components (Ausprunk, Boudreau and Nelson, 1981; Hashimoto and Prewitt, 1987).

The anastomosis of existing vessels and the coupling or recoupling of vessels within the wound space also occurs, leading to a well-developed blood supply within the granulation tissue. However, this state is not retained, as the granulation tissue is later remodelled into scar tissue. Capillary regression occurs, possibly in response to a loss of angiogenic stimuli, and is characterised by changes in the mitochondria of the endothelial cells, their gradual degeneration and necrosis, and final ingestion by macrophages.

Angiogenesis is stimulated and controlled through the action of many substances; these have been reviewed by Folkman and Klagsburn (1987), Madri and Pratt (1988) and Zetter (1988). Effects may be both direct and indirect, and arise from stimuli generated both at the time of injury and during the early stages of repair.

Wound contraction

Contraction, which is due to the centripetal movement of pre-existing tissue (Montadon, d'Andiran and Babbiani, 1977), is the process that reduces the size of a wound. Wound contraction is a major form of wound closure in loose-skinned animals such as rabbits and rats, and rarely leads to loss of function of the involved tissue. In humans, however, it is a 'double-edged sword': if there is too little contraction then wound closure is slow, allowing excess bleeding and possible infection, but too much contraction may lead to tissue contractures, possibly causing deformity and dysfunction. Alone, wound contraction rarely closes a human wound.

Wound contraction begins soon after injury and peaks at 2 weeks. Many theories have been posited as to the mechanisms involved. Recent work suggests that material within the wound may pull the wound margins inwards. Two theories are currently postulated for this process: they are the cell contraction theory, based on the actions of myofibroblasts (Gabbiani, Ryan and Manjo, 1971), and the cell traction theory, based on the action of fibroblasts (Ehrlich and Rajaratnam, 1990).

The cell contraction theory suggests that the contractile activity of myofibroblasts draws the edges of the wound together against the constant centrifugal tension of the surrounding tissues. Both actin and myosin have been identified in myofibroblasts, and it is suggested that the myofibroblasts attach themselves to collagen fibres and then retract, holding the collagen in place until it has stabilised its position. The theory suggests that the synchronised activity of the many myofibroblasts will lead to wound shrinkage (Skalli and Gabbiani, 1988).

The cell traction theory suggests that fibroblasts act as the agents of closure by exerting 'traction forces' on the extracellular matrix fibres to which they are attached; the process is analogous to the traction exerted by wheels on a surface. Traction forces are shear, tangential forces that are generated during cell activity. This process brings to mind the action of a traction engine.

Much argument surrounds these two theories. Current evidence suggests that wound contraction is cell mediated, and that the cells involved are of fibroblastic origin. Other studies suggest that wound contraction appears to start before many myofibrocytes are present in the area, again implicating fibroblastic activity (Darby, Skalli and Gabbiani, 1990; Ehrlich and Hembry, 1984). However, this does not preclude the suggestion that both mechanisms may be involved in the process in a sequential fashion (Hart, 1993).

Remodelling

Remodelling of the immature tissue matrix commences at about the same time as new tissue formation, although for clarity it is normally regarded as forming the third phase of healing. The matrix that is present at this stage is gradually replaced and remodelled over the subsequent months and years as the scar tissue matures.

Collagen is immature and gel-like in construction in the early stages of wound healing, and exhibits little tensile strength. Remodelling occurs over a period ranging from several months to years, with type III collagen being partly replaced by type I. Fibres reorientate themselves along the lines of stress applied to the lesion, thus resulting in greater tensile strength of the tissue. Wound breaking strength increases with the deposition of collagen, reaching approximately 20% of the normal strength

by day 21. The final strength attained will be in the region of 70–80% of the normal value.

REPAIR OF SPECIALISED TISSUES

The repair of certain specialised tissues may result in a number of modifications or additions to the normal healing process. A brief description follows of the processes that may occur when epidermal tissue, muscle, nerve and bone are damaged.

Epidermal tissue

Injuries to the skin may involve either the epidermis alone or both the epidermis and the dermis. When the skin is broken, rapid coverage of the surface is essential to reduce the hazards associated with environmental stress and contamination. While dermal healing is proceeding as described above, re-epithelialisation of the surface occurs to repair damage to the epidermis.

Re-epithelialisation is initiated within 24 hours of injury. Epidermal basal cells undergo changes which allow them to migrate toward the site of the lesion; they loosen their intercellular attachments (desmosomes), lose their cellular rigidity, and develop actinic pseudopodia—all of which facilitate cell mobility.

Epidermal cells migrate rapidly towards the base of a wound, travelling across the remaining viable basal lamina or the fibrin scaffolding of the blood clot formed in deeper lesions. Cells move across the wound surface in response to a number of substances in the wound matrix, including fibronectin, fibrin and collagen (type IV), which provide a structural network for migration (Hunt and Dunphy, 1980).

There is a certain lack of clarity about the factors that initiate and promote the restructuring process. However, they include chemotactic factors, structural macromolecules, degradative enzymes, tissue geometry (such as the free-edge effect), fibrin, collagen, fibronectin, thrombospondin and growth factors.

Epidermal differentiation follows migration. Mitotic activity, controlled by the cyclic adenosine monophosphate (cAMP) system, increases in the newly formed epithelium, resulting in thickening of the tissue and the development of a normal stratified appearance (Matoltsy and Viziam, 1970; Odland and Ross, 1977). Normal keratinisation follows, initially in the uppermost layers, followed by the development of a full stratum corneum.

Finally, the epidermis returns to normal. When the basement membrane is present and the re-epithelialisation complete, the cells resume their normal appearance and the hemidesmosomes re-form to link the basement membrane and the epidermal layer of cells. Where deficient, the basal lamina is synthesised by the epidermal cells over an infrastructure of newly formed collagen (Clark *et al.*, 1982b).

Muscle tissue

The degree to which regeneration takes place in muscle appears to depend both on the degree to which the basement membranes of the original fibres have been retained and on the vascular and nerve supply to the area (Carlson and Faulkner, 1983).

Muscle repair involves the removal of damaged cell components, the proliferation of satellite cells to form new muscle fibre building materials and the fusion of satellite cells to form new myotubes and muscle fibres (Fig. 3.2).

The processes involved in the early degenerative phase have been reviewed by Carpenter and Karpati (1984). Myofibrils lose their regularity and disorganisation of the Z disc occurs. Mitochondria become more rounded and lose their regular distribution within the cell. Actin and myosin filaments lose their regularity, glycogen particles disappear and tissue no longer stains positive for the enzymes, such as phosphorylase, which are used in glycogenolysis.

Proliferation of skeletal muscle satellite cells (or presumptive myoblasts) follows, and these provide a source of myonuclei for the regenerating muscle cells. Bischoff (1986, 1990) hoped to identify the factors which might initiate this process; he suggested that under normal conditions the sarcolemma exerted a negative control on satellite cells to prevent proliferation. This

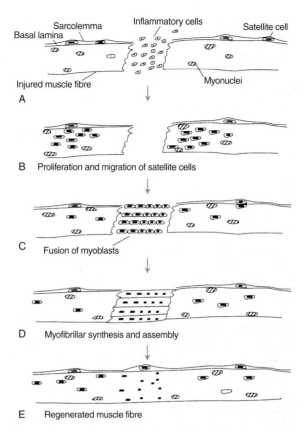

A

B Proliferation and migration of satellite cells

C Fusion of myoblasts

D Myofibrillar synthesis and assembly

E Regenerated muscle fibre

Figure 3.2 Muscle repair. A: Damaged cellular components are digested by cellular infiltration and inflammation. B: Satellite cells proliferate and then C fuse into myotubes to form new myofibrils. D: Myofibrillar proteins are synthesised to 'fill' new fibre resulting in E regenerated muscle fibre.

inhibition was removed following structural damage. Positive control through the action of mitogenic factors was also suggested by Bischoff (1990), although the nature of this is as yet unclear.

Regeneration subsequently follows the normal pattern of muscle development, with satellite cells aligning themselves along the basal lamina and fusing into myotubes. The presence of the basal lamina appears to influence this process, providing a substrate upon which alignment can occur; and expressing a number of extracellular matrix components. It is not, however, essential to the process, as reduced levels of regeneration occur in the absence of an intact lamina.

As the myotubules mature and differentiate they synthesise myofibrillar proteins and deposit them in the outer subsarcolemmal region. During this process, the muscle nuclei are normally pushed to the periphery, although a few remain centrally as testimony to the repair process.

Nervous tissue

When a peripheral axon is damaged it is sometimes possible for it to undergo repair, which allows normal conduction to resume. In mammals, however, repair of central axons is generally not possible, possibly owing to the absence of definite endoneurial tubes and the proliferation of macroglia cells. Considerable research is currently being conducted in this area to clarify matters.

When an axon is subject to trauma, changes occur on both sides of the injury. Distally, the axon swells and then disintegrates, with total degeneration and removal of the cytoplasmic matter occurring within the membrane of the axon. A similar process occurs in the proximal direction, gradually progressing toward the cell body. This normally leads to effects in the cell body such as changes in cytoplasmic RNA, dispersion of Nissl granules, production of protein-synthesising organelles, and positional reorganisation of both nucleoli and ribosomes (Fig. 3.3).

When regrowth of the axon is possible, as in the peripheral nervous system when the cell body has not been destroyed, an intact endoneurial sheath at or near to the site of damage helps to establish satisfactory contact with the peripheral receptors and end organs. Following degeneration of the myelin sheath, the Schwann cells proliferate and occupy the endoneurial tube. In addition, they form a bridge across any gap in the continuity of the axon. The proximal part of the axon develops a swelling which gives rise to a large number of axonal 'sprouts', and these spread out within the tissue surrounding the wound. Though many ultimately serve no useful purpose, one will enter the tube and grow distally, accompanied by the Schwann cells. When the axon finally makes successful contact with the end organs, the Schwann cells begin to synthesise a myelin sheath. Finally, the axonal diameter and the myelin-sheath thickness increase, leading to near-normal conduction behaviour.

Bone tissue

The repair of bone tissue follows the same basic pattern as that described in the section on the principles of healing, with an added osteogenic component. The process is described in full detail in many texts (e.g. Heppenstall, 1980; Williams et al., 1989).

Haemorrhage occurs immediately following injury. A clot forms, and the acute inflammatory phase of repair is initiated. Mast cells, polymorphonuclear leucocytes and macrophages move into the area and appear to be responsible for the release of factors which stimulate tissue repair. Dead and dying tissues are removed by macrophages and osteoclasts and a gradual

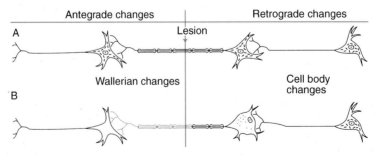

Figure 3.3 Repair of nervous tissue. A: Both antegrade and retrograde changes occur following damage to a neuron. B: Wallerian changes, which include generation of the myelin sheath and axon, occur in the antegrade direction. Cell body changes include movement of the nucleus to the periphery, removal of the protein synthesis apparatus and dispersion of Nissl granules.

ingrowth of granulation tissue occurs to replace the clot. This is completed normally by about 4 days.

Osteoblasts, whether derived from osteocytes, fibroblasts or a number of other sources, become active. They are stimulated into activity by a number of factors, including mast cell factors, decreased oxygen levels, and bone morphogenic substances. In addition, chondroblasts may become active under certain conditions, especially when oxygen levels are particularly poor. Small groups of cartilaginous cells appear within this early tissue, chiefly in the region of the peri-osteum. Osteoblasts deposit calcium both directly in the tissue matrix and in the islands of cartilage. The fracture is now united by a firm but pliable material known as *provisional* (or *soft*) *callus*.

Subsequently, both subperiosteal and endochondral ossification continues and, after about 2 months, the bone ends become united by primitive (or *woven*) bone, which is known as *hard callus*.

Finally, this woven bone is remodelled to form mature lamellar bone. Both osteoblasts and osteoclasts are involved in this process. The marrow cavity is restored, the contour of the bone smoothed, and the internal structure of the bone reorganised as the type of bone changes and the tissue responds to the normal external forces to which it is again submitted. Figure 3.4 illustrates the process of repair.

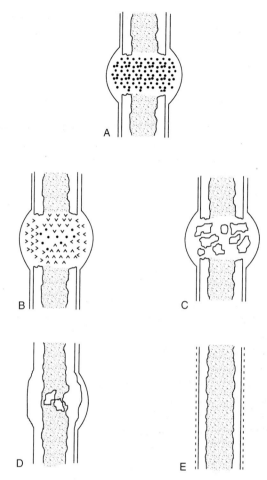

Figure 3.4 Repair of bone. A: Fracture leads to bleeding and blood clot. B: Granulation tissue forms. C: Calcification gradually occurs, leading to D new bone and E remodelling. (After *Gray's Anatomy*.)

REFERENCES

Ausprunk, DH, Boudreau, CL, Nelson, DA (1981) Proteoglycans in the microvasculature II. Histochemical localization in proliferating capillaries in the rabbit cornea. *American Journal of Pathology* **103**: 367–375.

Bischoff, R (1986) A satellite cell mitogen from crushed adult muscle. *Developmental Biology* **115**: 140–147.

Bischoff, R (1990) Interaction between satellite cells and skeletal muscle fibres. *Development* **109**: 943–952.

Carlson, BM, Faulkner, JA (1983) The regeneration of skeletal muscle fibres following injury: a review. *Medicine and Science in Sport and Exercise* **15**: 187–198.

Carpenter, S, Karpati, G (1984) *Pathology of Skeletal Muscle*. Churchill Livingstone, New York.

Clark, RAF (1985) Cutaneous tissue repair: basic biological considerations. *Journal of the American Academy of Dermatology* **13**: 701–725.

Clark, RAF (1988) Overview and general considerations of wound repair. In: Clark, RAF, Henson, PM (eds) *The Molecular and Cellular Biology of Wound Repair*. Plenum Press, New York.

Clark, RAF (1990a) Cutaneous wound repair. In: Goldsmith, LE (ed) *Biochemistry and Physiology of the Skin*. Oxford University Press, Oxford.

Clark, RAF (1990b). Fibronectin matrix deposition and fibronectin receptor expression in healing and normal skin. *Journal of Investigative Dermatology* 94, **6** (supplement): 128S–134S.

Clark, RAF (1991). Cutaneous wound repair: a review with emphasis on integrin receptor expression. In: Jansen, H, Rooman, R, Robertson, JIS (eds) *Wound Healing*. Wrightson Biomedical Publishing Ltd, Petersfield.

Clark, RAF, Della Pelle, P, Manseau, E, Lanigan, JM, Dvorak, HF, Colvin, RB (1982a) Blood vessel fibronectin increases in conjunction with endothelial cell proliferation and capillary ingrowth during wound healing. *Journal of Investigative Dermatology* 79: 269–276.

Clark, RAF, Della Pelle, P, Manseau, E, Lanigan, JM, Dvorak, HF, Colvin, RB (1982b) Fibronectin and fibrin provide a provisional matrix for epidermal cell migration during wound re-epithelialization. *Journal of Investigative Dermatology* 79: 264–269.

Czaja, MJ, Weiner, FR, Eghbali, M, Giambrone, MA, Eghbali, M, Zern, M (1987) Differential effects of interferon-gamma on collagen and fibrinectin gene expression. *Journal of Biological Chemistry* 262: 13348–13351.

Darby, I, Skalli, O, Gabbiani, G (1990) A smooth muscle actin is transiently expressed by myofibroblasts during experimental wound healing. *Laboratory Investigation* 63: 21–29.

Duncan, MR, Berman, B (1989) Differential regulation of collagen, glycosaminoglycan, fibronectin and collagenase activity production in cultured human adult fibroblasts by interleukin-1 alpha and beta and tumour necrosis factor alpha and beta. *Journal of Investigative Dermatology* 92: 699–706.

Ehrlich, HP, Hembry, RH (1984) A comparative study of fibroblasts in healing freeze and burn injuries in rats. *American Journal of Pathology* 117: 288–294.

Ehrlich, HP, Rajaratnam, JBM (1990) Cell locomotion forces versus cell contraction forces for collagen lattice contraction: an *in vitro* model of wound contraction. *Tissue and Cell* 22: 407–417.

Folkman, J, Klagsburn, M (1987) Angiogensic factors. *Science* 235: 442–447.

Gabbiani, G, Ryan, GB, Manjo, G (1971) Presence of modified fibroblasts in granulation tissue and their possible role in wound contraction. *Experientia* 27: 549–550.

Ginsberg, MH, Loftus, JC, Plow, EF (1988) Cytoadhesions, integrins and platelets. *Thrombosis and Haemostasis* 59: 1–6.

Hart, J (1993) *The effect of therapeutic ultrasound on dermal wound repair with emphasis on fibroblast activity*. PhD Thesis, London University, London.

Hashimoto, H, Prewitt, RL (1987) Microvascular changes during wound healing. *International Journal of Microcirculation: Clinical Experiments* 5: 303–310.

Heppenstall, RB (1980) Fracture healing. In: Heppenstall, RB (ed) *Fracture Treatment and Healing*. Saunders, Philadelphia.

Ho, Y-S, Lee, WMF, Snyderman, R (1987) Chemoattractant induced activation of *c-fos* gene expression in human monocytes. *Journal of Experimental Medicine* 165: 1524–1538.

Hosein, B, Mosessen, MW, Bianco, C (1985) Monocyte receptors for fibronectin. In: van Furth, R (ed) *Mononuclear Phagocytes: Characteristics, Physiology and Function*. Martinus Nijhoff, Dordrecht, Holland.

Hunt, TK (1987) Prospective: a retrospective perspective on the nature of wounds. In: Barbul, A, Pines, E, Caldwell, M, Hunt, TK (eds) *Growth Factors and Other Aspects of Wound Healing*. Liss, New York.

Hunt, TK, Dunphy, JE (1980) *Fundamentals of Wound Healing and Wound Infection: Theory and Surgical Practice*. Appleton-Century Croft, New York.

Ignotz, RA, Massague, J (1986) Transforming growth factor β stimulates the expression of fibronectin and collagen and their incorporation into the extracellular matrix. *Journal of Biochemistry* 260: 4337–4342.

Issekutz, AC (1981) Vascular responses during acute neutrophilic inflammation: their relationship to *in vivo* neutrophil emigration. *Laboratory Investigation* 45: 435–441.

Janssen, H, Rooman, R, Robertson, JIS (1991) *Wound Healing*. Wrightson Biomedical Publishing Ltd, Petersfield.

Kulozik, M, Heckmann, M, Mauch, C, Scharffeter, K, Krieg, Th (1991) Cytokine regulation of collagen metabolism during wound healing *in vitro* and *in vivo*. In: Jansen, H, Rooman, R, Robertson, JIS (eds) *Wound Healing*. Wrightson Biomedical Publishing Ltd, Petersfield.

Lark, MW, Laterra, J, Culp, LA (1985) Close and focal contact adhesions of fibroblasts to a fibrinectin-containing matrix. *Fed Proc* 44: 394–403.

Leibovich, SJ, Ross, R (1975) The role of macrophages in wound repair. *American Journal of Pathology* 78: 71.

Madri, JA, Pratt, BM (1988) Angiogenesis. In: Clark, RAF, Henson, PM (eds) *The Molecular and Cellular Biology of Wound Repair*. Plenum Press, New York.

Matoltsy, AG, Viziam, B (1970) Further observations on epithelialisation of small wounds: an autoradiographic study of incorporation and distribution of ^{3}H-Thymidine in the epithelium covering skin wounds. *Journal of Investigative Dermatology* 55: 20–25.

Mauch, C, Krieg, Th (1990) Fibroblast–matrix interactions and their role in the pathogenesis of fibrosis. *Rheumatic Disease Clinics of North America* 16: 93–107.

McCarthy, JB, Sas, DF, Furcht, LT (1988) Mechanism of parenchymal cell migration in wounds. In: Clark, RAF, Henson, PM (eds) *The Molecular and Cellular Biology of Wound Repair*. Plenum Press, New York.

Montadon, D, d'Andiran, G, Babbiani, G (1977) The mechanism of wound contraction and epithelialization. *Clinical Plastic Surgery* 4: 325.

Nicolas, JF, Gaycherand, M, Delaporte, E, Hartman, D, Richard, M, Croute, F, Thivolet, J (1991) Wound healing: a result of co-ordinate keratinocyte-fibroblast interactions. The role of keratinocyte cytokines. In: Janssen, H, Rooman, R, Robertson, JIS (1991) *Wound Healing*. Wrightson Biomedical Publishing Ltd, Petersfield.

Odland, G, Ross, R (1977) Human wound repair 1: epidermal regeneration. *Journal of Cell Biology* 39: 135–151.

Prostlethwaite, AE, Raghow, R, Stricklin, GP, Poppleton, A, Sayer, JM, Kang, AH (1988) Modulation of fibroblast function by interleukin-1 increased steady state accumulation of type I procollagen mRNA and stimulation of other functions but not chemotaxis by human recombinant interleukin-1α and β. *Journal of Cell Biology* 106: 311–318.

Proud, D, Kaplan, AP (1988) Kinin formation: mechanisms and roles in inflammatory disorders. *Annual Review of Immunology* 6: 49–83.

Repesh, LA, Fitzgerald, TJ, Furcht, LT (1982) Fibronectin involvement in granulation tissue and wound healing in rabbits. *Journal of Histrochemistry and Cytochemistry* 30: 351–358.

Riches, DWH (1988) The multiple role of macrophages in wound repair. In: Clark, RAF, Henson, PM (eds) *The Molecular and Cellular Biology of Wound Repair*. Plenum Press, New York.

Scharffetter, K, Heckmann, M, Hatamochi, A, Mauch, C, Stein, B, Riethmuller, G, Ziegler-Heitbrock, HB, Krieg, Th (1989) Synergistic effect of tumour necrosis factor-α and interferon gamma on collagen synthesis in human fibroblasts *in vitro*. *Experimental Cell Research* **181**: 409–419.

Skalli, O, Gabbiani, G (1988) The biology of the myofibroblast: relationship to wound contraction and fibrocontractive diseases. In: Clark, RAF, Henson, PM (eds) *The Molecular and Cellular Biology of Wound Repair*. Plenum Press, New York.

Terkeltaub, RA, Ginsberg, MH (1988) Platelets and response to injury. In: Clark, RAF, Henson, PM (eds) *The Molecular and Cellular Biology of Wound Repair*. Plenum Press, New York.

Toole, BP (1981) Glycosaminoglycans in morphogenesis. In: Hay, ED (ed) *Cell Biology of the Extracellular Matrix*. Plenum Press, New York.

Tsukamoto, Y, Helsel, JE, Wahl, SM (1981) Macrophage production of fibronectin, a chemoattractant for fibroblasts. *Journal of Immunology* **127**: 673–678.

Weeks, JR (1972) Prostaglandins. *Annual Review of Pharmacology and Toxicology* **12**: 317.

Williams, PL, Warwick, R, Dyson, M, Bannister, LH (eds) (1989) *Gray's Anatomy*. Churchill Livingstone, Edinburgh.

Williams, TJ (1988) Factors that affect vessel reactivity and leucocyte emigration. In: Clark, RAF, Henson, PM (eds) *The Molecular and Cellular Biology of Wound Repair*. Plenum Press, New York.

Zetter, BR (1988) Angiogenesis: state of the art. *Chest* **93**: 1595–1665.

4

Sensory and motor nerve activation

Oona Scott

INTRODUCTION

This chapter outlines basic muscle and peripheral nerve physiology. Particular attention is paid to the propagation of nerve and muscle action potentials, to differing characteristics of motor units and to the concept of nerve–muscle interaction.

Most of us are familiar with electrostatic charge and the sudden withdrawal we experience as we earth ourselves on a conducting surface. The ability to harness this response and therapeutic possibilities have developed over the past two hundred years since Luigi Galvani (1791) documented his observations of frog muscles contracting under the influence of what came to be called 'electricity'.

In 1833, Duchenne of Boulogne found that he could stimulate muscles electrically without piercing the skin and devised cloth-covered electrodes for percutaneous stimulation. Duchenne called his method of application 'localised currents' and he was the first to use 'faradism'—named for Michael Faraday, the pioneer of electrical engineering—for treatment. Duchenne observed that there were certain spots—motor points—along the surface of the body whose stimulation gave particularly strong muscle contraction. Differences in response between galvanic (unidirectional pulses lasting for more than 1 s and named after Galvani) and faradic (shorter pulses usually between 0.1 and 1 ms duration and applied at between 30 and 100 Hz) currents were recognised, with denervated muscle responding to galvanic rather than to faradic current. The duration of the current was the deciding factor in eliciting contraction.

Definition

Muscle- and nerve-stimulating currents are electrical currents which are capable of causing the generation of action potentials. They need to be of sufficient intensity and of an appropriate duration to cause depolarisation of the nerve or muscle membrane.

MOTONEURON TO MUSCLE ACTIVATION
Neural control of muscle

Smooth, coordinated movement is the output of a complex neuromuscular system. Skeletal muscle is capable of generating varying tensions and, at its very simplest, smooth, coordinated movement depends on the practical issue of contracting the required muscles in the right sequence at the right time. The control of coordinated movement is complex as different muscles combine in a variety of patterns. Appropriate combinations of excitation or of inhibition of different motoneurons in a dynamic series provide the required overall functional effect. There is much that is yet to be understood about the way in which the neural system devises these patterns of excitation and inhibition, about the interrelationship of the afferent and efferent neural systems, and not least about how motor units are selected to achieve a particular movement and about how firing patterns are updated as the movement evolves.

A brain uses stereotypical electrical signals—nerve action potentials—to process information received in the central nervous system (CNS) and analyses information at various levels. The signals consist of potential changes produced by electrical currents flowing across cell membranes, currents carried by ions such as those of sodium, potassium and chlorine (see Electrophysiological properties of nerves and muscles below). The coding of information depends principally on the frequency of impulses being transmitted along a nerve fibre, the number of fibres involved and on synaptic connections made within the spinal cord and higher levels of the central nervous system (CNS). Variability of response occurs at the level of neuronal synapses and the ability to modify processes of excitation and inhibition is thought to be critical to changes which occur in central control mechanisms.

The motor unit

The smallest unit of movement that a central nervous system can control is a *motor unit*, as defined by Sherrington in 1906. This unit consists of a motoneuron, together with its axon and dendrites, motor end plates and the muscle fibres it supplies. Motoneurons are the largest cells in the ventral horn of the spinal cord. The activity or firing frequency of these cells is dependent on their connections with afferent inputs from muscles, joints and skin, as well as their connections with other parts of the central nervous system.

Each motoneuron integrates excitatory (EPSP) and inhibitory postsynaptic (IPSP) potentials from thousands of synapses spread over the cell body or soma, and these influence whether or not it generates an action potential. When an action potential is discharged down the axon of a motoneuron, all the muscle fibres it supplies contract. This phenomenon, an *'all or nothing'* response, was first defined by Sherrington in 1906.

External electrical stimulation is used therapeutically to elicit skeletal muscle contraction supplementing or enhancing normal physiological processes and, to understand such uses, it is important to understand the underlying electrophysiological processes.

Electrophysiological properties of nerves and muscles

Conduction of action potentials along membranes of nerves and muscles occurs because there is a potential difference between the intracellular fluid and the extracellular fluid (Fig. 4.1). The *resting potential* is of the order of $-90\,$mV for skeletal muscle, and $-70\,$mV for lower motoneurons, the minus sign indicating that the inside of the cell has a negative potential relative to the exterior; this potential difference can be altered by passage of ions.

In cell membranes of both nerves and muscles, protein molecules are embedded in a double layer of lipid (fat) molecules which are arranged with their hydrophilic heads facing outward and hydrophobic tails extending into the middle of the layer (see Fig. 2.2, p. 34). Some protein molecules make contact with both the extracellular and the intracellular fluids. Protein molecules can have control functions with one region being a selectivity filter and another region providing a gate which can be open or closed.

The intracellular and extracellular fluids are in osmotic equilibrium. There is, however, a difference in the proportions of different ions in the two solutions: there is a higher concentration of potassium ions in the intracellular fluid, and higher concentrations of both sodium and chloride ions in the extracellular fluid.

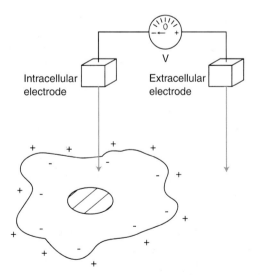

Figure 4.1 The potential difference across a cell membrane measured with an intracellular electrode and an extracellular electrode.

Movement of ions

Ions at high concentration tend to diffuse to areas of low concentration and their movement is also influenced by voltage gradients, with positive ions being attracted down the negative gradient, and vice versa. An outward movement of potassium ions down their concentration gradient would be expected but at the same time the inner surface of the membrane is at a negative potential with respect to the outside, and this tends to restrain the outward movement of positively charged ions.

The *equilibrium potential* of any ion is proportional to the difference between the logarithms of intracellular concentration and the extracellular concentration and is defined by the *Nernst equation*. The Nernst equation describes the equilibrium potential, which is the electric potential necessary to balance a given ionic concentration across a membrane so that the overall passive movement of the ion is zero.

It was proposed by Bernstein (1902) that only potassium ions could diffuse across the resting cell membrane. Later work by Hodgkin and Keynes (1955) showed that the cell membrane is permeable to other ions, including sodium ions, and that sodium ions are in a continuous state of flux across the membrane against both the concentration and the electrical gradients. Their findings supported the concept of an active transport system that uses energy supplied by the hydrolysis of adenosine triphosphate (ATP) to pump sodium ions out of the cell and to accumulate potassium ions within the cell. Evidence suggests that the expulsion of sodium ions to the influx of potassium ions is of the order of 3:2.

Generation and propagation of action potentials

The unequal distribution of ions across the cell membrane of both nerve and muscle cells forms the basis for generation and propagation of action potentials. Nerve and muscle cells are *excitable*—that is, they are able to produce an action potential after application of a suitable stimulus (see Threshold below). An *action potential* is a transient reversal of the membrane potential—a *depolarisation*. This lasts for about 1 ms in nerve cells and up to 2 ms in some muscle fibres.

Threshold

An initial opening of a few of the voltage-activated sodium channels occurs, followed by a rapid transient increase in sodium permeability. This allows sodium ions to diffuse rapidly into the cell, causing a sudden accumulation of positive charge on the inside surface of the neural or muscle fibre membrane. The increased permeability to sodium ions is followed by depolarisation via the opening of voltage-activated potassium channels; there is some hyperpolarisation beyond the resting potential.

The nature of the regenerating mechanism was demonstrated both in terms of the time course of the action potential and of ionic conductance by Hodgkin and Huxley (1952). Stimulus below the threshold required to produce an action potential reduces but does not reverse the membrane potential. As the stimulus is increased, the potential difference across the cell membrane is reduced until it reaches the critical threshold level. At this level, the stimulus will lead to the automatic generation of an action potential. The level of the threshold varies according to a number of factors, including how many action potentials the nerve fibre has conducted recently.

After an action potential, two changes occur that make it impossible for the nerve fibre to transmit a second action potential immediately. First, *inactivation* (the *absolute refractory period*) occurs during the falling phase of the action potential during which no amount of externally applied depolarisation can initiate a second regenerative response. After the absolute refractory period, there is a *relative refractory period* during which the residual inactivation of the sodium conductance and the relatively high potassium conductance combine to produce an increase in the threshold for action potential initiation.

To stimulate a nerve, the stimulus has to be both of sufficient intensity and of sufficient duration to depolarise the nerve membrane.

Action potentials can be initiated in peripheral nerves by the application of suitable electrical stimuli (pulses). The rate of change and frequency of stimuli are important. The graph in Figure 4.2 illustrates the relationship between the duration of an electrical stimulus and the intensity of stimulation (see Strength–duration curves in Ch. 19).

If the stimulus is applied very slowly—that is, its rise time is slow—then the rate of depolarisation is very slow. There is a steady flow of ions in one direction and no action potential is generated. A slow, steady, unidirectional current and a slow fall is typical of currents used in 'galvanic' treatment or iontophoretic treatments, and no stimulation of muscle or nerve occurs. If the stimulus is applied quickly and the duration of the stimulus is long enough, the nerve fibre is rapidly depolarised to the threshold and an action potential is generated. The slower the stimulus applied, the greater is the magnitude of depolarisation required to bring the fibre to threshold.

Neurons as conductors of electricity

Although permeability properties of cell membranes result in regenerative electrical signals, there are other factors to be considered. Many peripheral motor and sensory nerves are myelinated—*myelin* being an insulating material formed by Schwann cells and forming as many as 320 membranes in series between the plasma

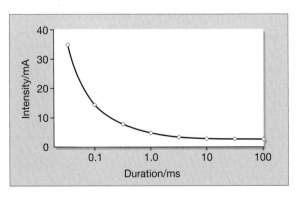

Figure 4.2 The relationship between strength and duration of a stimulus required to generate an action potential in a motor nerve fibre.

membrane of a nerve fibre and the extracellular fluid. This sheath of membranes is interrupted at regular intervals by the *nodes of Ranvier*, which are arranged such that the greater the diameter of the nerve fibre, the greater are the internodal distances. Because myelin is an insulator and ions cannot flow easily into and out of the sheathed internodal region, excitation skips from node to node (*saltatory conduction*), thereby greatly increasing the conduction velocity and, because ionic exchange is limited to the nodal regions, using less energy. While the excitation is progressing from one node to the next on the leading edge of the action potential, many nodes behind are still active. Myelinated nerve fibres exhibit a capability of firing at higher frequencies for more prolonged periods than other nerve fibres.

As a general rule, larger diameter nerves (group Aα motor nerves) conduct impulses more rapidly and have a lower threshold of excitability than the much smaller Aδ pain fibres (Table 4.1). This means that threshold and motor nerve conduction velocities can be tested without exciting the pain fibres (see Ch. 19). On stimulation, larger nerve fibres also produce larger signals, their excitatory response lasts for a shorter time and they have shorter refractory periods.

Within muscle, the axon of the motoneuron divides into many branches to innervate muscle fibres that are scattered throughout the muscle and together make up the motor unit. Each muscle fibre has one neuromuscular junction, lying usually about midway along the fibre.

Table 4.1   Classification of peripheral nerves according to conduction velocity and junction (with permission from *Human Neurophysiology* (2nd edn), Chapman and Hall)

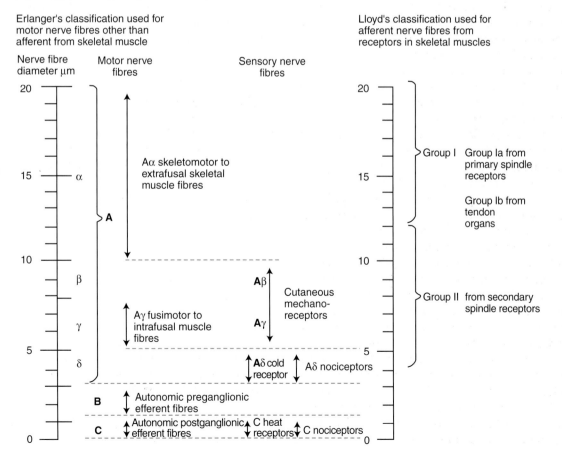

Synaptic transmission

Synapses are points of contact between nerve cells, or between nerves and effector cells such as muscle fibres. At electrical synapses, current generated by an impulse in the presynaptic nerve terminal spreads into the next cell through low-resistance channels. More commonly, however, synapses are chemical in action: the gap between the presynaptic and postsynaptic membrane is filled with fluid, and the nerve terminal secretes a chemical, a *neurotransmitter*, which activates the postsynaptic membrane. The postsynaptic junction or motor end plate is the specialised region on the muscle where the neuromuscular junction comes into close contact with the muscle fibre that it innervates.

Acetylcholine release

When an action potential arrives at a neuromuscular junction, it causes voltage-dependent calcium channels to open, and allows calcium ions to diffuse into the axon terminal. Acetylcholine from the synaptic vesicles in the nerve terminal diffuses across the synaptic cleft in multimolar packages (or quanta) to combine with the receptor sites on the motor end plate. This alters the end-plate membrane permeability to sodium and potassium and immediately depolarises the membrane. The end-plate potential (EPP) causes a local change in potential of the muscle membrane in close contact with it. This propagates a regenerative motor unit action potential (MUAP) in all directions along the adjacent muscle membrane using the mechanism already described for the propagation of action potentials along the axon membrane. The magnitude of a single MUAP is normally sufficient to cause contraction of all muscle fibres belonging to its motor unit—following the *all-or-none principle*.

The action of acetylcholine at the neuromuscular junction is terminated when an enzyme, acetylcholinesterase, is released. This enzyme, embedded in the basal lamina of the synaptic cleft of the motor endplate, hydrolyses acetylcholine and thereby prevents prolonged action of the transmitter. Along the length of the muscle fibre, the muscle cell membrane (the sarcolemma) has numerous infoldings forming a system of membranes called the transverse tubular system or T tubules. As the action potential goes along the sarcolemma, it passes close to the fibre down the T tubules (Figs 4.3 and 4.4).

Calcium release

Arrival of the action potential in the T tubules depolarises the sarcoplasmic reticulum, another complex membrane system in close contact with the myofibrils. The main function of the sarcoplasmic reticulum is to release and take up calcium during contraction and relaxation. Depolarisation of the transverse tubular system signals the release of calcium ions from the sarcoplasmic reticulum into the sarcoplasm and allows the actin–myosin cross-bridges to bond (see *Sliding-filament hypothesis*, p. 67). Calcium ions are then actively pumped back into the sarcoplasmic reticulum and contraction ceases (Fig. 4.4).

MUSCLES—BASIC CHARACTERISTICS, CLASSIFICATION AND THE INFLUENCE OF THE MOTONEURON
Gross structure and function

Muscles vary in function as well as in shape, size and in method of attachment to bone or to cartilage. A muscle may fulfil more than one function—stabilising, producing power and sustaining posture, as well as performing one or more specifically controlled movements during what is for the person a single sequence of movements.

The composition and structure of each muscle are often seen as a compromise between the different needs for speed of movement, force and economy of energy. There are, however, basic principles to the mechanical properties of muscle: the maximum force that can be produced by a muscle is generally proportional to its cross-sectional area and the maximum rate

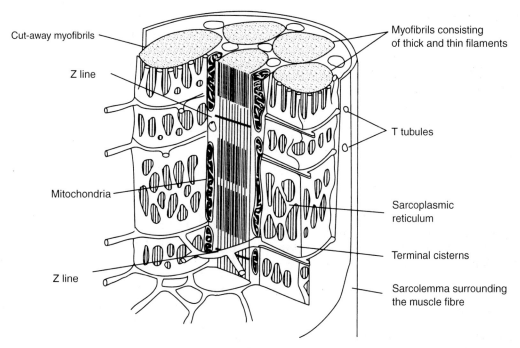

Cut-away myofibrils

Z line

Mitochondria

Z line

Myofibrils consisting
of thick and thin filaments

T tubules

Sarcoplasmic
reticulum

Terminal cisterns

Sarcolemma surrounding
the muscle fibre

Figure 4.3   A section of mammalian skeletal muscle. A single muscle fibre has been cut away to show the individual myofibrils and the thick myosin and thin actin filaments within a sarcomere. The sarcoplasmic reticulum is seen surrounding each myofibril, together with the T system of tubules in which the Ca^{2+} ions are stored and released during muscle contraction.

of contraction of a long muscle is greater than that of a short muscle.

As a rule, small muscles with precision tasks such as those in the hand are composed of motor units with few muscle fibres, whereas trunk and proximal limb muscles contain motor units with a large number of muscle fibres. At a simple level, two components are integrated in a single muscle: a contractile component, which is altered by stimulation and which can develop an active tension, and an elastic component, connective tissue, through which the contractile component transmits the generated force to the muscle tendon (Figs 4.3 and 4.4).

The response of a single motor unit to a single action potential is called a *twitch contraction* (Fig. 4.5). The muscle responds with a brief contraction and then returns to its resting state. If more than one impulse is given within an interval that is shorter than the contraction–relaxation cycle time of the motor unit, the muscle does not return to its resting state, and the forces produced by each impulse are said to *summate* or *fuse*.

At a sufficiently high frequency of stimulation, a fused, tetanic or smooth, contraction is produced as the force fluctuations of each impulse are indistinguishable in practical terms (Fig. 4.6). Because slow-contracting muscle fibres summate and produce a tetanic contraction at lower frequencies of nerve stimulation, investigators realised that slow muscles such as the soleus might be more suitable for sustained 'tonic' function at low levels of activation, whereas fast-contracting muscle fibres which fuse at higher frequencies of stimulation may be more appropriate for 'phasic' function, and for generating high forces for short periods of time.

Classification—matching motoneurons to the muscle fibres

The suggestion that mammalian muscle fibres had diverse functional properties occurred when Ranvier (1874) observed that the soleus muscle was a deeper red colour and contracted more slowly than other calf muscles.

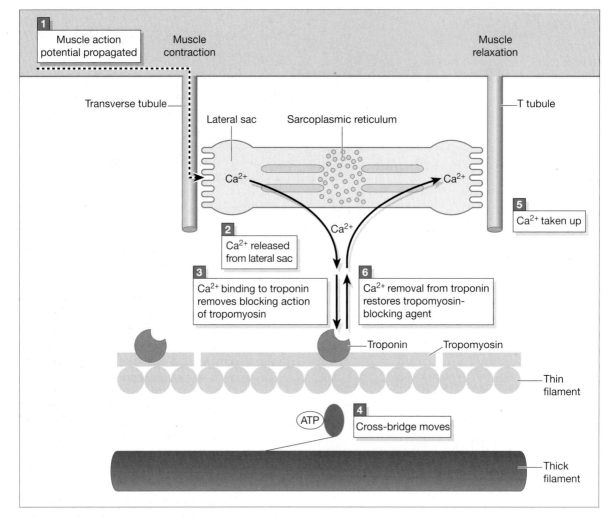

Figure 4.4   Sequence of calcium release and uptake during muscle contraction and relaxation. An action potential causes release of calcium ions from the sarcoplasmic reticulum into the sarcoplasm, which, in the presence of ATP, causes the interaction of the cross-bridges of the myosin filaments with the actin filaments and thus muscle contraction. When calcium is released from the sarcoplasmic reticulum, the myofibril contracts; when calcium is reabsorbed by the sarcoplasmic reticulum, the myofibril relaxes.

Eccles and his coworkers confirmed these observations in 1958 and classified motor units on the basis of the activity patterns of their motoneurons expressed in terms of firing frequency and an ability (or tonicity) to maintain firing. Fast-firing, so-called 'phasic', motoneurons innervated muscle fibres with fast contraction times and slow, 'tonic', motoneurons innervated muscle fibres with slow contraction times.

Edström and Krugelberg (1968) confirmed the similarity of muscle fibres belonging to a single motor unit by a method of glycogen depletion of individual motor units in response to prolonged stimulation of single motor nerve fibres. The finding that muscle fibres of individual motor units were homogeneous and that differences in properties did occur between fibres of different motor units suggested that the activity pattern

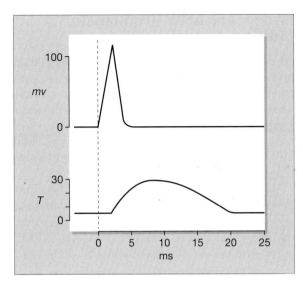

Figure 4.5 The electrical (mv=potential change) and mechanical (T=tension) response of a mammalian skeletal muscle fibre to a single action potential resulting in a twitch contraction.

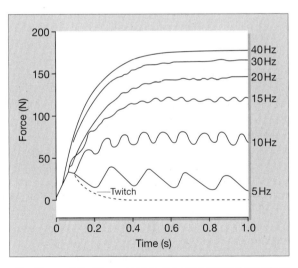

Figure 4.6 The response of human skeletal muscle to different rates of stimulation.

of the motoneuron was important in determining these properties.

The distribution of muscle fibres that make up a motor unit can be visualised using this method of glycogen depletion. Human muscle can be seen to be heterogeneous in that each is composed of a wide variety of different muscle fibres. Fibres belonging to any one motor unit are spread over a large territory rather than being clustered together. Edström and Krugelberg's finding has been modified (Martin *et al.*, 1988) as more sophisticated techniques showed that subtle differences do exist within individual motor units.

Speed of contraction and histological properties

The work of Burke and his colleagues (1973) on cat gastrocnemius muscle showed a close association between physiological or mechanical properties and histochemical ('histo = tissue', implying chemical reaction occurring in tissues themselves) properties of the muscle fibres in each motor unit. They identified three main types of motor units based on their speed of contraction and resistance to fatigue, and stated that each physiological category of muscle unit had a corresponding unique histochemical profile.

- **'FF' motor units.** These were fast contracting with short contraction times, developed relatively high tension, fatigued quickly and possessed high anaerobic glycolytic capacity but low oxidative capacity.
- **'FR' units.** These were also fast contracting, had similarly short twitch-contraction times but developed less tension than the 'FF' units, were less fatigable, possessed high glycolytic capacity and moderate-to-high oxidative capacity.
- **'S' units.** These were slow contracting with longer twitch-contraction times, developed least tension, and possessed high oxidative and low glycolytic capacity.

This classification by Burke *et al.* (1973) of motor units by their resistance to fatigue matched that based on enzyme histochemical characteristics of whole muscle fibre populations by Barnard *et al.* (1971) so that fast glycolytic (FG) fibres probably belong to the 'FF' (most fatigable) motor units, the fast oxidative glycolytic (FOG) to the 'FR' (less fatigable) units and the slow oxidative (SO) to the 'S' (fatigue-resistant) units. An additional fast-fibre subtype, type IIx (also known as type IId) has been identified more recently, by immunohistochemical analyses using antibodies raised against myosin heavy chains. Type IIx is intermediate to types IIa and IIb and is characterised as being more fatigue resistant than type IIb fibres.

In human studies, the histological method frequently used to distinguish muscle fibre types is based on staining techniques for myofibrillar actomyosin adenosine triphosphatase (mATPase) activity. The differences in the mATPase activity relate to specific myosin heavy-chain complements and make it possible to distinguish between specific muscle fibre types, called type I and type II for those fibres staining light and dark respectively.

Using differences in pH stability, type II fibres can be further subdivided into two major subgroups: IIa and IIb fibres (see Dubowitz, 1995); a further subgroup, IIc, has also been identified. Type IIc fibres, which are relatively infrequent, have been found predominantly in fetal and in diseased muscles. Bárány (1967) found that there was a close relationship between myosin ATPase activity and the speed of contraction, indicating that the activity of the myosin molecule correlated with the rate of muscle contraction.

Later work by Garnett and his colleagues (Garnett *et al.*, 1979; Garnett and Stephens, 1981), working at St Thomas's Hospital, showed that results with human subjects were comparable to those from other mammals. Using thin wire electrodes in human gastrocnemius muscle, they showed that it was possible to measure the time course of contraction of single motor units and to test their twitch-contraction time, using repeated tetani to measure fatigability. Finally, they were able to deplete the motor unit of glycogen (by stimulating repeatedly for 2 hours), whereupon serial sections of biopsies showed that FF fibres correlated with type IIb fibres, and SO fibres with type I fibres. They also reported that stimulation of sensory nerve endings changed the recruitment order of firing of the motoneurons, causing the larger motoneurons to fire before smaller motoneurons (see Ch. 8, Differences between electrical stimulation and exercise, p. 116).

Myosin and actin—contractile proteins

At the molecular level, the main elements visible under a light microscope are myofibrils, and these, arranged in parallel, make up a muscle fibre. Each myofibril has longitudinal myofilaments with the alternating light I (isotropic) and dark A (anisotropic) bands, which give skeletal muscle its typical striated or striped appearance (Figs 4.3, 4.7).

Under an electron microscope, it becomes apparent that each myofibril is composed of a series (end to end) of repeating units or *sarcomeres*, the functional unit of muscle contraction. Within each sarcomere are myofilaments composed

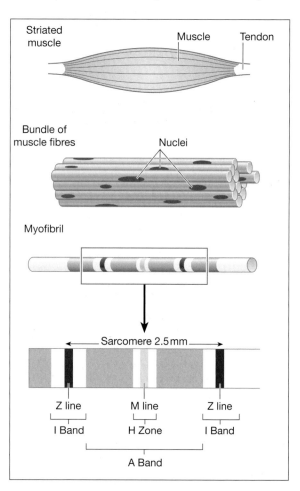

Figure 4.7 Schematic arrangements of contractile components.

mainly of either actin or myosin. Each sarcomere has two sets of thin actin filaments anchored at one end to a network of interconnecting proteins, called the Z line, and at the other end interdigitating with a set of thick myosin filaments. The myosin molecules, packed tail to tail, form the wide dark A band. The I band and the H zone are regions where there is no overlap between the actin and the myosin myofilaments; the I band has only the thin actin molecules and the H zone only the thick myosin myofilaments. Finally, in the centre of the H zone, is the M line, formed by proteins that bind all the myosin filaments together (Fig. 4.7).

Myosin molecules are relatively large proteins that consist of two globular heads or heavy myosin chain portions (HMM) and a single light myosin chain tail portion (LMM). Four light chains form the backbone or tail of the myosin molecule and are the thicker filaments in the sarcomere combining end to end with other tails. The portion extending from the backbone is the heavy-chain portion (HMM) of 2000 amino acids and consists of the flexible, so-called neck

portion—the S_2 portion—and the globular portion—or S_1 head portion—and two associated light chains. The composition of these light chains differs in fast and slow muscles, but so far their role has not been established. The globular portion contains the ATP-binding site and the actin-binding site (Figs 4.4 and 4.8).

Actin molecules polymerise to form two intertwined helical chains. Each actin monomer is relatively small and roughly spherical in shape. Two regulatory proteins, troponin and tropomyosin, are located on the actin. The two chains of tropomyosin molecules, each about the length of seven actin molecules, fit end to end along the strands of the actin double helix into a groove along the filament length, and they partially cover the myosin-binding site (Fig. 4.8).

The sliding-filament hypothesis

The force-generating mechanism appears to be cyclical, and the formation of cross-bridges between actin and myosin in the presence of ATP plays an essential role. Both this concept

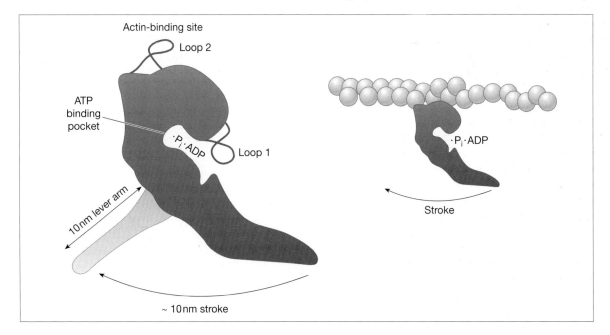

Figure 4.8 Myosin consists of two heads and a long α-helical tail. The figure shows a close-up of the S_1 (one of the two head portions) of the myosin molecule at the actin AM*·ADP·P_i state (see Fig. 4.9). The arrow shows the direction of the conformational movement. Loop 1 may set the rate constant for the ADP release rate while loop 2 interacts with the amino terminal of the actin molecule (after Spudich, 1994, with permission of *Nature* and Professor J.A. Spudich).

of cross-bridge action, and the model of myosin with a head that rotates and stretches a compliant portion of the molecule, follow from theories advanced by AF Huxley in 1957 and extended by Huxley and Simmons in 1971. They observed no change in length of either the thick myosin or the thin actin filaments and suggested that a sliding motion forces the thin actin filaments on either side of the sarcomere in the A band towards the M line, thereby shortening the sarcomere. Though the exact mechanism is still uncertain, recent work on molecular motors has provided considerable support for the mechanochemical actin-activated myosin–ATPase cycle. One form of this mechanism is illustrated in Figure 4.9.

In step one, the adenosine diphosphate (ADP) and inorganic phosphate (P_i) are bound to the myosin head. The myosin heads are free to bind to the actin molecules and form an actin–myosin–ADP–P_i complex (step 2). This binding triggers the release of energy, the myosin head rotates, and force is exerted between the two filaments. Movement occurs between the filaments if they are free to move and, if they are not, an 'isometric contraction' occurs. The link between the myosin and the actin molecules must be broken to allow the myosin cross-bridge to re-attach to a new actin molecule and repeat the cycle. Binding of a molecule of ATP breaks the link between actin and myosin (step 3). The ATP that is bound to the myosin then splits (step 4) forming the energised state of myosin, which can now reattach to a new site on the actin filament.

Role of calcium in contraction

At a critical calcium concentration, calcium binds to specific binding sites on troponin, one of the regulatory proteins. Troponin changes its conformation, moving the tropomyosin, and thereby exposing binding sites on the actin molecule (see Fig. 4.8). This enables the head of the myosin filament to interact with the binding sites on the actin molecule, forming cross-bridges cyclically and so developing force. Removal of calcium reverses this process and tropomyosin moves back into its blocking position.

Recruitment of motor units in voluntary contractions

In 1929, Adrian and Bronk introduced the concentric-needle electrode and showed that by inserting this electrode directly into the muscle it was possible to record the electrical events that cause contraction of the muscle fibres. They showed that voluntary muscle force could be

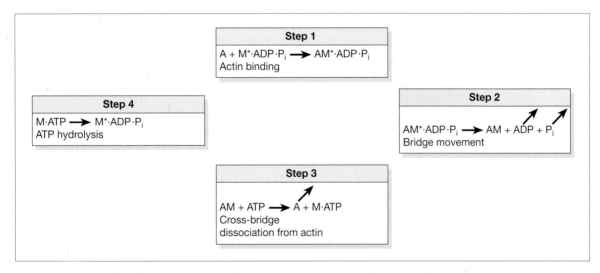

Figure 4.9 Chemical and physical events occurring during first four steps of the cross-bridge cycle.

increased both by increasing the firing frequency of motoneurons and by recruiting additional motor units. In the same year, Denny Brown (1929) found that the smaller motoneurons which innervate slow-contracting muscle fibres were more readily activated than the larger phasic motoneurons which innervate faster-contracting muscle fibres.

Denny Brown's finding supports the theory (see Gross structure and function earlier) that slow muscle fibres are used for sustained activities whereas faster-contracting muscle fibres are used when short bursts of high levels of force are required.

Henneman and Olson (1965) investigated the excitability of motoneurons and the order of their recruitment during movement. The size of the cell body of a motoneuron is related to the number of muscle fibres that it innervates. Large motoneurons have larger cell bodies, large diameter axons (and high conductance velocities) and a lower input resistance to an applied input current than do small neurons. For a similar input current, small motoneurons reach their threshold for firing sooner than large motoneurons. Henneman showed that the excitability or firing pattern of a motoneuron was directly correlated with its size and that, in any given movement, motoneurons were recruited in an orderly manner according to their size. It is now thought that this hierarchy of motor unit recruitment may be responsible for the heterogeneity of muscle fibres within the same muscle (see Pette and Vrbová, 1992, 1999).

In 1973, Milner-Brown, Stein and Yemm showed that slower-contracting motor units, in humans, were recruited first in both reflex and voluntary movements involving low tensions and that the larger, faster, motor units were activated 'only by rapid vigorous and briefly sustained contractions' with bursts of rapid firing. Patterns of firing and of recruitment of voluntary muscle force can be increased both by increasing the firing frequency of motoneurons and by recruiting additional motor units.

Only in very fast (ballistic) movements, where speed is of the essence, does the faster conduction speed of the large motoneurons play a part; the slow motor units, because of the slower conduction times of their axons, may fire after the faster motor units.

Normal frequencies of firing of motoneurons in human muscles rarely exceed 40 Hz and are rarely less than 6–8 Hz. Under most conditions, motor units fire asynchronously; they fire synchronously only during powerful contractions and during fatigue.

Influence of the motoneuron

The change of muscle properties in response to a change of neural input was first demonstrated by Buller and his colleagues in 1960 (Buller, Eccles and Eccles, 1960a,b). They sutured a nerve that normally supplied a slow-contracting muscle of a cat into the fast-contracting flexor digitorum longus (FDL). The soleus was innervated by suturing the nerve from FDL. This experiment showed not only that contractile properties of the two muscles exchanged but also that there were extensive sequential changes in their metabolic and histological properties.

The close association of a motoneuron's activity pattern and the contractile properties of the motor unit was underlined when it was shown, using chronic stimulation at 10 Hz, that it was possible to preserve the contractile characteristics of the soleus muscle of the rabbit following tenotomy (Vrbová, 1966).

The slow soleus would normally have become fast-contracting following section of its tendon and the spinal cord. However, when the muscle was stimulated chronically at 5–10 Hz for 8 hours each day, its contractile properties remained slow. If higher frequencies of stimulation were used (i.e. 20–40 Hz), the silenced soleus muscle became fast contracting (Salmons and Vrbová, 1969; Vrbová, 1966). This matching of the pattern of activity of motoneurons to the properties of the muscle fibres is fundamental. It underlies the hypothesis that activity has an impact on the phenotype of skeletal muscle (Pette and Vrbová, 1999) and provides an explanation for changes in skeletal muscle associated with clinical neurological situations (see Ch. 8).

AFFERENT INPUT TO THE CENTRAL NERVOUS SYSTEM

The ability to react to external stimuli depends on inputs of information from sources external to the CNS into the CNS. The nervous system receives information from a wide variety of receptors. There are receptors that respond to light, to sound, to mechanical stimuli, or to heat and to cold; some stimuli are perceived as pain; some chemical influences are perceived as smells or as tastes. Sensory nerve fibres are also called *afferent* nerve fibres.

Sensory pathways

The CNS not only receives information from sensory receptors but also acts upon them to modify their responses. Afferent neurons convey information from receptors at their peripheral endings to the CNS. Such neurons are sometimes called primary or first-order neurons because they are the first cells entering the CNS in the synaptically linked chains of neurons that handle the incoming information.

All information coming into the CNS is subjected to control mechanisms at synaptic junctions either by other afferent neurons or by descending pathways from higher regions such as the reticular formation and the cerebral cortex. These inhibitory controls are exerted at two main sites:

1. the axon terminals of the afferent nerves
2. the interneurons that are activated directly by the afferent neurons.

Motoneurons that innervate a particular muscle form a *motoneuron pool*, and α and γ motoneurons are mixed together in this pool, which is located in the ventral horn of one of several segments of the spinal cord. All motoneurons receive afferent fibres from all of the muscle spindles in the innervated muscle. The group Ia and group II afferent fibres make monosynaptic and polysynaptic excitatory connections to the motoneurons in the spinal cord.

The signals are either carried in ascending pathways to the brainstem and thalamus and then relayed to a specific area of the cerebral cortex, or the information is relayed from the interneurons along non-specific ascending pathways into the brain reticular formation and regions of the thalamus and cortex.

Transmission of impulses from receptors

Mathews in his book published in 1972 and more recently Jami in a comprehensive article (1992) reviewed their outstanding work on muscle stretch receptors. Skin is equipped with three categories of cutaneous receptor: *mechanoceptors* or pressure receptors, *thermoceptors* for sensing hot and cold, and *nociceptors* signalling damage to the skin.

Afferent neurons differ from motoneurons in that they have no dendrites and only one process or axon. On leaving the cell body, the axon divides into two branches: one, the peripheral process, which may end in a receptor and the other, the central process, enters the CNS and makes synaptic contact with its target neurons. In response to an adequate stimulus, the receptor generates a receptor potential that reflects the intensity, duration and location of the stimulus. A stimulus that is too weak to initiate nerve impulses is said to be *subthreshold*.

Adequate stimuli generate *receptor potentials*, which result in trains of action potentials that are propagated along afferent nerve fibres, some synapsing on motoneurons and some synapsing in the medulla. These stimuli have the same all-or-none nature of action potentials as described earlier for motoneurons. The greater the intensity of the stimulus the higher is the frequency of action potentials, and the more widespread the stimulus the greater is the number of receptors that are stimulated.

In a few cases, for instance the Pacinian, Meissner and Ruffini corpuscles (types of pressure receptors present in the skin), a single afferent neuron ends in one receptor. More commonly, the afferent neuron divides into fine branches, each terminating in a receptor, all of which are preferentially sensitive to the same type of stimulus or input. A single afferent neuron and all of its receptor endings make up a *sensory unit*, a concept similar to the motor unit described above. Sensory receptors act as transducers and the input stimulus is transformed into an electrical signal.

Adaptation

A stimulus that is applied and maintained results in different patterns of impulses depending on the particular receptor that is being stimulated. In some receptors, there is an initial burst of impulses on stimulation and then the discharge rate falls greatly or may cease altogether. This process is called *adaptation* and involves a decline in the intensity of response during stimulation that is sustained at constant intensity. Other receptors show no adaptation and the pattern of impulses accurately reflects the duration and intensity of the input stimulus. Adaptation of the subject to the sensory effects of electrical stimulation is important and is sometimes overlooked in evaluating tolerance to superimposed electrical stimulation (see sections on Pain and Low-frequency stimulation).

Classification of afferent nerve fibres

Sensory nerves, like motor nerves, may be myelinated and have been classified according to their function and the receptors that they innervate. Two methods of classification have been used (see Table 4.1). Lloyd and Chang (1948) proposed a system of classification of grades, I–IV for muscle afferents based on fibre diameter, which is inversely related to conduction velocity. The largest and fastest-conducting sensory nerves are group Ia afferents (12–20 μm in diameter) and have the lowest threshold of any sensory nerves to electrical stimulation. Their terminals are found in the central parts of both bag and chain fibres (Fig. 4.10) and form the primary endings. They correspond to α motoneurons having conduction velocities that range from 50 to 70 m/s. Group Ib afferents are slightly smaller and come from Golgi tendon organs. The smaller Group II (6–12 μm in diameter) afferents come from terminals found in less central positions of the muscle spindles, where they form secondary endings (Fig. 4.10). The other afferent nerves share Erlanger's A, B and C classification based on the conduction velocities for the motor nerves (Table 4.1). The A group have a wide spectrum of fibre diameter

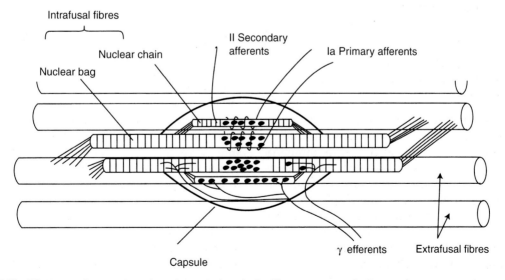

Figure 4.10 Diagrammatic representation of a muscle spindle. The two types of afferent sensory ending (group Ia and group II) are shown on the upper chain, and bag fibres and the efferent endings on the lower fibres.

(1–20 μm). Erlanger and Gasser (1937) were the first to realise that the compound action potential of a peripheral nerve in a frog shows several distinct peaks. For convenience, these were divided according to their conduction velocity; peak A is subdivided into α, β, γ and δ. Each peak contains nerve fibres with particular functions. The Aα and γ peaks include efferent nerve fibres that supply extrafusal and intrafusal muscle fibres.

Sensory receptors in skeletal muscle

Skeletal muscle contains the following sensory receptors: free nerve endings, Golgi tendon organs, Pacinian corpuscles and muscle spindles. Receptors in skeletal muscles are sophisticated, and their response to stretch is moderated by the central nervous system. (For a detailed review see Jami 1992.)

Free nerve endings are found in association with every structure in muscle; they are the endings of all non-myelinated afferent fibres and the smallest myelinated nerve endings—type Aδ fibres. Types of stimuli that excite these endings are pressure, pain, increase in osmolarity, tetanus and infusion of potassium ions—all conditions that might be expected to exist in exercising or stimulated muscle.

Golgi tendon organs are mechanoreceptors found at the points of attachment of muscle fibres to tendinous tissue. They are encapsulated structures composed of collagen bundles innervated by large, myelinated (8–12 μm diameter) Ib afferent fibres. Golgi tendon organs, originally believed to be high-threshold stretch receptors, actually have a low threshold and a dynamic sensitivity which signals small and rapid changes in contractile forces in the muscle. Their widespread distribution at the musculotendinous junction enables monitoring of contractions of every portion of muscle. In addition to ascending pathways, activation of Ib axons from the tendon organs produces inhibition of homonymous and synergic motoneurons and excitation of antagonist motoneurons. *Pacinian corpuscles* are usually found in association with Golgi tendon organs and are supplied by group II (3 μm diameter) myelinated fibres.

Muscle spindles are highly complicated receptors and are found in greatest number in skeletal muscles, which undergo small length variation requiring precision movement. Figure 4.10 shows a schematic diagram of a spindle. The spindles are structures of about 10 mm in length which lie parallel to the extrafusal muscle fibres. They are attached at either end to extrafusal fibres or to tendinous insertions and consist of a bundle of specialised muscle fibres or intrafusal fibres. They have a rich nerve supply, the role of which is not yet fully established. The central part of the spindle is contained within a thick connective tissue capsule. There are two types of intrafusal muscle fibres in the spindle: two or three bag fibres, and up to eight chain fibres. Bag fibres can be further subdivided into bag$_1$ and bag$_2$ fibres.

The large, Ia afferent fibres (12–20 μm diameter) have primary spiral endings on all of the muscle fibres in a spindle. These endings are on the most central region of each fibre. On either side of them, there may be up to five secondary spiral endings of the Group II afferent neurons, lying mainly on the bag$_2$ and chain fibres. The primary and secondary afferent endings differ in their responses to stretch and to vibration.

The primary endings respond with a rapid discharge during actual extension, have a slower rate of discharge during static stretch, and do not fire during the release of stretch. The secondary endings fire during static stretch. The primary endings are more highly sensitive to vibration than the secondary endings.

The motor supply to the spindles is provided mainly by small motor nerves (2–8 μm in diameter) fusimotor or γ fibres, which are found at the poles of the spindles within the capsule. There are two main classes of γ efferent motor fibres. One group, γ_δ, innervate the dynamic bag fibres, whereas γ_σ innervate ends on static bag$_2$ fibres and chain fibres. Stimulation of the fusimotor nerves elicits no increase in muscle tension but produces an increase in sensory Aβ discharge. More recently it has been recognised that some of the motor supply to the spindles comes from branches of the motoneuron supplying extrafusal muscles.

The primary endings are very sensitive to stretch and are thought to be the mechanical response of the bag_1 fibre, and these endings are thought to be length and velocity sensitive.

Nociceptive systems and pain

The pain receptors are free nerve endings without specialised accessory structures. Information about noxious or painful stimuli is passed to the spinal cord by two distinct sets of fibres. The myelinated Aδ axons (1–4 μm in diameter) conduct at 6–24 m/s. They are stimulated by sharp, pricking, well-localised pain, respond to noxious stimuli such as burning and cutting, and are mechanothermal receptors. The non-myelinated C axons at 0.1–1 μm in diameterconduct more slowly (at 0.5–2 m/s) and provide the second wave of pain, which is associated with a burning or aching sensation and is poorly localised.

These afferent fibres form synapses with second-order cells in the dorsal horn, sending their axons to the contralateral side and ascending in the spinothalamic tracts to the thalamus. The subject of pain modulation has received considerable attention and will be addressed in detail in Chapter 5. Many experiments have shown that no noxious stimulus can fail to activate other receptors responding to touch, pressure, displacement, stretch and cooling, and much interest in the treatment of pain by stimulation of the afferent system is based on these findings.

REFERENCES

Adrian, ED, Bronk, DW (1929) The discharge of impulses in motor nerve fibres II, the frequency of discharge in reflex and voluntary contractions. *Journal of Physiology* **67**: 119–151.

Bárány, M (1967) ATPase activity of myosin correlated with speed of muscle shortening. *Journal of Genetics and Physiology* **50**: 197–218.

Barnard, RJ, Edgerton, VR, Furukawa, T, Peter, JB (1971) Histochemical, biochemical and contractile properties of red, white and intermediate fibres. *American Journal of Physiology* **220**: 410–414.

Bernstein, J (1902) Untersuchungen zur Thermodynamik der bioelktrishen Strome. *Pflügers Archiv* **92**: 521–562.

Buller, AJ, Eccles, JC, Eccles, RW (1960a) Differentiation of fast and slow muscles in the cat hind limb. *Journal of Physiology* **150**: 399–416.

Buller, AJ, Eccles, JC, Eccles, RW (1960b) Interactions between motoneurones and muscles in respect of the characteristic speeds of their responses. *Journal of Physiology* **150**: 417–439.

Burke, RE, Levine, DN, Tsiaris, P, Zajac, FE (1973) Physiological types and histochemical profiles in motor units of the cat gastrocnemius. *Journal of Physiology (Lond)* **234**: 723–748.

Denny Brown, D (1929) The histological features of striped muscle in relation to its functional activity. *Proceedings of the Royal Society (Series B)* **104**: 371–411.

Dubowitz, V (1995) Muscle disorders in childhood. W.B. Saunders, London.

Eccles, JC, Eccles, RN, Lundberg, A (1958) The action potentials of the alpha neurones supplying fast and slow muscles. *Journal of Physiology* **142**: 275–291.

Edström, L, Krugelberg, E (1968) Histochemical composition, distribution of units and fatigeablity of single motor units. *Journal of Neurology, Neurosurgery and Psychiatry* **31**: 424–433.

Erlanger, J, Gasser, HS (1937) *Electrical Signs of Nervous Activity*. University of Pennsylvania Press, Philadelphia, PA.

Erlanger, J, Gasser, HS (1970) *Human Neurophysiology* 2nd edition. Chapman and Hall, London.

Galvani, L (1791) De *Viribus Electricitatis*. Translation 1953 by R Green, Cambridge.

Garnett, RAF, O'Donnavan, MJ, Stephens, JA et al. (1979) Motor unit organisation of human gastrocnemius. *Journal of Physiology* **287**: 33–43.

Garnett, RAF, Stephens, JA (1981) Changes in the recruitment threshold of motor units produced by cutaneous stimulation in man. *Journal of Physiology* **311**: 463–473.

Henneman, E, Olson, C (1965) Relations between structure and function in the design of skeletal muscles. *Journal of Neurophysiology* **28**: 581–598.

Hodgkin, AL, Keynes, RD (1955) Active transport of cations in giant axons from Sepia and Lologo. *Journal of Physiology* **128**: 28–60.

Hodgkin, AL, Huxley, AF (1952) Currents carried by sodium and potassium ion through the membrane of the giant axon of Loligo. *Journal of Physiology* **116**: 449–472.

Huxley, AF (1957) Muscle structure and theories of contraction. *Progress in Biophysics* **7**: 255–318.

Huxley, AF, Simmons, RM (1971) Proposed mechanism of force generation in striated muscle. *Nature* **233**: 533–538.

Jami, L (1992) Golgi tendon organs in mammalian skeletal muscle: Functional properties and central actions. *Physiology Review* **72**: 623–666.

Lloyd, DPC, Chang, HT (1948) Afferent nerves in muscle nerves. *Journal of Neurophysiology* **11**: 488–518.

Martin, TP, Bodine-Fowler, S, Roy, RR, Eldred, E, Edgerton, VR (1988). Metabolic and fibre size properties of cat tibialis anterior motor units. *American Journal of Physiology* **255**: C43–C50.

Mathews, PBC (1972) *Mammalian Muscle Receptors and their Central Actions*. Edward Arnold, London.

Milner-Brown, HS, Stein, RB, Yemm, R (1973) The orderly recruitment of human motor units under voluntary isometric contractions. *Journal of Physiology* **230**: 371–390.

Pette, D, Vrbová, G (1992) Adaptation of mammalian skeletal muscle fibres to chronic electrical stimulation. *Review of Physiology and Biochemistry* **120**: 116–202.

Pette, D, Vrbová, G (1999) What does chronic electrical stimulation teach us about muscle plasticity? *Muscle and Nerve* **22**: 666–677.

Ranvier, L (1874) De quelques faits relatifs a l'histologie et la physiologie des muscles striès. *Archives of Physiology and Normal Pathology* **6**: 1–15.

Salmons, S, Vrbová, V (1969) The influence of activity on some contractile characteristics of mammalian fast and slow muscles. *Journal of Physiology* **201**: 535–549.

Sherrington, CS (1906) *The Integrative Action of the Nervous System*, reprinted 1961 ed. Yale University Press, New Haven, CT.

Spudich, JA (1994) How molecular motors work. *Nature* **372**: 515–518.

Vrbová, G (1966) Factors determining the speed of contraction of striated muscle. *Journal of Physiology* **185**: 17P–18P.

5

Physiology of pain

Leslie Wood

INTRODUCTION

Ask any group of people to define what is meant by the word 'pain' and they will invariably each come up with a different set of words and terms to describe it. This reflects the general difficulty shared by scientists in trying to come up with a meaningful and accurate definition of what pain is and, perhaps more importantly, what it means in the context of the normal functioning of the human body. In addition, the relationship between the physiological events occurring in the body and the psychological state of the subject during the experience of pain is an important one.

As a starting point, therefore, it may be useful to provide a loose definition of pain as being the subjective sensations which accompany the activation of nociceptors (pain receptors) and which signal the location and strength of actual or potential tissue-damaging stimuli. As will be discussed later, this definition does not always apply in situations where pain may be experienced without apparent nociceptor activation.

Despite the difficulty in arriving at an acceptable definition of pain, most people would agree that it can be of a variable quality, ranging from mild irritation, through itching, burning and pricking sensations to more intense stabbing and throbbing sensations and finally to agonising, intractable pain which for some subjects can be beyond endurance. In most cases these sensations are associated with the activation of nociceptors and the sensation of pain, but the differences in the subjective responses reflect both the strength and severity of the nociceptor activation and subjects' individual psychological and emotional responses to this information. As will be discussed later, these differences can be important in the modulation of pain in certain circumstances.

There are also circumstances, however, where subjective pain may be felt by a subject in the absence of any tissue damage or nociceptor activation. In these cases, the pain arises due to changes in the sensitivity of cells within the central nervous system (see later).

PERIPHERAL ASPECTS

Nociceptors are generally free nerve endings embedded throughout the tissues, with variations in the density of these receptors in different tissues. The free nerve endings are no more than simple nerve endings without any associated accessory structures, which might be found with other sensory nerve endings (Fig. 5.1). The free nerve endings have a relatively high threshold to activation and are sensitive to potentially tissue-damaging stimuli such as mechanical, thermal, electrical and chemical stimuli.

These free nerve endings give rise to small diameter afferent nerve fibres which convey action potentials to the spinal cord and higher centres in the central nervous system. These afferent fibres are classed as either myelinated Aδ fibres, with conduction velocities of between 5 and 30 m/s, or non-myelinated C fibres, which conduct action potentials at velocities between 0.5 and 2 m/s (N.B. Aδ fibres are also sometimes referred to as group III fibres, and C fibres as group IV fibres). These two types of afferent fibres are responsible for what is termed 'fast' and 'slow' pain, the properties of which are outlined in Table 5.1.

These two pain *modalities* underlie the concepts of transient and prolonged pain sensations. Transient pain is the first sensation to accompany a noxious stimulus and usually involves only minimal tissue damage. It is of short duration and has no real long-term consequences for the subject. The Aδ afferent nerve fibres which are responsible for these sensations are also involved in the withdrawal reflex

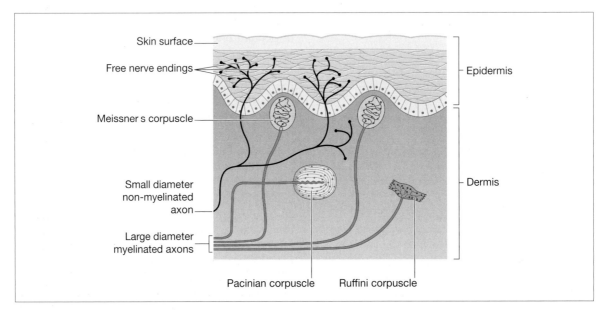

Figure 5.1 Types of sensory endings found in the skin. The endings giving rise to large diameter afferents are those serving the sensations of touch, vibration, pressure and temperature. The non-myelinated afferents from the free nerve endings convey nociceptive information to the central nervous system.

Table 5.1   Properties of 'fast' and 'slow' pain fibres

Properties	Fast pain	Slow pain
Receptors	Free nerve endings	Free nerve endings
Afferents	Aδ (group III) fibres	C (group IV) fibres
Action potential conduction velocity	Relatively slow; 5–30 m/s	Very slow; 0.5–2 m/s
Subjective sensation	Sharp, pricking pain	Dull, burning, throbbing pain
Onset of sensation	Short latency, quick onset	Long latency, slow onset
Localisation	Well-localised, easily identified	Poorly localised, diffuse
Duration of sensation	Short lasting	Long lasting
Subjective response	Reflex withdrawal, less emotional involvement	Difficult to endure, possible emotional and automatic response

(see below). Prolonged pain is associated with activation of the group C afferent nerve fibres and usually accompanies a greater degree of tissue damage. This damage to the tissue cells results in the release of chemical mediators, such as *bradykinin, substance P, histamine, 5-hydroxytryptamine* (5-HT) and *prostaglandins*, both from the damaged cells themselves and from activated nociceptor nerve endings. These chemical mediators can activate nociceptive nerve terminals directly and can also sensitise the nociceptors' response to normal stimuli by altering the transduction properties of the free nerve endings. As well as activating group C nociceptive endings, these chemical mediators are also responsible for initiating the inflammatory responses in the damaged tissue. Figure 5.2 summarises how tissue damage and the release of chemical mediators can activate nociceptors and transmit this information to the central nervous system.

The subjective involvement of both transient and prolonged pain can be best illustrated by referring to the pain sensations which accompany an injury such as stubbing a toe. Initially, there is a sharp pain associated with the physical contact of the toe with a hard object—the transient pain—followed by a duller, throbbing pain which lasts for a much longer time. This is the prolonged pain caused by the ongoing release of chemical mediators from the damaged tissue in the toe.

As part of this process, the injured area may become much more sensitive to what were

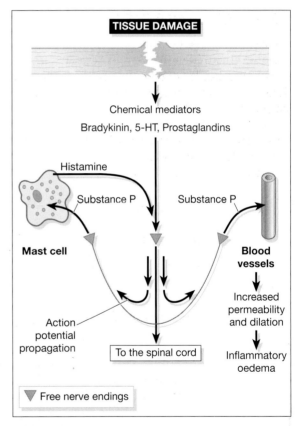

Figure 5.2   The role of chemical mediators in the activation of nociceptors and in the generation of inflammatory processes. Action potentials generated in the nociceptive afferents can travel towards the spinal cord, but they can also travel along axonal branches to cause the release of the neurotransmitter substance P from other terminals. This, in turn, can influence mast cells, causing them to release histamine, which further activates the free nerve endings and also causes vasodilation and increased permeability of nearby blood vessels.

previously innocuous stimuli and these stimuli now may produce painful sensations. This sensitisation may take place either at the free nerve endings themselves (peripheral sensitisation; see above) or in the neurons of the dorsal horn of the spinal cord (central sensitisation; see later). This increase in sensitivity is termed hyperalgesia, and is also associated with allodynia (tenderness) attributed to the affected tissue.

CENTRAL ASPECTS

Information from the nociceptive afferent nerves is transmitted to the spinal cord where it subsequently influences reflex activity, or is further transmitted via specific pathways to higher brain centres. Nociceptive afferents enter the spinal cord via the dorsal root and make synaptic connections with other neurons located in the dorsal horn of the spinal cord grey matter. The dorsal horn is the site of convergence of several inputs relating to nociception, including the peripheral afferents described above, spinal interneurons and also descending neurons from higher centres in the brain.

The main reflexes involving nociceptive afferents are the flexor withdrawal and crossed extensor reflexes. These are polysynaptic reflexes and involve several muscle groups as well as operating over several spinal segmental levels. Nociceptive inputs make excitatory polysynaptic connections with motoneurons supplying flexor muscle groups and inhibitory polysynaptic connections with extensor motoneurons on the ipsilateral side. When these pathways are activated, they produce flexion in the limb where the original noxious stimulus arose while simultaneously switching off activity in the extensor muscles of this limb. These actions serve to move the limb away from the initial stimulus and, therefore, act in a protective fashion by removing the area from potential damage. At the same time, different polysynaptic connections from the same nociceptive afferents excite extensor motoneurons and inhibit flexor motoneurons in the *contralateral* limb. This action serves to stabilise the body during flexion

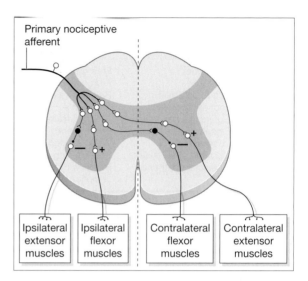

Figure 5.3 Spinal reflex pathways for the flexor withdrawal and crossed extensor reflexes. Excitatory interneurons are shown in white, and inhibitory interneurons in black.

of the ipsilateral limb. Figure 5.3 summarises these connections.

The nociceptive afferents entering the spinal cord grey matter terminate in the dorsal horn, where they make synaptic connections either with interneurons serving the reflexes described above, or with second-order neurons (so-called transmission cells, or T cells). These cross the midline of the spinal cord to transmit information to the higher centres via the lateral spinothalamic pathways on the contralateral side of the spinal cord (Fig. 5.4). The axons travelling in these pathways are therefore always second-order neurons which have their cell bodies in the marginal zone or substantia gelatinosa (SG) of the spinal cord grey matter. Some of these second-order axons will ascend ipsilaterally for a few spinal segments before crossing the midline, while others will cross immediately. When these ascending neurons reach the ventrobasal nucleus of the thalamus, they terminate on third-order neurons, which then convey the information on the noxious stimulus to the cerebral cortex.

In addition, information is also passed to higher centres via the multisynaptic spinoreticular tract. This pathway sends projections from several brainstem terminations via the

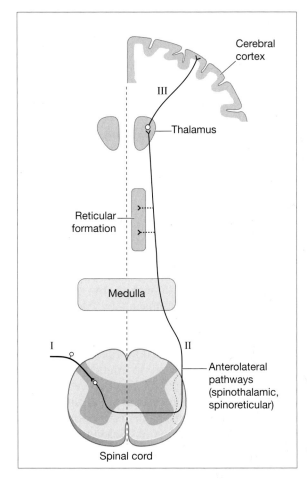

Figure 5.4 Ascending pathways conveying nociceptive information to higher centres. Primary nociceptive afferents (I) enter the dorsal horn where they synapse with second-order neurons, which cross the midline to ascend in the anterolateral pathways (II). Some axons terminate in the reticular formation of the pons and medulla (dashed lines) while other axons ascend to the thalamus where they synapse with third-order neurons (III), which ascend to the somatosensory cortex.

intralaminar nucleus of the thalamus to areas such as the hypothalamus, the frontal lobe and the limbic system of the brain. These areas coordinate the autonomic, psychological and emotional responses to pain.

MODULATION OF PAIN TRANSMISSION

It is in the spinal cord, though, that the possibility exists for the modulation of transmission of nociceptive information to higher centres. To understand how this operates, it is useful to look in a bit of detail at what happens in the dorsal horn of the spinal cord grey matter. As we have already noted, primary nociceptive afferents terminate on second-order neurons, which then transmit the nociceptive information to higher centres.

The excitability of this pathway can be altered by other interneurons present in the dorsal horn. Cells of the substantia gelatinosa (SG cells) have an inhibitory influence on the transmission cells. This is achieved by presynaptic inhibition of the nociceptive afferent terminals at the point where they synapse with the transmission cells (Fig. 5.5A). However, the SG cells are inhibited when the nociceptive afferents are activated (Fig. 5.5B), reducing the presynaptic inhibition of the nociceptor afferent terminal and thereby allowing nociceptive information to be passed to higher centres.

The SG cells are also influenced by other inputs, however. Activation of low-threshold, large diameter mechanosensitive afferents stimulates the SG cells via an excitatory synapse, and therefore increases the amount of presynaptic inhibition acting on the nociceptor afferent terminals and preventing the transmission of nociceptive information to higher centres (Fig. 5.5C). It should be noted here that the large diameter afferents also have excitatory inputs on to the T cells, but that this is also inhibited by presynaptic inhibition of these terminals (Fig. 5.5C).

In addition to these inputs to SG cells from peripheral afferents, descending inputs from higher centres also have excitatory connections to the SG cells (Fig. 5.5D), thereby allowing descending control on the overall excitability of the T cells (see below). The important point to note is that activation of the SG cells will inhibit pain transmission to higher centres.

The overall balance of excitation and inhibition impinging on the T cells is therefore of great importance in determining whether or not nociceptive information is relayed to the higher cognitive centres of the brain. By altering the balance in favour of inhibition via the SG inhibitory interneurons, transmission of

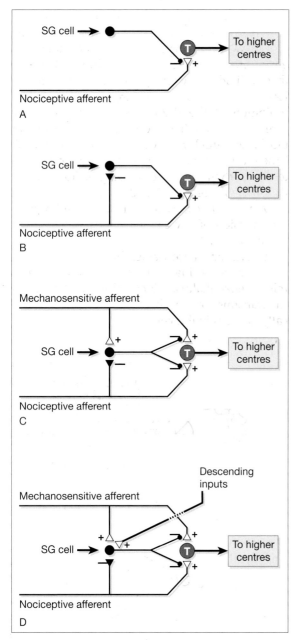

Figure 5.5 A–D: Neural circuits in the dorsal horn which influence pain transmission to higher centres. See text for detailed explanation. (SG = substantia gelatinosa; T = transmission cell.)

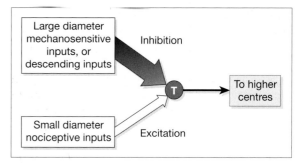

Figure 5.6 Inhibition of pain transmission is achieved by altering the balance of inputs to the transmission cells such that it favours those from large diameter mechanosensitive afferents or from descending inputs. When this happens, the larger amount of inhibitory input (large arrow) overrides the excitatory input generated by the nociceptive afferents (small arrow). (T = transmission cell.)

transmission cells is known as the *gate control theory*, which was established by Melzack and Wall in 1965. In its simplest form, this mechanism can be regarded as a system in which the 'gate' is either open, to allow nociceptive information to be passed on to higher centres, or closed, preventing this information from being transmitted. In terms of producing analgesia, it is the goal of the therapist to ensure that the balance of inputs is always in favour of closing the gate.

Since the SG cells receive inputs both from large diameter mechanosensitive afferents and from descending inputs, activation of these inputs will provide a mechanism whereby pain transmission can be modulated. Large diameter mechanosensitive afferents can be activated by a number of means, including direct, simple mechanical stimulation of receptors in the skin, muscles and joints, as well as being activated artificially by electrical stimulation.

This therefore has implications for the management of pain in physiotherapy. Any technique which activates these afferents has the potential to modulate pain transmission in the spinal cord. Techniques such as massage, joint manipulation, traction and compression, thermal stimulation and electrotherapy all have the capability to produce sensory inputs from low-threshold afferents, which can ultimately inhibit pain transmission in the spinal cord by 'closing the gate', i.e. inhibiting T cell activity via the SG

nociceptive information to higher centres can be reduced or abolished (Fig. 5.6).

This modulation of pain transmission by altering the influences of the different inputs to the cells. Transcutaneous electrical nerve stimulation (TENS) can be used to stimulate the large diameter afferents in the skin directly and when administered in an appropriate area and at an appropriate voltage can therefore influence pain transmission in the relevant spinal segments. In this way, both the therapist and the patient can have control over pain modulation and can adjust the levels of this at any time.

The descending influences on the T cells are also important. These inputs come principally from the *periaqueductal grey matter* (PAGM, the grey matter surrounding the cerebral aqueduct, located in the midbrain) and the *raphe nucleus* (located in the medulla). These both have excitatory effects on the inhibitory interneurons of the substantia gelatinosa in the dorsal horn of the spinal cord, and so have the ability to reduce pain transmission at the level of the spinal cord. These descending pathways are thought to exert their effects on the SG cells by releasing monoaminergic neurotransmitters such as noradrenaline and 5-HT. Under normal circumstances, though, these pathways are usually *inactive* due to further influence of inhibitory interneurons from other areas of the brain. These inputs therefore turn off or reduce the activity of the cells of the PAGM or raphe nucleus.

In certain situations this inhibition of the PAGM and the raphe nucleus can be removed. This is achieved by the actions of neurons projecting from other areas of the central nervous system associated with pain modulation. These neurons arise from the *limbic system*—a term used collectively to describe structures such as the hypothalamus, the hippocampus and the amygdala—as well as from other areas within the PAGM itself. The limbic areas are involved in emotion and mood and can have wide-ranging influences on other aspects of nervous control, including the control of pain.

Activity in these areas stimulates the production of naturally occurring (endogenous) opioids (opiate-like chemicals). There are three families of endogenous opioids—the *enkephalins*, the *endorphins* and the *dynorphins*. Neurons containing and utilising these opioids have clearly distinct distributions throughout the brain and

spinal cord and have different roles to play in the modulation of pain transmission. The actions of the endogenous opioids on their target neurons are generally inhibitory. Therefore these opioids allow excitation of the descending PAGM neurons by inhibiting the background inhibition of the PAGM cells, rather than by direct excitation (i.e. these opioids turn off, or block, the inhibition of the PAGM neurons). When this happens, these cells are now free to exert their own descending influences on the SG cells of the dorsal horn of the spinal cord grey matter, which, in turn, will inhibit transmission of nociceptive information via the T cells (Fig. 5.7).

In addition, these descending pathways may also activate spinal cord interneurons, which release enkephalins, which subsequently inhibit the transmission cells both pre- and postsynaptically at the spinal level.

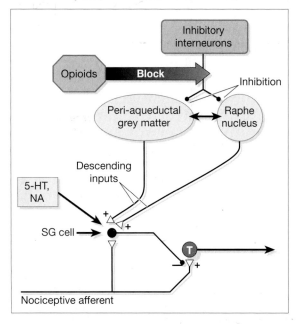

Figure 5.7 Descending influences on substantia gelatinosa (SG) cell activity. The periaqueductal grey matter (PAGM) and raphe nucleus inputs are normally held in check by the actions of inhibitory interneurons. Release of endogenous opioids blocks this inhibition, leading to activation of these descending pathways, which exert excitatory effects on the SG cells utilising 5-hydroxytryptamine (5-HT) and noradrenaline (NA). (T = transmission cell.)

It is thought that these effects of the endogenous opioids are associated with producing analgesia related only to the prolonged aspects of pain, rather than the initial, faster pain responses produced when an injury first occurs—that is, the inhibitory effects of PAGM and raphe nucleus activation influence only the transmission of pain mediated by C fibres and not that by Aδ fibres.

There is, however, an alternative theory for the role of the descending pathways in pain modulation. There is some evidence to suggest that the descending pathways are activated by nociceptive inputs and actually *enhance* pain transmission in the spinal cord. The effects of the release of endogenous opioids is therefore to suppress the activity in these descending pathways and thereby reduce the transmission of pain to higher centres. Research is ongoing to establish a clearer understanding of the nature of the descending modulation of pain transmission.

Whatever the mechanism of descending pain modulation, it is clear that higher cognitive centres in the brain can have some influence on these processes. Fear, stress, excitement and even pain itself can all reduce, or even abolish, the feelings of pain associated with injury. A well-known example of this is the so-called *'battlefield analgesia'*, where a soldier may have sustained a severe injury to part of the body but is initially unaware of it until some time later, usually after reaching safety. Similar reduced responses to pain are observed in many sports, with players or athletes managing to continue despite having sustained what would otherwise be a debilitating injury. This higher suppression of pain sensation is probably mediated from the cerebral cortex via the limbic system to the descending pain control systems described above.

Such mechanisms can also be of importance for therapeutic interventions at a psychological, rather than physiological, level. The fact that patients may simply be receiving attention from a therapist, regardless of the techniques being employed, may be sufficient to induce an emotional or psychological response which may modulate the pain they are experiencing. Figure 5.8 summarises the possible influences of the therapist on pain modulation.

SENSITISATION

We have already noted the possibility of increased sensitivity of the free nerve endings due to the action of chemical mediators (*peripheral sensitisation*). We should also note that, following activation by group C afferents, the excitability of the dorsal horn transmission cells

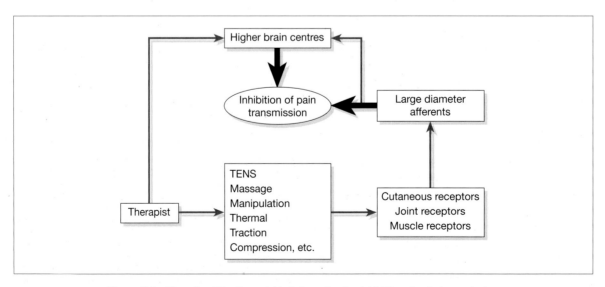

Figure 5.8 The role of the therapist in influencing the inhibition of pain transmission.

can remain elevated for several hours, via alterations in intracellular second messengers in these cells. This leads to changes in membrane channels and membrane receptors which, in turn, increase both the excitability of the neurons and their sensitivity to synaptic transmitters. This is termed *central sensitisation*.

The altered sensitivity of the transmission cells means that they now respond abnormally to inputs from the large diameter mechanosensitive afferents, which can now elicit flexor withdrawal reflexes as well as pain sensations.

The consequences of these abnormal responses of the transmission cells to innocuous afferent input are that any clinical pain reduction treatment aimed at preventing or reducing nociceptive input to the spinal cord will not be sufficient to prevent pain sensations in the subject, since these can now be elicited by simple stimulation of the large diameter mechanosensitive afferents. Such alterations to the sensitivity of the dorsal horn cells can last for several hours or more. These mechanisms help to explain the phenomena of hyperalgesia and allodynia.

In some cases, injury and the subsequent sensitising effects on spinal cord neurons may produce more lasting changes in the synaptic connections of the neurons in the dorsal horn, resulting in reorganised neural circuitry in the pathways mediating pain transmission. In such cases the reorganisation may be such that the sensitisation of the pain transmission pathways becomes permanent and irreversible, leading to persistent abnormal responses to peripheral stimuli which are subjectively interpreted as pain.

PAIN STATES

It should be apparent by this stage that the delivery of nociceptive information to higher centres is highly dependent on the state of the nervous pathways serving the transmission processes. Put simply, these pathways can be in the normal state, the suppressed state or the enhanced, sensitised state. These three states therefore equate with the concepts of *'normoalgesia'*, *'hypoalgesia'* and *'hyperalgesia'*. In each of these three different possible states, the same stimulus intensity may produce different subjective sensations of pain depending on how the nociceptive information is delivered to, and processed by, the central nervous system. For example, a particular stimulus intensity may produce a painful sensation in the normoalgesic state whereas the same stimulus intensity would not elicit any subjective pain in the suppressed, hypoalgesic state. Similarly, an innocuous stimulus may not elicit pain in either the normoalgesic or hypoalgesic states but will produce subjective pain in the hyperalgesic state. The reasons for this are summarised diagrammatically in Figure 5.9.

In this figure we can see that the threshold for eliciting a subjective painful sensation is altered depending on how readily the nervous pathways respond to the incoming afferent information. In the suppressed, hypoalgesic state (Fig. 5.9B), the threshold is reached only at higher stimulus intensities, whereas it is reached at lower (often innocuous) intensities in the enhanced, hyperalgesic state (Fig. 5.9C).

For these reasons, it is important for therapists to be aware that stimuli applied to a patient as part of a therapeutic treatment programme may not, in fact, result in the desired outcome of pain relief and may instead exacerbate a painful condition.

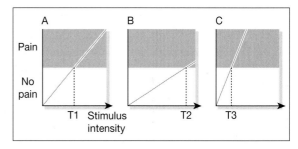

Figure 5.9 Generation of subjective pain sensations in three pain states—normoalgesia, hypoalgesia and hyperalgesia. A: Normoalgesia—increasing stimulus intensity eventually reaches a threshold level (T1), which crosses the boundary between no pain sensation and pain. B: Hypoalgesia—suppressed pain transmission (reduced slope) means that greater stimulus intensities are required to reach the threshold level (T2 higher than T1), i.e. it is more difficult to elicit pain sensations. C: Hyperalgesia—sensitised pain transmission (increased slope) means that the threshold level is reached much sooner (T3 lower than T1), i.e. pain sensations are elicited with weaker stimuli.

Table 5.2 Sites of referred pain and their sites of origin

Origin of pain	Site of referred pain and spinal segments involved
Heart (angina pectoris)	Chest, left shoulder, left arm (T1–T5)
Gallbladder and bile ducts	Right upper quadrant of abdomen, below right shoulder (T7, T8)
Diaphragm	Top of shoulder (C3–C5)
Stomach	Upper central region of abdomen (epigastrium) (T7, T8)
Duodenum (e.g. duodenal ulcer)	Anterior abdominal wall above umbilicus (T9, T10)
Kidneys and ureter	Loin and groin (L1, L2)
Appendix	Umbilicus initially, then to lower right quadrant of abdomen when peritoneum becomes inflamed (T10)

REFERRED PAIN

Pain which arises from deep structures in the body—visceral pain—is often felt by the subject in locations that are far removed from the site of origin. Such translocation of pain sensation is known as *referred pain*. An example of this is the pain associated with angina pectoris. Here, the organ that is affected is the heart, but the pain is often described as arising in (or referred to) the upper chest, left shoulder and arm. Other sites of referred pain and their sites of origin are given in Table 5.2.

The explanation for the pattern of referred pain lies in the pattern of convergence of afferent nerve fibres in the dorsal horn of the spinal cord. Dorsal horn neurons, including those which act as transmission cells, receive inputs from a wide variety of sources that are innervated by the same spinal segments (T1–T4 in the case of the heart and left arm). These convergent inputs may include nociceptive inputs from both cutaneous areas and visceral areas (Fig. 5.10A).

As previously described, these transmission cells pass this nociceptive information to higher centres where it is perceived and interpreted as pain sensation. However, the higher centres cannot distinguish the source of this information as being either cutaneous or visceral in origin since they receive inputs only from single transmission cells. Peripheral nociceptive input from cutaneous or skeletal muscle receptors normally predominates in normal, everyday circumstances (rather than nociceptive input from the heart) and so the higher centres incorrectly ascribe the information passed on by the transmission cells as coming from their usual source of the skin or muscles, rather than the deeper, visceral organ, the heart.

There is also some evidence that, in some cases, referred pain might arise owing to bifurcations in the peripheral neurons which converge on the transmission cells in the dorsal horn—that is, single peripheral afferents may split to supply both skin areas and deeper visceral areas (Fig. 5.10B).

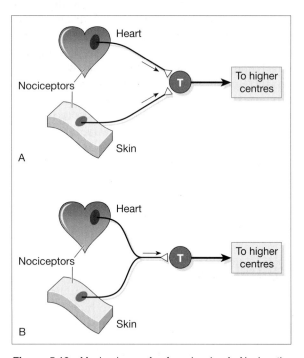

Figure 5.10 Mechanisms of referred pain. A: Nociceptive afferents from two different locations (here the heart and the skin) converge on the same transmission cell in the dorsal horn of the spinal cord. B: the nociceptors from the two different areas share the same primary afferent axon entering the spinal cord.

It is important for the therapist to be aware of the possible patterns of referred pain (see Table 5.2), since the patient might describe pain as arising in a structure which has no underlying lesion, misleading the therapist as to the real source of the complaint.

PHANTOM LIMB PAIN

When a limb has been amputated or the sensory nerves from a limb have been destroyed, the sensation of the limb still being present can exist in some cases (phantom limb) and sometimes pain referred to the missing limb can be perceived. Pain associated with a missing limb is known as *phantom limb pain*. Phantom limb pain is often described as burning, electric or cramping sensations, and may persist for many years after the loss of the limb.

The source of this phantom limb pain may be the severed ends of the peripheral nerves that were cut during the amputation or injury. This may set up abnormal patterns of discharge in the peripheral nerve fibres, particularly nociceptive afferents, which are then relayed to higher centres and perceived as pain sensations arising in the areas these nerves formerly supplied. Additionally there may be altered activity in the neurons of the dorsal horn associated with pain transmission (see Sensitisation above). This altered activity may arise as a result of afferent degeneration inducing postsynaptic changes in the dorsal horn neurons.

Recent research has suggested a further cause of phantom limb pain. This proposes that phantom limbs and the sensations associated with them are a consequence of activity in neural networks in higher centres of the brain. These neural networks form a so-called *neuromatrix*, the structure and functioning of which may be genetically determined, and which is susceptible to inputs from peripheral structures. This neuromatrix is not localised, but widespread throughout the brain. It provides a neural framework which underpins subjects' experience of their own body as a physical entity which 'belongs' to them. Sensory inputs from all areas of the body can manipulate and modify the activity of the neuromatrix. It has been suggested that phantom limb pain arises as a result of abnormal or absent modulating input to this neuromatrix and missing channels of output from the neuromatrix to the muscles. Interestingly, more recent research has proposed a novel method of relieving phantom limb pain in some patients. This effectively involves fooling the patients' central nervous system by allowing patients to 'see' the phantom limb using a mirror reflection of their intact opposite limb. When this is done, manipulation or movement of the intact limb is viewed in the mirror and is transposed by the brain on to the phantom limb. In certain circumstances this simple technique can be used to remove painful sensations arising from the phantom limb.

REFERENCE

Melzack, R, Wall, PD (1965) Pain mechanisms—a new theory. *Science* **150**: 971–979.

BIBLIOGRAPHY

Basbaum, AI, Fields, HL (1984) Endogenous pain control systems—brainstem spinal pathways and endorphin circuitry. *Annual Review of Neuroscience* **7**: 309–338.
Bear, MF, Connors, BW, Paradiso, MA (1996) *Neuroscience—exploring the brain*. Williams & Wilkins, Baltimore, MD.
Cohen, H (1999) *Neuroscience for Rehabilitation*, 2nd edn. Lippincott, Williams & Wilkins, Baltimore, MD.
Dickenson, AH (1991) Mechanisms of the analgesic actions of opiates and opioids. *British Medical Bulletin* **47**(3): 690–702.

Kandel, ER, Schwartz, JH, Jessell, TM (2000) *Principles of Neural Science*, 4th edn. McGraw-Hill, New York.

Kiernan, JA (1998) *Barr's The Human Nervous System—an Anatomical Viewpoint*, 7th edn. Lippincott–Raven, New York.

Melzack, R (1990) Phantom limbs and the concept of a neuromatrix. *Trends in Neuroscience* **13**: 88–92.

Melzack, R, Wall, PD (1996) *The Challenge of Pain*, 2nd edn (updated). Penguin, London.

Rang, HP, Bevan, S, Dray, A (1991) Chemical activation of nociceptive peripheral neurons. *British Medical Bulletin* **47**(3): 534–548.

Ramachandran, VS, Blakeslee, S (1998) *Phantoms in the Brain*. Fourth Estate, London.

Shipton, EA (1999) *Pain—Acute and Chronic*. Arnold, London.

Wall, PD, Melzack, R (eds) (1994) *Textbook of Pain*, 3rd edn. Churchill Livingstone, New York.

Wells, PE, Frampton, V, Bowsher, D (1994) *Pain—Management by Physiotherapy*, 2nd edn. Butterworth Heinemann, Oxford.

Woolf, CJ (1991) Generation of acute pain—central mechanisms. *British Medical Bulletin* **47**(3): 523–533.

Scientific basis of therapy

SECTION CONTENTS

6

Thermal effects

Sheila Kitchen

INTRODUCTION

Chapter 1 presented the basic scientific principles underpinning the way in which changes in temperature affect materials. This chapter will examine in more detail the effects that are produced in biological materials, particularly when these are part of a functioning body.

THERMAL HOMEOSTASIS

In health, humans maintain internal and external heat exchanges and preserve a constant body temperature by means of a highly efficient thermoregulatory system. This process of homeothermy is defined as 'a pattern of temperature regulation in which cyclic variation in deep body (core) temperature is maintained within arbitrary limits of $\pm 2°C$ despite much larger variations in ambient temperature' (International Union of Physiological Sciences, 1987). Thus, with a normal body temperature of about 37°C, hyperthermia may be regarded as a core temperature in excess of 39°C and hypothermia a temperature below 35°C. At rest, and in a neutral environment, core temperature can be kept within a much more narrow band of control ($\pm 0.3°C$) in accord with the body's intrinsic diurnal temperature rhythm. Claude Bernard's concept of thermal homeostasis depicting a virtual straight-line constancy is shown to be not so precise, since spontaneous rhythmic variations in body temperature occur with diurnal, monthly (e.g. ovulatory) and seasonal temperature cycles.

Body temperature

The body is usually considered to consist of two thermal compartments: the core or central compartment, and the shell or superficial layer. The core temperature is controlled at a constant level by physiological mechanisms. The shell, at the interface between the body and the environment, is subject to much greater variation in temperature. Although the core temperature is kept within a narrow range around 37°C, it must not be regarded as a simple fixed entity, for there are significant temperature gradients within the anatomical core. Organs such as the liver and active skeletal muscles, for example, have a higher rate of metabolic heat production than other tissues and therefore maintain a higher temperature. Similarly, there are temperature gradients within the vascular compartment perfusing both the core and the shell.

The diurnal (circadian) core temperature rhythm is one of the most stable of biological rhythms, with a well-marked intrinsic component (Fig. 6.1). Body temperature is lowest in the early morning and highest in the evening, though in a small minority of people the phase is reversed. The diurnal range of variation is usually about 0.5–1.5°C in adults, depending on other external factors such as the effects of meals, activity, sleep and ambient temperature (which can sometimes influence the oral temperature). Different intrinsic biological rhythms are often in phase with each other. There is evidence that desynchronisation of different rhythms is deleterious to function; for example desynchronisation of the sleep–wake cycle and the core temperature cycle by continuous light exposure can bring about impairment of thermoregulatory function (Moore-Ede and Sulzman, 1981).

Across approximately 1 cm of the body shell, from the skin surface to the superficial layer of muscle, there is a temperature gradient that varies according to the temperature of the core and the external environment. The gradient is not uniform, but changes with the thermal conductivity of the tissue layers and the rate of blood flow in the different regions (Fig. 6.2). Skin temperatures differ widely over the body surface, especially in hot or cold conditions. When an individual is in a comfortable environment of, say, 24°C, the skin of the toes may be

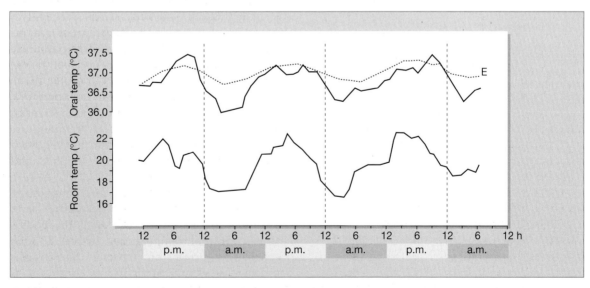

Figure 6.1 Diurnal variation in body temperature showing the influence of ambient (room) temperature on the oral temperature when meals and physical activity are kept constant. (E = intrinsic temperature rhythm.)

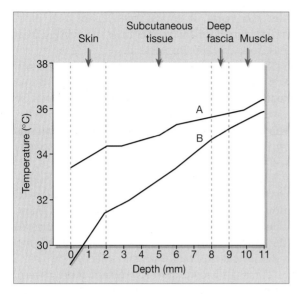

Figure 6.2 Temperature gradients in the forearm between the skin surface and deep tissues in A: comfortably warm conditions and B: cold conditions.

27°C, the upper arms and legs 31°C, the forehead 34°C, while the core is maintained at 37°C.

Body temperature measurement

Core temperature is measured conventionally by a mercury-in-glass thermometer placed in the mouth. The instruments for clinical use comply with the British and EC Standards (British Standards, 1987). The Standards also apply to subnormal temperature, ovulation and dual scale (Fahrenheit and Celsius) thermometers. Electronic thermometers are widely used, but apart from the increase in range of measurement they are no quicker or more accurate than mercury thermometers. Errors in taking the oral temperature arise with any thermometer if there is mouth breathing or talking during measurement, or if hot or cold drinks have just been consumed, or if the tissues of the mouth are affected by a hot or cold external environment. The rectal temperature is a slowly equilibrating but often more reliable measurement of core temperature and is on average about 0.5°C higher than the mouth temperature. However, cold blood from chilled legs or warmed blood from active leg

muscles can affect the rectal temperature. The reading will also depend on the position of the probe in relation to the rectal venous plexus of vessels influenced by blood from the lower limbs. The temperature of the urine is also a reliable measure of core temperature, provided that it is possible to void a stream of 50–100 ml or more. For accurate and fast recording, measurement can be made in the ear canal (near to but not touching the tympanic membrane) by thermistor or thermocouple, but unless this is done in a warm environment and with lagging placed over the ear then errors are introduced because of heat conduction from the ear canal to the colder pinna. It is possible to overcome this problem by employing a zero-gradient self-correcting electronic thermometer (Keatinge and Sloane, 1975). Oesophageal temperature also provides an accurate measurement of core temperature, but placement of the thermistor probe is important in order to avoid cooling from the trachea and warming from the stomach. Telemetric monitoring is sometimes appropriate for measuring intestinal temperature by a temperature-sensitive pill that is easily swallowed. Internal temperature is thus continuously transmitted to an external receiver.

Average values for skin temperature can be obtained by applying a number of separate thermistors or thermocouples over the skin surface and applying weighting factors for the different areas of skin represented. Contact temperatures of this nature are, however, prone to errors, notably from changes in skin temperature produced by the probe and tape, the effect of pressure on the skin, sweating, and heat transfer from the detector to the air. Regional variations can be visualised and an integrated mean skin temperature computed by infrared thermography.

Temperatures in the shell and in deeper tissues of the body can be determined locally by inserting thermocouples or thermistors into the tissues. Thermocouples can be made very small and probes inserted in 29-gauge needles. Techniques for constructing probes of the order of 10 μm diameter have been described. This is an invasive procedure, but non-invasive thermometry has become possible by thermal tomography, a technique that is particularly relevant for monitoring hyperthermia treatments. Most existing systems have, however, inherent inaccuracies in their temperature sensitivity and spatial discrimination that require care in interpretation.

Thermal balance

Whilst the core temperature remains constant, there is an equilibrium between internal heat production and external heat loss. This is expressed in the form of a *heat balance equation*:

$$M \pm w = \pm K \pm C \pm R - E \pm S$$

where:

- M is the rate of metabolic heat production
- w is the external work performed by or on the body
- K, C and R are the loss or gain of heat by conduction, convection and radiation respectively
- E is the evaporative heat loss from the skin and respiratory tract
- S is the rate of change of body heat storage (resultant $= 0$ at thermal equilibrium).

Metabolic heat production (M) can be derived from the measurement of total body oxygen consumption. Basal metabolic rate during complete physical and mental rest is about $45\,W/m^2$ (i.e. watts per square metre of body surface) for an adult male of 30 years and $41\,W/m^2$ for a female of the same age. Maximum values of heat production occur during severe physical work and may be as high as $900\,W/m^2$ for brief periods. Heat production can increase at rest in cold conditions by involuntary muscle contractions that produce shivering. A small increase in M follows the eating of a meal, the thermogenic response to food.

Heat loss or gain by conduction (K) depends on the temperature difference between the body and the surrounding medium, on the thermal conductivities and on the area of contact. Little heat is normally lost by conduction to the air since air is a poor heat conductor. The amount of subcutaneous fat is an important factor determining tissue cooling by providing tissue insulation

(the reciprocal of conductance) and it is especially important for preventing conductive heat loss in cold water immersion.

Normally, the surface temperature of a person is higher than that of the surrounding air so that heated air close to the body moves upwards by natural convection as colder air takes its place. The value of *convective heat exchange* (C) depends on the nature of the surrounding fluid (i.e. air) and the existing characteristics of its flow.

Radiant heat transfer (R) depends on the nature of the radiating surfaces, their temperature and the geometrical relationship between them. Extending the arms and legs effectively increases the surface area over which convective and radiant heat exchange can take place.

At rest in a comfortable ambient temperature, an individual loses weight by evaporation of water diffusing through the skin and from the respiratory tract. This is described as insensible water loss, normally at a rate of about $30\,g$ per hour, which produces a heat loss of about $10\,W/m^2$. Sweating (sensible water loss) contributes a much greater potential *evaporative heat loss* (E). Complete evaporation of 1 litre of sweat from the body surface in 1 hour will dissipate about $400\,W/m^2$.

The specific heat of the human body is $3.5\,kJ/kg$. If a person of $65\,kg$ increases mean core temperature by $1°C$ over a period of 1 hour, the *rate of heat storage* (S) becomes $230\,kJ/h$, or $64\,W$. S can be positive or negative, but when determining heat storage the difficulty is to assess the change in mean body temperature. The change in mean core temperature is not sufficient for assessment because different weightings are contributed by the core and shell. During cold exposure, for example, the volume of the core of the body is effectively reduced, thereby altering the skin–core weighting coefficients. Various formulae have been suggested, for example 0.90 core temperature $+ 0.10$ skin temperature in hot conditions; and 0.67 core temperature $+ 0.33$ skin temperature in cold conditions.

In recent years, thermotherapy has developed numerical methods for quantitatively analysing the complex interactions between diathermy energy and the tissues by computer modelling (Emery and Sekins, 1990). It has particular applications in hyperthermia treatment of malignancies where there are critical thresholds for cell viability. (Temperatues of 43°C are typically maintained for 60 minutes.) Thermal modelling by computer has similarly led to an increased understanding of safe exposure times and the processes of heat exchange in whole-body exposures to hot and cold temperatures (Wissler, 1988).

Control of body temperature

Thermoregulation is integrated by a controlling system in the central nervous system that responds to the heat content of tissues as signalled by thermoreceptors. These receptors are sensitive to heat and cold thermal information arising in the skin, in the deep tissues and in the central nervous system itself. They provide feedback signals to central nervous structures situated mainly in the hypothalamus of the brain in a servo- or loop-system (Fig. 6.3). The temperature of the blood perfusing the hypothalamus is a major physiological drive to thermoregulation, in addition to the neural inputs from thermoreceptors. The hypothalamus thus monitors ambient thermal load or deficit in the heat balance of the body and initiates appropriate physiological responses (vasodilatation and sweating in hot conditions, or vasoconstriction and shivering in cold) that counteract any deviation of the core temperature. Apart from these involuntary responses, thermal information is also transmitted by afferent nerves to other regions of the brain controlling endocrine functions, and to the cerebral cortex signalling thermal sensations and inducing behavioural thermoregulation.

An essential role in processing thermal signals is ascribed to the preoptic region of the anterior hypothalamus and to a region in the posterior hypothalamus, described respectively as the 'heat loss' and 'heat gain' centres, since they are considered to exert the primary control on vasodilatation/sweating in the heat and vasoconstriction/shivering in a cold environment. The integration of incoming and outgoing information, and the 'set-point' or 'gain' at which the hypothalamic centres operate, is the basis on which present views of thermoregulatory control are constructed (Collins, 1992; Hensel, 1981).

PHYSIOLOGICAL EFFECTS OF THERMAL CHANGES

The physiological effects of thermal changes to tissue are largely independent of the agent used to produce the change. Those related to

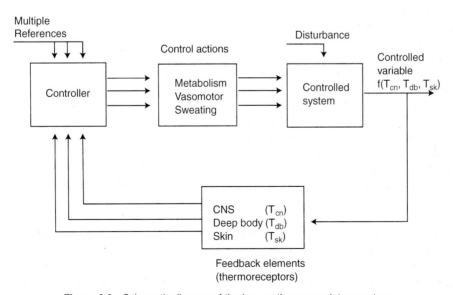

Figure 6.3 Schematic diagram of the human thermoregulatory system.

heating and cooling of tissue are therefore described in some detail here; the individual chapters following highlight any differences and issues of efficacy related to individual agents.

Physiological effects of heat

Local effects

Once energy is absorbed it is immaterial as to how the heat was delivered. There are no *different* heats, only different means of generating the same heat. The different effects of heating are the consequence of such factors as:

- the volume of tissue absorbing the energy
- the composition of the absorbing tissue
- the capacity of the tissue to dissipate heat—largely a factor of blood supply
- rate of temperature rise
- the temperature to which the tissue is raised.

Cell activity. Chemical reactions involved in metabolic activity are increased by a rise in temperature (Van't Hoff's law). Metabolic rate may increase by about 13% for each 1°C rise in tissue temperature, the increase in metabolism being greatest in the region where most heat is generated. As a result, there is an elevated tissue demand for oxygen and nutrients and enhanced output of metabolic waste products.

Accelerated cellular metabolism can produce many beneficial therapeutic effects to treat injury or infection. However, some components of enzyme systems, such as proteins, are heat sensitive and increasingly destroyed by raising the temperature beyond a threshold value. Rising tissue temperature first produces an increase in enzyme activity to a peak value, followed by a decline, and then finally abolition of enzyme activity. As an example, a specific destructive enzyme such as collagenase (found to have an important role in rheumatoid arthritis) brings about an increase in collagenolysis at 36°C when compared with that at 30°C in tissue experiments (Harris and McCroskery, 1974).

Clinically, it has been demonstrated that normal knee joints have a temperature of 30.5–33°C, whereas joints with active synovitis have temperatures between 34 and 37.6°C. It might be anticipated that had the joint temperature been raised to, say, the range 40–45°C, the destructive collagenase may be inactivated. The problem is, of course, that in vivo other enzyme systems with lower thresholds may also be destroyed. At temperatures of about 45°C, so much protein damage occurs that there is destruction of cells and tissues. At this temperature, skin burns occur if contact is maintained for long enough. It has been found that 'heat-shock proteins' accumulate in cells and tissues exposed to high temperatures, the function of which, though not yet clearly agreed, is thought to confer a degree of protection to cells upon subsequent heat exposure. Temperature has an all-pervasive influence on cellular function, and heat damage can occur at multiple sites. Cell membranes are particularly sensitive; the lipoprotein structure of membranes may become more fluid with increasing temperature and cause a breakdown in permeability (Bowler, 1987).

A number of studies have demonstrated cellular effects with specific agents, though this does not means that others will not produce the same effect. Kligman (1982) showed that prolonged exposure (15 minutes, three times a week over 45 weeks) of guinea pigs to infrared radiation at an intensity of $12.45\,J/cm^2$ (giving rise to a skin temperature of about 40°C) can result in an increase in elastic fibres in the upper dermis and a large increase in ground substance. This effect is particularly noticeable when the infrared is combined with ultraviolet light.

Infrared radiation may also cause an alteration in the amino acid composition of proteins, which then appear to become more resistant to heat. This means that thermal tolerance develops and results in a reduction in the physiological effects of subsequent doses (Westerhof et al., 1987). This effect is overcome by allowing a period of between 36 and 72 hours to elapse between treatments.

Abnormal cells are also affected by short periods of heating. Whilst normal cells are unaffected, the effects of *mild* hyperthermia (around 40°C) on cancer cells can include the inhibition of the synthesis of ribonucleic acid (RNA), deoxyribonucleic acid (DNA) and proteins (Westerhof *et al.*, 1987). This can cause irreversible structural damage to cell membranes and the disruption of organelles.

Blood flow. When the skin is heated, the surface reddens (erythema) and blood vessels become vasodilated leading to increased blood flow. A good blood supply is essential for healing and, if there is infection, the increased number of white cells and fluid exudate available assist in destroying bacteria. The vasodilatation is caused by several mechanisms. First, the temperature elevation has a direct effect on the state of dilatation of arterioles and venules by acting on the smooth muscle of the vessels. If any local tissue damage occurs during heating, further dilatation may be produced by the release of histamine-like and tissue dilator substances such as bradykinin. Vasodilatation may also be produced in the skin by a local axon reflex in which stimulation of sensory cutaneous nerve endings produces antidromic nerve impulses in branches of the sensory nerves arborising around skin blood vessels. Increased skin blood flow occurs in areas remote from the heated tissue owing to long spinal nervous reflexes (Kerslake and Cooper, 1950). Increased levels of certain metabolites in the blood—the result of increased metabolic activity arising from the increased temperatures—also have a direct effect on vessel walls, stimulating vasodilation.

Veins commonly run close to arteries, which allows a ready exchange of heat between the vessels. By a countercurrent exchange, heat flows from the arterial blood to the cooler venous blood, thus returning some of the heat to the core. Its effect is to reduce body convective heat transfer by the blood but, in a warm environment, its effect is considerably diminished because of dilatation in the large superficial veins. Much of the variation in skin blood flow, however, is due to the presence of arteriovenous anastomoses deep below the skin capillaries. When these vessels open, the fall in temperature along the artery is reduced, thus raising skin temperature and increasing heat loss.

Increased blood flow in the deeper organs and tissues has been shown to occur as a consequence of heating, but it is usually less marked than in the skin. Part of the overall circulatory response in thermoregulation involves a redistribution of circulating blood in favour of the skin blood vessels for the purpose of heat exchange and at the expense of blood supply to the core. There is consequently a complex blood flow response in deeper tissues, involving direct vasodilatation due to heat, increased blood flow due to increased metabolic activity (e.g. in skeletal muscle) and a reduced blood flow because of a relative vasoconstriction brought about by thermoregulation.

It is unlikely that skeletal blood flow will be greatly influenced by superficial heating methods, but the presence of chemical mediators such as bradykinin and histamine, which are associated with heating, may affect capillary and postcapillary venule permeability. This, together with the increase in capillary hydrostatic pressure, may result in oedema. It is for this reason that the application of local heat in the early stages of trauma should be avoided (Feibel and Fast, 1976). This view is further supported by experimental evidence derived from animal models; acute and chronic inflammatory conditions were created in the paws of rats. It was found that the application of heat depressed the chronic inflammatory response but aggravated acute inflammation (Schmidt *et al.*, 1979). Similarly, clinical research has demonstrated an increase in oedema together with a prolonged healing time in acute injuries treated with heat (Wallace *et al.*, 1979).

As suggested above, slight differences in circulatory changes may occur with superficial (e.g. infrared irradiation or contact methods) and deep-heating methods of heating (e.g. short-wave and microwave diathermy), though only due to depth of penetration. Infrared radiation has been shown to cause an increase in blood flow in the cutaneous circulation (Crockford and Hellon, 1959; Millard, 1961; Wyper and McNiven, 1976). These changes are not reflected in the deeper tissues of the body such as the underlying muscle tissue and no significant changes are seen in body core temperature and blood pressure, even when the whole of one aspect of the body is exposed to a source of infrared.

In contrast, short-wave and microwave diathermy are thought to penetrate further and affect deeper structures. The effects of short-wave diathermy are examined in some detail in Chapter 11. Evidence suggests that microwave irradiation will significantly increase skin and muscle temperature and blood flow in dogs (Kemp, Paul and Hines, 1948; McMeeken and Bell, 1990a; Richardson et al., 1950; Siems et al., 1948), pigs (Sekins et al., 1980) and humans (de Lateur et al., 1970; McMeeken and Bell, 1990b; Sekins et al., 1984).

In a study investigating the effects of microwave irradiation to the forearm in 21 healthy individuals, forearm temperature increased from $30.3 \pm 0.2°C$ (average ± standard deviation) to $40.3 \pm 0.5°C$, and blood flow increased from $6.0 \pm 0.6°C$ to $44.9 \pm 9.8\,ml/100\,g/min$ (McMeeken and Bell, 1990b). The maximum blood flow increase to the forearm was achieved in a mean time of 15 minutes and hyperaemia was sustained for at least 20 minutes after the microwave irradiation ceased. The sustained increase in flow appears to be due to an increase in metabolic rate in the irradiated tissues.

Collagen. The properties of specific tissues may be changed by heating. For example, tendon extensibility can be increased by raising the temperature with the result that a stretch of a given intensity will produce greater elongation when heat is applied. Joint temperature influences the resistance to movement, with low temperature increasing and higher temperature reducing the resistance. These changes in joint movement can be in part attributed to changes in viscosity of the synovial fluid.

A number of researchers have suggested that an increase in temperature is, therefore, of value prior to the application of passive or active stretch designed to mobilise scars or lengthen contractures. Most have examined the behaviour of animal collagen tissue under passive stretch and have used a variety of heating methods, including hot water baths. Gersten (1955) showed an increase in the extensibility of frog Achilles'

tendons following heating with ultrasound, whilst Lehmann et al. (1970) heated rat-tail tendons to a temperature of 41–45°C, using a hot water bath. At these temperatures the viscous properties of tendon were evident, leading to a reduction in tensile strength. The stress–strain relationship was altered and residual elongation occurred following the application of a designated force at temperatures of 45°C. No such effects occurred at normal body temperatures. Similarly, Warren, Lehmann and Koblanski (1971, 1976), using rat-tail collagen heated in a water bath, demonstrated that tissue rupture occurred at similar levels of stress in collagen heated to 45°C and in material tested at normal body temperatures; at 39°C, however, rupture occurred at loads of 30–50% of normal. This temperature relates to the transition phase of collagen.

Such studies provide useful information about the behavior of collagen under stress at different temperatures, but it is important to remember that caution must be used when attempting to extrapolate from the experimental to clinical environments. The passive stretch applied by a physiotherapist on tissue is probably in the region of about one-third of the force used in vitro to produce deformation. Similarly, stresses applied during active exercise vary widely, but are also unlikely to reach experimental levels. In addition, the role played by reflexes, especially when pain is present, and the behaviour of muscle under stretch must also be taken into account. Thus, clinical results may not mimic experimental data.

Neurological changes. These effects primarily include changes to muscle tone and levels of pain. These two are closely interrelated, effects on the one possibly leading to changes in the other.

Muscle tone. It is noted in clinical practice that increased muscle tone, secondary to underlying pathology, can sometimes be relieved through the use of heat. Though the physiological basis for this is still poorly understood, a number of possibilities have been investigated. Lehmann and de Lateur (1990a) describe work which demonstrated that heating tissue to therapeutic temperatures of between 40°C and 45°C results in a reduction of spasm, and that stimulation of skin in the neck region could result in increased muscle relaxation.

The response of muscle spindles, secondary afferents and Golgi tendon organs to heating have all been investigated. The Ia afferents of muscle spindles have been shown to increase their firing rate with a moderate rise in temperature (Mense, 1978), whilst most (though not quite all) secondary afferents demonstrate decrease firing with temperature increases (Lehmann and de Lateur, 1999). In addition, there is increased firing from Golgi tendon organs, resulting in increased inhibition. All these factors are likely to reduce tone, assuming that secondary muscle spasm is largely a tonic phenomenon.

There is also some evidence that heating of the skin results in reduced tension, probably due to γ fibre activity affecting the muscle spindles (Fischer and Solomon, 1965). Thus superficial heating, such as contact heating and infrared, can reduce tone as well as the deeper-penetrating modalities that can affect deeper tissues directly.

Though an increase in temperature is most likely to be effective in reducing tone due to local problems, such as pain, there is some evidence that increased tone associated with upper motoneuron lesions can also be reduced by heating. These effects are only short term, however, and the use of cold may be a more effective method of treatment in this instance as the temperature of muscle returns to normal less rapidly following cooling than heating; this is discussed further later in the chapter.

Pain relief. Heat is often used to relieve pain in a variety of disorders, though the mechanism is uncertain, and supporting research evidence limited. In some cases, pain may be relieved by reducing secondary muscle spasm (see above). Pain alleged to be related to ischaemia may be reduced by heat-induced vasodilatation, with cells and chemicals brought to the area to assist healing and remove the breakdown products of injury.

Heat has also been claimed to act as a 'counterirritant'. It has been suggested that such responses might be explained on the basis of the pain gate theory, in that the transmission of thermal sensations may take precedence over nociceptive impulses. Counterirritant effects may be mediated through the effects of the morphine receptors in the central nervous system and the role of the enkephalins and endorphins in moderating pain (Doubell, Mannon and Woolf, 1999; Fields and Basbaum, 1999). (see Ch. 5 for more detail.)

Alterations in nerve conduction velocity may also be a factor. Kramer (1984) utilised infrared as a control when evaluating the heating effect of ultrasound in nerve conduction tests on normal subjects. Both infrared and ultrasound were applied separately to the distal humeral segment of the ulnar nerve in dosages that generated a rise in tissue temperature of 0.8°C; an increase in the post-treatment ulnar nerve conduction velocity was found in both cases. The workers attributed this velocity change directly to the increases in temperature. The studies of Halle, Scoville and Greathouse (1981) and Currier and Kramer (1982), again on human subjects, supported this work, suggesting possible implications with respect to motor and sensory conduction.

An increase in motor conduction can result in an increase in speed of a reflex response and possibly the speed of muscle contraction. Current theories suggest that an increase in sensory conduction may influence sensory responses via an increase in endorphins, which could affect the pain gate mechanism, though there is no firm evidence for this view at present. However, it has also been suggested that the counterirritant effects discussed above may be more important (Currier and Kramer, 1982; Lehmann and de Lateur, 1999).

Whatever the details of the underlying physiology, there is subjective evidence that people with pain consider heat to be beneficial. Barbour, McGuire and Kirchott (1986) conducted a subjective evaluation of methods of pain relief used by patients suffering from cancer. He found that 68% used heat in some form to help control pain.

Muscle performance. Both muscle strength and endurance may be affected by an increase in temperature. Following immersion of the lower limbs in a water bath at 44°C for 45 minutes, Edwards *et al.* (1970) demonstrated a reduction in the ability of subjects to sustain an isometric contraction. Similarly, an immediate reduction in the strength of the quadriceps muscle following the application of heat through the use of short-wave diathermy has also been demonstrated (Chastain, 1978). In this study, a temperature of 42.4°C at a depth of 3.22 cm was reported. However, Chastain (1978) also noted that over the ensuing 2 hours the muscle strength increased and remained above pretreatment levels. These findings are important in clinical practice, and should be considered both when making objective measurements of muscle strength in order to evaluate treatment efficacy and when implementing exercise programmes.

Tissue healing. Although it is important to remember that heating can be detrimental to tissue repair in the early stages as it can increase bleeding, oedema and chemical activity, which may all lead to increased pain, it has a number of beneficial effects in the later stages.

Positive changes can arise from an increase in the chemical reaction rates. There is an increase in oxygen uptake associated with a muscle temperature of about 38.6°C (Abramson *et al.*, 1958). The right-sided shift of the oxygen dissociation curve that occurs with an increase in temperature means that oxygen is more readily available for tissue repair. Haemoglobin releases twice as much oxygen at 41°C as at 36°C, and this also occurs twice as quickly (Barcroft and King, 1909). The increase in blood flow means that there are likely to be a greater number of white cells and more nutrients available for the healing process. Heat has secondary pain-relieving effects as the vasodilation accelerates the removal of pain-inducing metabolites or inflammatory products, and the heat reduces congestion and associated tissue tension.

There is conflicting evidence arising from animal studies regarding the efficacy of heating in the management of haematomas. Fenn (1969) showed a greater resolution of artificially induced haematomas in rabbit ears accompanying the application of short-wave diathermy compared with a control group. Lehmann *et al.* (1983) aslo reported benefits; they studied the effect of 327 mm (915 MHz) microwaves on the dispersal of haematomas created by the injection of radio-labelled blood into the thigh of six pigs. The treated side showed more rapid resolution of the haematoma and it was suggested that microwave diathermy would assist in the management of haematomata in muscle injuries. In contrast, a randomised, controlled study by Brown and Baker (1987) treated experimental haematomas in rabbits with pulsed short-wave diathermy (PSWD). No differences in the rate of healing between the treated and control animals were found. However, the clinical relevance of this study must be questioned as treating two animals with one machine must have distorted the PSWD field shape, and thus the distribution of imparted energy.

Systemic effects

Local heating causes a rise in temperature of tissues and reflex vasodilatation in remote areas of the body, but if heating is extensive and prolonged then a general rise in core temperature can ensue. Blood heated by the local tissues carries heat throughout the circulation. The hypothalamic centres are thus stimulated both by reflex mechanisms arising from peripheral thermoreceptors and from the direct blood-borne heat stimulus.

The immediate systemic response is a generalised skin vasodilatation, which serves to transport heat by conduction and convection from the core to the shell. There is a concomitant reduction in splanchnic blood flow resulting in reduced hepatic clearance rate and reduction in urine flow. If the heat stress is great, the skin temperature rises and approaches 35°C over the whole of the body. At or near this point, the body temperature becomes stabilised by the stimulation of sweat glands, which secrete hypotonic sweat on to the body surface so that increased evaporative cooling may take place. High radiant temperatures can be tolerated for many minutes if the environment is dry (as in a sauna). An increase in ambient humidity makes these conditions immediately unbearable. This is because the vapour pressure gradient between the skin and air is reduced, allowing sweat to run off the body instead of dissipating heat by evaporation.

Heat illness may occur with sudden increases in heat stress, most readily in those who are not adapted (acclimatised) to heat. Generalised skin vasodilatation may cause swelling of the feet and ankles (heat oedema) or syncope during postural change or prolonged standing. Prickly heat, a papulovesicular rash accompanied by a dermal prickling sensation when sweating is provoked, occurs in some people when areas of the skin are continuously wetted by sweat. More serious heat illnesses such as heat exhaustion from water deficiency or salt deficiency are due to imbalance of body water and salt respectively with excessive sweating and lead to collapse. Left untreated, they may result in potentially fatal heat stroke when the core temperature reaches high levels of 41°C and above and the central heat-regulatory mechanisms fail (Khogali and Hales, 1983).

Physiological effects of cold

Local effects

As is the case with an increase in temperature, once cooling has occurred it is immaterial as to how it was brought about. The different effects of cooling are the consequence of such factors as:

- the volume of tissue
- the composition of the tissue
- the capacity of the tissue to moderate the effects of cooling—largely a factor of blood supply
- the rate of temperature fall
- the temperature to which the tissue is lowered.

Cell activity. It is generally, but not universally, true that chemical and biological processes slow down with decreasing temperature. Since most enzyme systems operate at an optimal temperature, lowering the temperature results in a slow

inactivation of chemical processes. Cell viability is critically dependent on membrane transport systems involving active biochemical pumps and passive leaks in membranes, which maintain intracellular ionic composition. The failure of pumps at low temperatures relative to the leaks brings about a gain in Na^+, Ca^{2+} and loss of K^+ at reduced temperature in the cells of many species; that is, membranes lose their selective permeability in cold conditions.

Freezing damage to cells occurs when the local temperature drops to zero. Viscosity increases, ice crystallises and the remaining solution in the cells is reduced in volume as water leaks into the interstitial space. A characteristic feature of cold injury is the vascular damage which occurs with intravascular aggregation of platelets and red blood cells and the formation of occlusion masses in the vessels.

Blood flow. Cooling the skin causes an immediate vasoconstriction, which acts to diminish body heat loss. Thermoreceptors in the skin are stimulated and produce an autonomic reflex vasoconstriction over the body surface. In addition, there is a direct constrictor effect of cold on the smooth muscle of arterioles and venules. Countercurrent heat exchange helps to reduce heat transfer to the periphery. This is most effective in the limbs because of the relatively long parallel pathways between the deep arteries and veins. In this way, body core temperature is prevented from falling rapidly. Arteriovenous anastomoses that open to allow more blood flow to the skin in hot conditions are constricted in the cold.

Although immersion of the hands in water at 0–12°C at first causes the expected vasoconstriction, this is followed after a delay of 5 minutes or more by a marked vasodilatation. This is then interrupted by another burst of vasoconstriction and subsequent waves of increased and decreased local blood flow. This phenomenon is known as cold-induced vasodilatation (CIVD) and demonstrates a hunting reaction of the vessels that can be measured simply by thermocouple readings on the cooled skin (Fig. 6.4). At first, CIVD was thought to be caused by a local neurogenic axon reflex or the local release of vasodilator hormones into the tissues, or both. However, later work on isolated strips of vascular tissue revealed that CIVD is most likely to be due to the direct effect of low temperature causing paralysis of smooth muscle contraction in the blood vessels (Keatinge, 1978). The reaction may provide protection to tissues from damage caused by prolonged cooling and relative ischaemia.

Muscle blood flow is not much influenced by thermal reflexes but is determined largely by local muscle metabolic rate. During exercise there is a large increase in muscle blood flow due to accumulation of metabolites, and stress release of adrenaline also causes substantial vasodilatation in the muscle vessels. A striking feature of attempts at muscle cooling in cryotherapy is the prolonged period taken to reach maximum cooling. Muscles are generally shielded from temperature changes at the skin surface by the insulative layer of subcutaneous fat.

There is a marked difference in the appearance of the *skin erythema* due to CIVD as compared with that produced by skin heating. In CIVD the skin has a brighter red colour owing to the presence of more oxyhaemoglobin and less of the reduced haemoglobin in blood. It is apparent in the skin of babies who appear bright pink instead of pale when they are hypothermic or suffering from cold injury. The reason for this is that at low temperatures there is a shift in the oxygen dissociation curve so that

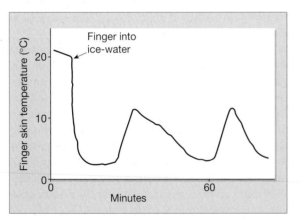

Figure 6.4 Cold vasodilatation in the finger immersed in ice-water, measured by skin temperature changes.

the blood tends to hold on to its oxygen, with oxyhaemoglobin dissociating less readily. One result of this is that, although cooling is immediately useful for haemostasis, cryotherapy probably does not benefit healing.

Collagen. As would be expected, collagen tends to become stiffer when cooled. This has been shown to occur both in experimental conditions, using excised collagen tissue, and in joints. For example, subjects with rheumatoid arthritis experience an increase in stiffness as temperatures are reduced.

Neurological changes. As with a decrease in temperature, a reduction in both muscle tone and pain can occur.

Muscle tone. Though the underlying physiology is not totally understood, cold is often used to reduce muscle tone. Effects may be due to changes in activity of muscle spindles, Ia and secondary afferents, α motor neurons, γ fibres, neuromuscular junctions or the muscle itself (when increased twitch-contraction and half-time relaxation may result).

Muscle spindles respond more rapidly than other neural and muscular structures as the reduction in temperatures required to produce changes in activity are not so great. With reduced temperatures, muscle spindle sensitivity drops in proportion to the degree of cooling, possibly as a result of a direct effect on the sensory terminal, or as the firing rate of Ia afferents is decreased, or both (Eldred, Lindsey and Buchwald, 1960; Ottoson, 1965). To achieve this a thorough cooling of muscle appears to be necessary, presumably to ensure cooling of the spindles which are embedded in the muscle structure. Miglietta (1973) and Trnavsky (1983) showed that prolonged cooling was needed to reduce clonus, and suggesting that the intramuscular temperature needed to be low to produce clinical effects. This was confirmed by Price *et al.* (1993) who demonstrated a significant reduction in spasticity at the ankle (secondary to head injury) following the application of liquid ice in a bag to the gastrocnemius muscle, after thorough cooling for 20 minutes.

Whilst the authors of these papers suggest that the effect seen is most likely to be due to effects on muscle spindles, it is also possible that greater degrees of cooling can affect other tissues, such as those listed above. Effects may be due to a slowing of conduction in both the muscle and motor nerves, a reduction in the sensitivity of the muscle spindle, or impaired conduction in the γ or α efferents.

However, because rapid responses are also seen on skin cooling (30 s after the application of ice) other explanations have been sought. It is postulated that reflexes from the cold skin may inhibit the dominant excitatory stimuli which operate in the region of the anterior horn neurons of the spinal cord, causing spasticity and spasm (Lehmann and De Lateur, 1990b). In addition, following an acute injury a reduction in muscle spasm may be attributed partly to the reduction of pain which has been described above.

Despite all these inhibitory effects, it is important to note that cooling may result in an immediate increase in tone for a short period; in line with other researchers, Price *et al.* (1993) noted that two of the patients treated with cold to reduce tone exhibited an aggravated response, which was attributed to the effects of tactile stimulation. Lehmann and de Lateur (1999) suggest that evidence points to an initial increase in excitability of the α motor neurons. An increase in tone has also been demonstrated with the use of ice massage.

Thus it is important to use an appropriate method of cooling to produce either excitation (e.g. a brief stimulus such as ice massage), or inhibition (more prolonged cooling such as with an ice pack). The response to cold may be rapid, occurring in a matter of seconds, but it is clinically important that the muscle is cooled thoroughly and for at least 30 minutes in order to achieve a longer-lasting effect.

Pain relief. Cold applied to the skin stimulates *cold* and *pain sensation.* If the cold is sufficiently intense, both sensations are suppressed because of inhibition of nerve conduction.

The reduction in pain that accompanies cooling can be due to either direct or indirect factors. Cold may be used as a counterirritant; as with heating, it has been suggested that such responses might be explained on the basis of the pain gate theory. Effects may also be mediated through the effects of the morphine receptors in the CNS, and the role of the enkephalins and endorphins (Doubell, Mannon and Woolf, 1999; Fields and Basbaum, 1999) (see Ch. 5 for more detail).

It has been demonstrated that peripheral nerve conduction is slowed by cold (Lee, Warren and Mason, 1978) and that fibres vary in their sensitivity according to their diameter and whether they are myelinated. Animal studies have demonstrated that the small diameter myelinated fibres (i.e. Aδ fibres), which conduct pain, are most responsive to cold. Although it would be unwise to extrapolate these findings directly to humans, evidence suggests that nerve conduction drops successively with increasing cold in humans, finally ceasing altogether. It is possible that this is a mechanism for the analgesic effects of cooling. It is, therefore, reasonable to suggest that effects on nerve fibres and free nerve endings lead to a reduction in pain.

Pain may sometimes be due to particular tissue irritants. For example, a number of studies have suggested that patients with arthritis may experience pain relief owing to the adverse effects of cooling on the activity of destructive enzymes within the joints (Harris and McCroskery, 1974; Pegg Littler and Littler, 1969).

Changes in perception of pain occurs both in normal subjects and in those with clinical pain; an elevation of the pain threshold has been demonstrated in normal subjects (Benson and Copp, 1974) and in patients with rheumatoid arthritis (Curkovic *et al.*, 1993). It occurs almost immediately following treatment but declines within 30 minutes.

Muscle performance

Muscle strength. The effect of temperature on muscle strength is a complex issue involving the effects of cold on the contractile process and the effects of temperature on neuromuscular transmission and circulatory oxygen. Some muscle properties have a large thermal dependence whereas others are barely influenced by temperature (Bennett, 1985). An additional point to consider is the actual temperature achieved in the muscle, as this will vary enormously.

When muscle strength is diminished by cooling, it is probably because of increased fluid viscosity and reduced metabolism, but there is evidence that strength may increase over its initial value approximately 1 hour after cooling has ceased.

A number of experimental studies have been conducted to examine these effects. For example, Davies and Young (1983) examined the effects of cooling the triceps surae muscle by immersion at 0°C for 30 minutes, which resulted in a deep muscle temperature drop of 8.4°C. They reported a reduction in maximal voluntary contraction and peak power output, components of muscle performance which are thought to be most temperature sensitive. Clinical studies support these findings (e.g. Oliver et al., 1979) but there is evidence that muscle performance improves above pretreatment levels during the hours following cooling.

The ability to sustain a maximal muscle contraction is also temperature dependent and is optimum at 27°C. Above 27°C the increase in muscle metabolism leads to a build-up in metabolites, which produces an early onset of fatigue. Below this temperature, the mechanisms described above come into play and the muscle may be further impaired by an increase in viscosity, which hampers repetitive exercise (Clarke, Hellon and Lind, 1958). Short-term increases in strength have been reported following brief application of ice, but the mechanism for this remains unclear.

Agility. Evans et al. (1995) examined the effect of cooling by immersion (20 minutes at 1°C) of the foot and ankle on agility measures (carioca manoeuvre, cocontraction test and shuttle run). Results indicated that, though mean agility scores were slightly lower, the time taken was similar to control runs. It is therefore unlikely that the temperatures used in normal clinical practice will affect agility.

Exercise-induced muscle damage. Muscle damage can result especially from strenuous or eccentric exercise, and it has been suggested that cooling after exercise may affect the symptoms. Easton and Peters (1999) examined the effect of cooling following maximal reciprocal contractions of the elbow flexors in a randomised controlled trial. Immersion at a temperature of 15°C immediately after activity and at 12 hour intervals for 3 days demonstrated that there was no difference in perception of tenderness and strength loss in the treated group, although the authors suggest that there was some indication of reduced muscle stiffness and damage.

Tissue healing. The fundamental process of tissue repair (see Ch. 3) is not enhanced by cooling as it slows down the cellular activity required for repair; however, a reduction in temperature can bring about changes that ultimately may be beneficial in the process. These include a reduction in bleeding, reduced swelling at the site of acute trauma, pain relief and a reduction in local muscle spasm. (These indirect effects are largely addressed above under circulatory and neurological changes.)

The reduction in swelling that accompanies the application of cold therapy following acute injury can be attributed to the immediate vasoconstriction of the arterioles and venules, which reduces the circulation to the area and therefore reduces the extravasation of fluid into the interstitium. This effect is enhanced by the reduction in both cell metabolism and vasoactive substances, such as histamine, which are also associated with cooling. It is important to note that the period of vasoconstriction lasts between 10 and 15 minutes and is then followed by the cycle of CIVD followed by vasoconstriction known as the 'hunting reaction'. This means that the beneficial aspects of vasoconstriction may be utilised for only a limited period of time.

It is of interest that experimentally induced swelling in animals has shown a variable response to the application of cooling, although the techniques used to produce cooling are not necessarily representative of current practice. Several of these studies have demonstrated an increase in swelling following ice therapy (e.g. Farry and Prentice, 1980) and it may be that this is due to the effects of CIVD or possibly to thermal injury of the lymphatic system (Meeusen and Lievens, 1986). However, a recent randomised controlled study by Dolan et al. (1997) reported a significant reduction ($P < 0.05$) in the volume of injured rat limbs following immersion in cold water (12.8–15.6°C). They concluded that immediate cooling following injury was effective in curbing the development of oedema.

In contrast, a number of clinical studies support the empirical evidence for the use of ice to reduce swelling (e.g. Basur, Shephard and Mouzos, 1976). It is, however, important to note that cooling in clinical practice is often accompanied by compression, which means that it is difficult to ascribe the benefits to cooling alone.

In addition, it is possible that cooling may lead to a reduction in bleeding; again this may be due to a reduction in blood flow and is most likely to occur during the early phase of treatment.

Systemic effects

A generalised vasoconstriction develops over the skin surface when a cold stimulus is applied. The effect on heat transfer may be judged from calculations showing that $60\,W/m^2$ can be transferred across the shell of the body when peripheral blood vessels are fully dilated, compared with $10\,W/m^2$ in the vasoconstricted state. Skin vasoconstriction and increased blood viscosity raise peripheral resistance and produce an increase in the arterial blood pressure.

As the skin temperature decreases, the drive to internal heat production grows. This is brought about by an involuntary increase in muscle tone (preshivering tone) that eventually develops into shivering. Voluntary movement and muscular exercise tend to inhibit shivering, mostly by helping to raise the body temperature and reduce the central nervous drive. Behavioural responses such as adopting a contracted posture with arms and legs drawn up to the body can reduce the surface area exposed for heat loss by up to 50%. Many animals possess another mechanism for thermogenesis in the cold that involves the biochemical uncoupling of metabolic pathways within the mitochondria of cells of brown fat tissue. The human neonate relies strongly on this process of non-shivering thermogenesis to balance body heat loss, but there is usually little evidence of this tissue in the adult as brown fat disappears during development.

Severe local cooling of the limbs can induce non-freezing cold injury in the extremities. Cooling for short periods below 12°C may cause sensory and motor paralysis of local nerves. 'Trench foot' is due to prolonged cooling of the feet in mud or water resulting in damage to nerve and muscle tissue with subsequent long-term diminution of function when normal body temperature and blood flow is restored. Hypothermia is a condition of low core temperature, defined as a deep body temperature below 35°C (Collins, 1983). It is potentially life threatening and often develops insidiously without the subject being aware of the threat. As the body temperature falls below 35°C there are increasing disturbances of brain and cardiac function. Consciousness is lost at a body temperature between 33 and 26°C with considerable variability between individuals.

REFERENCES

Abramson, DI, Kahn, A, Tuck, S et al. (1958) Relationship between a range of tissue temperature and local oxygen uptake in the human forearm. I. Changes observed under resting conditions. *Journal of Clinical Investigation* **37**: 1031–1038.

Barbour, LA, McGuire, DS, Kirchott, KT (1986) Non-analgesic methods of pain control used by cancer outpatients. *Oncology Nursing Forum* **13**: 56–60.

Barcroft, J, King, W (1909) The effect of temperature on the dissociation curve of blood. *Journal of Physiology* **39**: 374–384.

Basur, R, Shephard, E, Mouzos, G (1976) A cooling method in the treatment of ankle sprains. *Practitioner* **216**: 708.

Bennett, AF (1985) Temperature and muscle. *Journal of Experimental Biology* **115**: 333–344.

Benson, TB, Copp, EP (1974) The effects of therapeutic forms of heat and ice on the pain threshold of the normal shoulder. *Rheumatology and Rehabilitation* **13**: 101–104.

Bowler, K (1987) Cellular heat injury: are membranes involved? In: Bowler, K, Fuller, BJ (eds) *Temperature and Animal Cells*. Company of Biologists, Cambridge, pp 157–185.

Brown, M, Baker, RD (1987) Effects of pulsed shortwave diathermy on skeletal muscle injury in rabbits. *Physical Therapy* 67: 208–214.

British Standards (1987) BS 691 *Specification for Solid Stem Clinical Maximum Thermometers (Mercury in Glass)*. British Standards Institution, London.

Chastain, PB (1978) The effect of deep heat on isometric strength. *Physical Therapy* 58: 543.

Clarke, RSJ, Hellon, RF, Lind, AR (1958) The duration of sustained contractions of the human forearm at different temperatures. *Journal of Physiology* 143: 454–473.

Collins, KJ (1983) *Hypothermia the Facts*. Oxford University Press, Oxford.

Collins, KJ (1992) Regulation of body temperature. In: Tinker, J, Zapol, WM (eds) *Care of the Critically Ill Patient*, 2nd edn. Springer-Verlag, London, pp 155–173.

Crockford, GW, Hellon, RF (1959) Vascular responses of human skin to infra-red radiation. *Journal of Physiology* 149: 424–432.

Curkovic, B, Vitulic, V, Babic-Naglic, D, Durrigl, T (1993) The influence of heat and cold on the pain threshold in rheumatoid arthritis. *Zeitschrift für Rheumatologie* 52: 289–291.

Currier, DP, Kramer, JF (1982) Sensory nerve conduction: heating effects of ultrasound and infrared. *Physiotherapy Canada* 34: 241–246.

Davies, CTM, Young, K (1983) Effect of temperature on the contractile properties and muscle power of triceps surae in humans. *Journal of Applied Physiology* 55: 191–195.

de Lateur, BJ, Lehmann, JF, Stonebridge, JB *et al.* (1970) Muscle heating in human subjects with 915 MHz microwave contact applicator. *Archives of Physical Medicine and Rehabilitation* 51: 147–151.

Dolan, MG, Thornton, RM, Fish, DR, Mendel, FC (1997) Effects of cold water immersion on edema formation after blunt injury to the hind limbs of rats. *Journal of Athletic Training* 32: 233–237.

Doubell, P, Mannon, J, Woolf, CJ (1999) The dorsal horn: state dependent sensory processing, plasticity and the generation of pain. In: Wall, PD, Melzack, R (eds) *Textbook of Pain*, 4th edn. Churchill Livingstone, New York, pp 165–182.

Easton, R, Peters, D (1999) Effect of cold water immersion on the symptoms of exercise induced muscle damage. *Journal of Sports Sciences* 17: 231–238.

Edwards, R, Harris, R, Hultman, E *et al.* (1970) Energy metabolism during isometric exercise at different temperatures of m. quadriceps femoris in man. *Acta Physiologica Scandinavica* 80: 17–18.

Eldred, E, Lindsey, DF, Buchwald, JS (1960) The effects of cooling on the mammalian muscle spindle. *Experimental Neurology* 2: 144–157.

Emery, AF, Sekins, KM (1990) Computer modeling of thermotherapy. In: Lehman, JF (ed) *Therapeutic Heat and Cold*, 4th edn. Baltimore, MD, Williams & Wilkins, pp 113–149.

Evans, TA, Ingersoll, C, Knight, KL, Worrell, T (1995) Agility following the application of cold therapy. *Journal of Athletic Training* 30: 231–234.

Farry, PJ, Prentice, NG (1980) Ice treatment of injured ligaments: an experimental model. *New Zealand Medical Journal* 9: 12.

Feibel, H, Fast, H (1976) Deep heating of joints: A reconsideration. *Archives of Physical Medicine and Rehabilitation* 57: 513–514.

Fenn, JE (1969) Effect of pulsed electromagnetic energy (Diapulse) on experimental haematomas. *Canadian Medical Association Journal* 100: 251.

Fields, HL, Basbaum, AI (1999) Central nervous system mechanisms of pain. In: Wall, PD, Melzack, R (eds) *Textbook of Pain*, 4th edn. Churchill Livingstone, New York, pp 309–330.

Fischer, E, Solomon, S (1965) Physiological responses to heat and cold. In: Licht, S (ed) *Therapeutic Heat and Cold*, 2nd edn. E Licht, New Haven, CT, pp 126–169.

Gersten, JW (1955) Effect of ultrasound on tendon extensibility. *American Journal of Physical Medicine* 34: 362–369.

Halle, JS, Scoville, CR, Greathouse, DG (1981) Ultrasound's effect on the conduction latency of the superficial radial nerve in man. *Physical Therapy* 61: 345–350.

Harris, ED Jr, McCroskery, PA (1974) The influence of temperature and fibril stability on degradation of cartilage collagen by rheumatoid synovial collagenase. *New England Journal of Medicine* 290: 1–6.

Hensel, H (1981) *Thermoreception and Temperature Regulation*. Monographs of the Physiological Society no. 38. Academic Press, London.

International Union of Physiological Sciences (1987) Commission for Thermal Physiology. A glossary of terms for thermal physiology. *Pflugers Archives* 410: 567–587.

Keatinge, WR (1978) *Survival in Cold Water*. Blackwell, Oxford, pp 39–50.

Keatinge, WR, Sloane, REG (1975) Deep body temperatures from aural canal with servo-controlled heating to outer ear. *Journal of Applied Physiology* 38: 919–921.

Kemp, CR, Paul, WD, Hines, HM (1948) Studies concerning the effect of deep tissue heat on blood flow. *Archives of Physical Medicine* 29: 12–17.

Kerslake, D McK, Cooper, KE (1950) Vasodilatation in the hand in response to heating the skin elsewhere. *Clinical Science* 9: 31–47.

Khogali, M, Hales, JRS (1983) *Heat Stroke and Temperature Regulation*. Academic Press, London.

Kligman, LH (1982) Intensification of ultraviolet-induced dermal damage by infrared radiation. *Archives of Dermatological Research* 272: 229–238.

Kramer, JF (1984) Ultrasound: evaluation of its mechanical and thermal effects. *Archives of Physical Medicine and Rehabilitation* 65: 223–227.

Lee, JM, Warren, MP, Mason, SM (1978) The effects of ice on nerve conduction velocity. *Physiotherapy* 64: 2–6.

Lehmann, JF, De Lateur, BJ (1990a) Therapeutic heat. In: Lehmann, JF (ed) *Therapeutic Heat and Cold*, 4th edn. Baltimore, MD, Williams & Wilkins, p 444.

Lehmann, JF, De Lateur, BJ (1990b) Cryotherapy. In: Lehmann, JF (ed) *Therapeutic Heat and Cold*, 4th edn. Baltimore, MD, Williams & Wilkins, pp 590–632.

Lehmann, JF, de Lateur, B (1999) Ultrasound, shortwave, microwave, laser, superficial heat and cold in the treatment of pain. In: Wall, PD, Melzack, R (eds) *Textbook of Pain*, 4th edn. Churchill Livingstone, New York, pp 1383–1397.

Lehmann, JF, Masock, AJ, Warren, CG, Koblanski, JN (1970) Effects of therapeutic temperatures on tendon extensibility. *Archives of Physical Medicine in Rehabilitation* 51: 481–487.

Lehmann, JF, Dundore, DE, Esselman, PC *et al.* (1983) Microwave diathermy: Effects on experimental muscle haematoma resolution. *Archives of Physical Medicine and Rehabilitation* 64: 127–129.

McMeeken, JM, Bell, C (1990a) Effects of microwave irradiation on blood flow in the dog hindlimb. *Experimental Physiology* 75: 367–374.

McMeeken, JM, Bell, C (1990b) Microwave irradiation of the human forearm and hand. *Physiotherapy Theory and Practice* 6: 171–177.

Mense, S (1978) Effects of temperature on the discharges of motor spindles and tendon organs. *Pflugers Archives* 374: 159–166.

Meussen, R, Lievens, P (1986) The use of cryotherapy in sports injuries. *Sports Medicine* 3: 398–414.

Miglietta, O (1973) Action of cold on spasticity. *American Journal of Physical Medicine* 52: 198–205.

Millard JB (1961) Effects of high frequency currents and infrared rays on the circulation of the lower limb in man. *Annals of Physical Medicine* 6: 45–65.

Moore-Ede, MC, Sulzman, FM (1981) Internal temporal order. In: Asch-off, J (ed) *Handbook of Behavior Neurobiology.* Plenum, New York, pp 215–241.

Oliver, RA, Johnson, DJ, Wheelhouse, WW *et al.* (1979) Isometric muscle contraction response during recovery from reduced intramuscular temperature. *Archives of Physical Medicine in Rehabilitation* 60: 126.

Ottoson D (1965) The effects of temperature on the isolated muscle spindle. *Journal of Physiology* 180: 636–648.

Pegg, SMH, Littler, TR, Littler, EN (1969) A trial of ice therapy and exercise in chronic arthritis. *Physiotherapy* 55: 51–56.

Price, R, Lehmann, JF, Boswell-Bessette, S, Burleigh, S, de Lateur, B (1993) Influence of cryotherapy on spasticity at the human ankle. *Archives of Physical Medicine in Rehabilitation* 74: 300–304.

Richardson, AW, Imig, CJ, Feucht, BL *et al.* (1950) The relationship between deep tissue temperature and blood flow during electromagnetic irradiation. *Archives of Physical Medicine* 31: 19–25.

Schmidt, KL, Ott, VR, Röcher, G, Schaller, H (1979) Heat, cold and inflammation. *Rheumatology* 38: 391.

Scowcroft, AT, Mason, AHL, Hayne, CR (1977) Safety with microwave diathermy: A preliminary report of the CSP working party. *Physiotherapy* 63: 359–361.

Sekins, KM, Dundore, D, Emery, AF *et al.* (1980) Muscle blood flow changes in response to 915 MHz diathermy with surface cooling as measured by Xe^{133} clearance. *Archives of Physical Medicine and Rehabilitation* 61: 105–113.

Sekins, KM, Lehmann, JF, Esselman, P *et al.* (1984) Local muscle blood flow and temperature responses to 915 MHz diathermy as simultaneously measured and numerically predicted. *Archives of Physical Medicine and Rehabilitation* 65: 1–7.

Siems, LL, Kosman, AJ, Osborne, SL (1948) A comparative study of shortwave and microwave diathermy on blood flow. *Archives of Physical Medicine and Rehabilitation* 29: 759.

Trnavsky G (1983) Die Beeinflussing des Hoffman-Reflexes durch Kryoangzeittherapie. *Wiener Medizinische Wochenschrift* 11: 287–289.

Wall, PD, Melzack, R (eds) (1999) *Textbook of Pain.* 4th edn. Churchill Livingstone, New York.

Wallace, L *et al.* (1979) Immediate care of ankle injuries. *Journal of Orthopaedic and Sports Physical Therapy* 1: 46.

Warren, CG, Lehmann, JF, Koblanski, JN (1971) Elongation of rat tail tendon: effect of load and temperature. *Archives of Physical Medicine in Rehabilitation* 52: 465–475.

Warren, CG, Lehmann, JF, Koblanski, JN (1976) Heat and stretch procedures: an evaluation using rat tail tendon. *Archives of Physical Medicine in Rehabilitation* 57: 122–126.

Westerhof, W, Siddiqui, AH, Cormane, RH, Scholten, A (1987) Infrared hyperthermia and psoriasis. *Archives of Dermatological Research* 279: 209–210.

Wissler, EH (1988) A review of human thermal models. In: Mekjavic, IB, Banister, EW, Morrison, JB (eds) *Environmental Ergonomics.* Taylor & Francis, London, pp. 267–285.

Wyper, DJ, McNiven, DR (1976) Effects of some physiotherapeutic agents on skeletal muscle blood flow. *Physiotherapy* 62: 83–85.

7

Low-energy treatments: non-thermal or microthermal?

Sheila Kitchen
Mary Dyson

INTRODUCTION

Chapter 6 outlined the thermal changes which can arise both locally and generally in the human subject following the use of electrophysical agents such as infrared irradiation and shortwave diathermy. Heating is not, however, the only way in which physiological changes can be brought about in body tissues by electrophysical agents. Other effects include the use of low-frequency currents to produce stimulation of muscle or nervous tissue and the use of the predominantly non-thermal effects of high-frequency agents such as ultrasound and light to facilitate tissue repair, or reduce pain, or both. Chapter 8 addresses the former aspects whilst this chapter addresses the latter.

The term 'non-thermal' is frequently used in clinical practice to mean a treatment which does not result in the patient being conscious of any thermal sensations. It must be remembered, however, that almost all forms of energy can degrade ultimately into heat energy. 'Non-thermal' treatments may, therefore, still involve the production of low levels of heat, which it may be possible for the tissues to convert to chemical changes within the cell. In addition to any such microthermal changes, some agents are known to produce specific effects which do not depend primarily on heat for their occurrence. All of these will be discussed in this chapter.

Although there is clear evidence of the non-thermal effects of agents such as ultraviolet irradiation, visible light, X-rays and gamma rays, there is currently much controversy surrounding the possible existence of such effects from the use of low-intensity, non-ionising radiations and mechanical waves in physiotherapy practice. Arguments for and against their existence arose early in the development and evaluation of a number of agents (including ultrasound and pulsed short-wave diathermy) and the controversies have continued into recent times. For example, in 1990 Frizzell and Dunn believed there to be no evidence at that time to support the idea that biological effects are produced through the use of low-energy ultrasound; however, evidence is also available which repudiates this (Mortimer and Dyson, 1988). Barker and Freestone (1985) and Barker (1993) had similar reservations with respect to pulsed short-wave diathermy. Although the Food and Drug Administration (FDA) of the USA have yet to be convinced of the efficacy of low-level laser therapy, experimental work is in progress in the USA to test this, and was reported in 1999 at the inaugural meeting of the North American Laser Therapy Association held at the FDA offices in Rockville. It has been suggested by some that almost all effects are mediated through thermal changes, albeit at microthermal levels, whilst others have indicated that additional mechanisms may be active.

A variety of suggestions has been made about the ways in which predominantly non-thermal effects may occur. Many of those postulated are based on the suggestion that electrophysical agents can influence the mechanisms which lead to cell communication. Tsong (1989) suggests that cells communicate both *directly* through chemical means and *indirectly* through the influence of electrical, physical and acoustic signals, and it is thought that electrophysical agents may produce some physiological changes through these mechanisms.

INTERACTIVE TARGETS

'Interactive targets' are cellular components that may be receptive to interventions. These interactive targets include the cell itself, its plasma membrane, and intracellular structures such as the intracellular membranes, microtubules, mitochondria, chromophores, cell-associated ions and the nucleus.

Plasma membrane

The cell was described in terms of its electrical structure and function in Chapter 2, and it will be recalled that the plasma membrane consists of a bilayered, phospholipid structure which surrounds the cell, and is studded with transmembranous proteins (see Fig. 2.2, p. 34). These proteins have a number of functions: they strengthen the membrane, they transport substances such as proteins, sugars, fats and ions across the membrane, and they form specialist receptor sites for proteins (such as hormones and neurotransmitters) and enzymes. In addition, the plasma membrane is electrically charged, possessing a negative charge on its internal surface and a positive charge on its external surface. The resulting potential difference of approximately $-70\,mV$ is maintained through the passive and active movement of ions across the cell membrane.

A number of electrophysical agents are thought to effect changes at the level of the plasma membrane. For example, Adey, in 1988, postulated the transduction of a pulsed magnetic field (PMF) signal across the cell membrane and regarded this structure as the primary site of interaction between the oscillating electrical field and the cellular components of the tissue. He suggested that a large amplification of an initial weak trigger can occur as the result of the binding of hormones, antibodies and neurotransmitters to their specific binding sites on the cell membrane owing to the effects of magnetic fields.

Other workers, such as Tsong (1989), Westerhoff *et al.* (1986) and Astumian *et al.* (1987) have postulated that proteins can undergo conformational changes owing to interaction with an oscillating electrical field. For this to occur with any degree of efficiency, the frequency of the field must match the kinetic characteristics of the reaction and be at an optimum field strength (Tsong, 1989). This reaction can lead to pumping effects, with substances being actively transported across the cell membrane, leading to subsequent ATP synthesis. Though none of these researchers has specifically examined the effects of pulsed shortwave diathermy, it may be that it also acts upon cells in one or more of these ways.

Mechanical energy may also effect changes in cell membrane behaviour; such changes have been shown to occur when therapeutic levels of ultrasound are applied to cells in vitro. Hill and ter Haar (1989) state that acoustic cavitation results in sound energy being converted into other forms of energy, including shear energy. The sound energy induces the oscillation of minute bubbles within the tissues, which in turn induce microstreaming of liquids both around the bubbles themselves and around the cell walls (further details are provided in Ch. 14). Some writers, such as Repacholi (1970) and Repacholi et al. (1971), suggest that microstreaming may alter membrane permeability and secondary messenger activity and be responsible for changes in the surface charge of cells, resulting in the transduction of signals. This view has been reinforced by both Dyson (1985) and Young (1988), who have suggested that microstreaming (at therapeutic doses) may influence cell function by reversibly affecting the permeability of the plasma membrane and modifying the local environment through mechanisms such as altered cell metabolite gradients. Mortimer and Dyson (1988) have demonstrated that therapeutic levels of ultrasound can induce permeability changes to calcium ions, and that this is associated with cavitation.

Finally, writers such as Smith (1991a, b) have suggested that low-level laser radiation of certain types may initiate reactions at the cell membrane level, possibly through photophysical effects on Ca^{2+} channels.

Intracellular membranes

Intracellular membranes surround the internal organelles of the cell and exhibit similar electrical characteristics to cell membranes. One of their functions is to exercise control over the movement of substances into and out of these structures (Alberts et al., 1994; Frohlich, 1988) and thereby control the behaviour and actions of the organelles and ultimately of the entire cell. Similar effects to those induced at the cell surface may occur across these membranes, resulting in changes in activity of the organelles.

Microtubules

Microtubules are elongated cylinders made of protein that are present within cells. Electrically, they consist of dimers, which are charged dipole units—their internal ends being negatively charged relative to the periphery. This arrangement results in the cell having similar electrical properties to electrets, which are insulators carrying a permanent charge analogous to permanent magnets. These properties include the ability to exhibit piezoelectric and electropiezo effects and, in addition, such dipole units rotate under the influence of oscillating fields. However, they do not respond equally to all frequencies of energy, but instead have preferred resonant frequencies, which are governed by their moment of rotation (Frohlich, 1988).

Such dipole units may respond to the alternating magnetic and electrical fields produced by short-wave diathermy equipment. In general, it seems likely that such motion will give rise to *microthermal* changes, and Muller (1983) has suggested that an oscillation in temperature might allow a biological system to absorb free energy. Westerhoff et al. (1986) note that an electrical field is a 'thermodynamic quantity' and suggest that it may be the oscillation in this parameter which results in changes in the cyclical enzymatic activity of cells.

Mitochondria

It has been suggested that mitochondria may be stimulated directly by the application of electrophysical energy, and a number of researchers have suggested that laser radiation of certain wavelengths may initiate changes at this site in the cell. Karu (1988) has postulated the following sequence of events: certain wavelengths of red light, when absorbed by components of the respiratory chain within the mitochondria, cause a brief activation of that chain; oxidation of the nicotinamide adenine dinucleotide (NAD) pool occurs, leading to changes in the redox status of the mitochondria and cytoplasm; these changes lead to altered membrane permeability, and consequently to changes in the transport of ions across the cell wall. For example, changes in the $Na^+ : H^+$ ratio across the membrane occurs, and there are subsequent increases in Na^+K^+–ATPase activity. The Ca^{2+} flux is consequently altered, resulting in modulation of DNA and RNA synthesis and consequent changes in cell growth and proliferation. Smith (1991a, b) has suggested that other wavelengths (e.g. infrared radiation), not absorbed by mitochondrial cytochromes may be absorbed by cytochromic components of the cell membrane, producing direct changes in calcium flux at this site.

Ions

Ions are electrically charged particles that are present in both intracellular and extracellular fluids. Being electrically charged, they respond to oscillating electrical fields and ionic vibration is likely to occur (Frohlich, 1988). Such movement again may lead to changes in ionic distribution within the cells, affecting the cells' activity.

Nucleus

The interaction of electromagnetic fields with the nucleus of the cell has been reviewed by Nicolini (1985) and Frohlich (1988), who note that relatively little is known about these effects. Hiskenkamp et al. (1978) and Takahashi et al. (1986) are amongst those who believe that direct effects on the nucleus may occur, and they have suggested that pulsed magnetic fields may influence DNA synthesis and transcription. Adey (1988), however, postulates that any changes that have been noted are more likely to be the result of the presence of secondary messengers such as cAMP and Ca^{2+} ions, which may exert such an influence at the membrane level.

Chromophores

Chromophores are molecules that absorb specific wavelengths of electromagnetic radiation. They include melanin, nucleic acids and proteins, and are therefore distributed widely in the tissues and cells of the body. Ultraviolet radiation, visible light and infrared radiation may be absorbed by these structures.

When energy is absorbed by chromophores, an atom of the molecule affected becomes temporarily excited, resulting in the movement of an electron to a higher energy level. It subsequently degrades, releasing energy which may be passed on to other molecules, be used to effect a variety of biochemical changes or degrade into heat.

Cells

If free to move and subjected to ultrasonically induced standing waves, entire cells can be transported in a predominantly non-thermal fashion to pressure nodes spaced at half-wavelength intervals (Dyson et al., 1974). Although this is generally a reversible phenomenon, it can be irreversibly damaging in certain circumstances and should therefore be avoided (see Ch. 14).

THE EFFECT OF DOSAGE PARAMETERS

Though it has been suggested that many forms of energy (including electrical, mechanical and chemical) may initiate changes in cell behaviour, it is becoming increasingly clear that the dosage parameters of the energy imparted to the cell are likely to affect the end result. For example, Frohlich (1988) has suggested that ion oscillation and dipole rotation are dependent upon the frequency and amplitude of the electrical field in question. In addition, enzyme activity depends on the availability of specific charge sites on membrane surfaces which, Frohlich (1988) suggests, may be unlocked by the application of electrical signals of an 'appropriate type'. Tsong (1989) states that 'in principle, each class of protein is adapted to respond to an oscillating force field (electrical, sonic or chemical potential) of a defined frequency and strength'. Smith (1991a, b) has suggested that laser radiations of different wavelengths may affect different structures; he postulates that radiation at 633 nm may initiate activity at the mitochondrial level, as suggested by Karu (1987), whereas at 904 nm it may initiate reactions at the cell membrane level, possibly through photophysical effects on Ca^{2+} channels. In addition, it is known that ultraviolet irradiation of certain frequencies is more likely to produce erythematous changes ('sunburn') and carcinogenic changes than others.

Currently, there is little published information about the precise dosage parameters of many of these agents which are most likely to achieve therapeutic effects in clinical practice. The Arndt–Schultz law applies with ultrasound and light, too little energy having no measurable effect, too much being damaging, while energy levels between these extremes can be therapeutic. Though there is some evidence that low intensities are adequate to stimulate cell activity in vitro, more work is needed to establish the most effective wave bands and pulsing frequencies and to confirm this in clinical environments. It should, however, be appreciated that many therapeutic forms of energy act as stimuli at the cellular level, whether in vitro or in vivo. The cells transduce these stimuli and amplify them, so the energetic output of the cells far exceeds the energetic input, an extremely efficient mode of activity which would not occur should the changes be of a purely thermal nature.

CONCLUSION

This overview has highlighted the many theories which are currently being explored with respect to the ways in which the electrotherapy agents used by physiotherapists may effect therapeutically significant changes in cell behaviour. As this discussion has shown, it is possible that a number of similarities exist between the mechanisms whereby physiological changes are induced by the use of agents such as low-level ultrasound, pulsed non-thermal levels of short-wave diathermy and laser radiation. However, concrete evidence both of the mechanisms of interaction and of the physiological effects which occur in living, injured tissue is limited, a fact which should be borne in mind as the various agents are studied and used in clinical practice.

Later chapters in this book will examine in further detail the effects and efficacy of a number of agents used by physiotherapists at predominantly non-thermal intensities to treat soft tissue lesions and reduce pain.

REFERENCES

Adey, WR (1988) Physiological signalling across cell membranes and co-operative influences of extremely low frequency electromagnetic fields. In: Frohlich, H (ed) *Biological Coherence and Response to External Stimuli*. Springer-Verlag, Heidelberg.

Alberts, B, Bray, D, Lewis, J, Raff, M, Roberts, K, Watson, JD (1994) *Molecular Biology of the Cell*, 2nd edn. Garland Publishing, New York.

Astumian, RD, Chock, PB, Tsong, TY, Westerhoff, HV (1987) Can free energy be transduced from electrical noise? *Proceedings of the National Academy of Science, USA* **84**: 434–438.

Barker, AT (1993) Electricity magnetism and the body. *IEE Science, Education and Technology Division* **December**: 249–256.

Barker, AT, Freestone, IL (1985) Medical applications of electric and magnetic fields. *IEE Electronics and Power* **October**: 757–760.

Dyson, M (1985) Therapeutic applications of ultrasound. In: Nyborg, WL, Ziskin, MC (eds) *Biological Effects of Ultrasound (Clinics in Diagnostic Ultrasound)*. Churchill Livingstone, New York.

Dyson, M, Pond, J, Woodward, B, Broadbent, J (1974) The production of blood cell stasis and endothelial damage in the blood vessels of chick embryos treated with ultrasound in a stationary wave field. *Ultrasound in Medicine and Biology* **1**: 133–148.

Frizzell, LA, Dunn, F (1990) Biophysics of ultrasound. In: Lehmann, JF (ed) *Therapeutic Heat and Cold*, 4th edn. Williams and Wilkins, Baltimore, MD, pp. 362–397.

Frohlich, H (1988) *Biological Coherence and Response to External Stimuli*. Springer-Verlag, Heidelberg.

Hill, CR, ter Haar, G (1989) Ultrasound. In: Suess MJ, Benwell-Morison, DA (eds) *Nonionizing Radiation Protection*, 2nd edn. WHO.

Hiskenkamp, M, Chiabrera, A, Pilla, AA, Bassett, CAL (1978) Cell behaviour and DNA modification in pulsing electromagnetic fields. *Acta Orthopaedica Belgica* **44**: 636–650.

Karu, TI (1987) Photobiological fundamentals of low power laser therapy. *IEEE Quantum Electronics* **23**: 1703–1717.

Karu, TI (1988) Molecular mechanism of the therapeutic effects of low intensity laser radiation. *Lasers in Life Science* **2**: 53–74.

Mortimer, AJ, Dyson, M (1988) The effect of therapeutic ultrasound on calcium uptake in fibroblasts. *Ultrasound in Medicine and Biology* **14**: 499–506.

Muller, AWJ (1983) Thermoelectric energy conversion could be an energy source of living organisms. *Physics Letters A* **96**: 319–321.

Nicolini, C (1985) Cell nucleus and EM fields. In: Chiabrera, A, Nicolini, C, Schwan, HP (eds) *Interactions between Electromagnetic Fields and Cells*. Plenum Press, London.

Repacholi, MH (1970) Electrophoretic mobility of tumour cells exposed to ultrasound and ionising radiation. *Nature* **227**: 166–167.

Repacholi, MH, Woodcock, JP, Newman, DL, Taylor, KJW (1971) Interaction of low intensity ultrasound and ionising radiation with the tumour cell surface. *Physics in Medical Biology* **16**: 221–227.

Smith, KC (1991a) The photobiological basis of the therapeutic use of radiation from lasers. In: Ohshiro T, Calderhead RG (eds) *Progress in Light Therapy*. John Wiley, Chichester.

Smith, KC (1991b) The photobiological basis of low level laser radiation therapy. *Laser Therapy* **3**: 19–24.

Takahashi, K, Kaneko, I, Date, M, Fukada, E (1986) Effects of pulsing electromagnetic fields on DNA synthesis in mammalian cells in culture. *Experientia* **42**: 185–186.

Tsong, TY (1989) Deciphering the language of cells. *TIBS* **14**: 89–92.

Westerhoff, HV, Tsong, TY, Chock, PB, Chen, Yi-der, Astumian, RD (1986) How enzymes can capture and transmit free energy from an oscillating electrical field. *Proceedings of the National Academy of Science, USA* **83**: 4734–4738.

Young, SR (1988) *The Effect of Therapeutic Ultrasound on the Biological Mechanisms Involved in Dermal Repair*. PhD Thesis, London University.

8

Stimulative effects

Oona Scott

INTRODUCTION

This chapter reviews some recent reports of
changes in contractile characteristics of human
skeletal muscles associated with immobilisation, ageing, neuromuscular disease and neurological pathology. Differences between electrical
stimulation and exercise are considered, as is
the physiological basis for therapeutic use of
low-frequency electrical stimulation.

In the neuromuscular system, performance
capabilities are affected by the amount and types
of daily physical exercise (Komi, 1986). A person
who exercises on a regular basis will have a
leaner body mass and greater strength than a
person who takes little or no exercise. Detraining
effects have been shown to affect cardiorespira-
tory endurance, muscle endurance, muscle
strength and power. An individual confined to
bed for a few weeks or who has a limb immobilised in a cast will experience muscle atrophy
and loss of muscle strength.

Early studies of human muscle function were
limited to evaluating maximum strength or
maximum voluntary force (MVC) and estimating energy metabolism during work. In the
1970s, advances in histochemical techniques
(see Ch. 4), together with more acceptable
methods of taking muscle biopsies (Edwards
et al., 1977), were complemented by examination
of contractile properties using electrophysiological techniques.

Over the past 20 years, advances in molecular
biochemistry and genetic coding have been

accompanied by monitoring individual or group muscle performance in either isometric or iso-kinetic contractions or using kinemetric technology. Whole-muscle cross-sectional area can now be measured with ultrasonography and computerised axial tomography (CAT). Increasingly studies are undertaken that enable both clinicians and researchers to measure and to monitor changes in the molecular, physiological and biomechanical components of living human muscle. At the same time, neuroscientists have been making significant advances in understanding the control systems underlying normal movement.

CHANGES IN CONTRACTILE CHARACTERISTICS OF HUMAN SKELETAL MUSCLES

There is now substantive evidence of adaptation in human skeletal muscles accompanying chronic changes in neural activity. It is reasonable to assume that we are on the threshold of significant advances in recognising and ameliorating such changes. Appropriate electrical stimulation and exercise regimens are two of the ongoing challenges in rehabilitation in the twenty-first century.

Effect of immobilisation

Periods of 5 to 6 weeks without weight bearing in animals result in a decrease in protein synthesis, loss of muscle mass and loss of muscle strength with changes in fibre types. Studies of bed rest in normal healthy subjects for a similar period suggest that there is an increase in muscle fibres in a 'transitional state' from type 1 slow-contracting muscle fibres to faster-contracting type IIa and IIx together with overall fibre atrophy (Andersen *et al.*, 1999).

The position of immobilisation affects changes observed in muscles. Animal muscles immobilised in a shortened position atrophy faster and to a greater degree than stretched muscles (Williams and Goldspink, 1973). There also appears to be an increase in connective tissue as a result of immobilisation in a shortened position (Williams and Goldspink, 1984) which

could be modified by stretching and by electrical stimulation (Williams *et al.* 1986; Williams 1988).

Enoka (1997), reviewing neural adaptations with chronic physical activity, cited evidence from two separate human studies on limb immobility. A study by Duchateau and Hainaut (1990) on the effects of plaster cast immobilisation on the adductor pollicis showed loss of strength and e.m.g. and an inability to activate fully on voluntary command after 6 weeks of immobilisation, with a rapid return to normal activity on remobilisation. A similar experiment of immobilisation by Yue *et al.* (1994) for 4 weeks resulted in loss of strength and an inability to activate the elbow flexor muscles.

Studies by Snyder-Mackler, Binder-Macleod and Williams (1993) on the activity of the quadriceps femoris muscle following anterior cruciate reconstruction using a modified Burke fatigue test (see Ch. 19) showed weakness of the involved muscles but a less marked rate of fatigue over the first 60 seconds of the test than occurred in the stronger uninvolved muscles. These were surprising results and suggest that there had been selective type II fibre atrophy in the involved muscles.

Other investigators have examined both maximum voluntary strength and changes in contractile characteristics of various groups of normal subjects, ranging from very young to fit, active, elderly subjects. Comparative studies have been undertaken to monitor these changes in patient groups with spinal cord lesions, multiple sclerosis and children with neuromuscular diseases (Gerrits *et al.*, 1999; Lenman, Tulley and Vrbová, 1989; Scott *et al.*, 1990) and more recently in patients recovering from brain injury and stroke patients (Bateman *et al.*, 1998; Cramp *et al.*, 1995). Changes in the contractile properties often accompany muscle atrophy and loss of strength. These changes are thought to be associated with alterations in neuronal activity (see Ch. 4).

Muscle weakness and endurance in elderly people

Age-related declines in muscle strength and power, an inactive lifestyle, increasing difficulty with functional tasks requiring rapid power output, such as climbing stairs or rising from a chair, and an increased incidence of falls have been well documented in older people (for a review see Thomson *et al.*, 1994). Loss of strength is most marked in the lower limb muscles. Studies of the quadriceps femoris show age-related reductions in muscle mass although there is some doubt about the ability of elderly people to activate this muscle fully (for an explanation of activation see Ch. 19).

The differences in strength between young and fit elderly women have been associated with increased fatigue resistance together with slowing of relaxation times but with no differences in their ability to activate their quadriceps femoris muscles fully (O'connor *et al.*, 1993). Roos and his colleagues (1999), in a study of the muscles of young and old men, reported a similar 50% loss of strength, slower contractile speeds and higher tetanic fusion at lower frequencies of stimulation with full activation of quadriceps femoris muscles in the older men. They found no age-related difference in motor unit firing rates. This suggests that the loss of strength was not related to central activation or changes in motoneuron firing rates but rather to detraining through lack of exercise.

Progressive resistance training has been shown to be an effective means of improving muscle strength in very elderly people; the 'neural' changes specific to the training tasks played an important role in the initial strength gains (Harridge *et al.*, 1999). None of the women were able to activate the quadriceps femoris muscles fully either before, or indeed after, progressive exercise training. However there was an increase in muscle mass after training together with increased strength and ability to lift weights.

Changes in contractile properties following spinal cord injury

Studies by Gerrits *et al.* (1999) compared the contractile properties and fatigability of seven spinal-cord-injured (SCI) patients with those of 13 able-bodied control individuals. The SCI muscles demonstrated faster rates of contraction and relaxation as well as greater fatigability compared with controls—results which are in agreement with a characteristic preponderance of fast glycolytic muscle fibres.

Changes in contractile properties following stroke

Muscle weakness is an immediate consequence of stroke with both agonist and antagonist muscles usually demonstrating corresponding degrees of weakness. Muscle weakness is particularly evident in the extensors of the upper limb and flexors of the lower limb. Distal muscles are more affected than proximal muscles. There is much variation in individual patterns of weakness on the opposite side to the brain lesion. Weakness is also observed in the ipsilateral limb.

Recent studies have looked at recovery of muscle strength together with alterations in contractile properties and central control mechanisms following stroke (Cramp, 1998). As expected, affected muscles were weaker than unaffected muscles and reciprocal inhibition mediated by Ia recovery was reduced in affected limbs in the early stages after stroke. Changes were seen in fatigue resistance, and similar patterns of change were seen in affected and unaffected muscles of stroke patients suggesting that extraneous factors such as inactivity may affect muscle function. This view was supported by the observed differences in muscle strength, fatigue resistance and reciprocal inhibition between patients with good walking function (and who were assumed to be more active) and those with poor walking function (Cramp, 1998).

Muscle spasticity, or an increased resistance to passive movement, is not an inevitable consequence. In physiological terms, spasticity can be defined as a motor disorder characterised by a velocity-dependent increase in tonic stretch reflexes with exaggerated tendon jerks resulting from hyperexcitability of the stretch reflex. There is some evidence that changes in muscle structure, as a consequence of defective muscle activation or disuse, may be responsible for the increased resistance associated with muscle spasticity. Dietz *et al.* (1986) found fibre-type transformation, type II atrophy and structural changes in spastic gastrocnemius medialis muscle and muscle changes correlated with alterations in muscle activation. O'Dwyer *et al.* (1996) found that increased resistance to passive stretch was associated with muscle contracture but not with reflex hyperexcitability in 24 patients with stroke. There is a general opinion that both neural and non-neural mechanisms may underlie the development and presence of spasticity in stroke patients.

Changes in muscle properties in children with neuromuscular diseases

'As children grow older, they become stronger'— this well-established fact is characterised in the linear relationship between the strength of the trunk and the limb musculature in fit healthy young children. Interestingly the muscles of young children before puberty show a high resistance to fatigue with a significant slowing of relaxation time during electrically stimulated fatigue testing (see Ch. 19).

In contrast, children with Duchenne muscular dystrophy (DMD), a progressive muscular disease, show no increase in strength of their muscles as they grow older. Histochemically there is a predominance of type I fibres and few if any type II fibres. Immunocytochemical techniques have shown the persistence of fetal and slow myosin in many of these fibres. As in healthy children's muscles, dystrophic muscles have a high resistance to fatigue but, unlike the muscles of healthy children, do not show any change in their contractile characteristics during or after fatigue testing (Scott *et al.*, 1986, 1990).

BASIS FOR THE THERAPEUTIC USE OF ELECTRICAL STIMULATION

Excitability of nerve and muscle tissue provides a basis for therapeutic application of electrical stimulation, which was used throughout the twentieth century. Early studies used interrupted galvanic (unidirectional pulses lasting for more than 1 s) currents to produce contraction in denervated muscles. More recently, electrical stimulation has been used to supplement exercise programmes and, in the past 20 years, the ability of skeletal muscle to alter both its functional and contractile properties in response to long-term or chronic low-frequency stimulation has been investigated in clinical practice.

To achieve an electrically elicited contraction, two electrodes are placed on the skin over the muscle. One electrode (the cathode has proved to be the more comfortable) is placed over the motor point of the muscle (see Ch. 4) and the other (the anode) is placed elsewhere on the body, generally more distally on the muscle belly. Placement over the motor point of a muscle means identifying the point on the skin where maximum muscle contraction can be achieved. It is often associated with the point at which the nerve supplying a muscle enters its muscle belly. Frequently located at the junction of the proximal one-third with the distal two-thirds of the muscle belly, this is the position where it is possible to influence the greatest number of motor nerve fibres. If the peripheral nervous system is intact, stimulation is achieved by the intramuscular branches of the nerve supplying that muscle. If not, then direct stimulation can be applied to the muscle, though there are doubts about the efficacy of this procedure in human subjects (Low and Reed, 2000).

DIFFERENCES BETWEEN ELECTRICAL STIMULATION AND EXERCISE

It is well known that muscle strength can be increased by almost any method provided that the frequency of the exercise and loading intensities sufficiently exceed those of the normal or current level of activation of an individual muscle (Komi, 1986). In electrical stimulation, activity is restricted to the stimulated muscle. The muscle is less influenced by other training effects that occur during exercise. Superimposed electrical stimulation bypasses the central neuronal control mechanisms. Provided that stimuli (pulses) are of sufficient intensity and duration to depolarise the nerve membrane, action potentials are generated, the motor units are activated synchronously and muscle contraction occurs. There is now overwhelming evidence (see Long-term (chronic) electrical stimulation of skeletal muscle later in this chapter) that an important factor in determining the properties of a skeletal muscle is the amount of neuronal or impulse activity relative to the activity that is usual for that muscle. Electrical stimulation manipulates the output activity pattern from the motoneuron by adding to its inherent activity; in contrast, during voluntary exercise individual motor units are activated in a graded and hierarchical manner (see Recruitment of motor units in voluntary contractions in Ch. 4).

Training effects

Training at high forces (i.e. with loads greater than 60–70% of maximum strength) repeated as few as 10 times per day, where each contraction is held for 2–5 s, recruits both high- and low-threshold motor units and increases maximum voluntary strength by about 0.5–1% per day. In lower-intensity training regimens of about 30% of maximum strength, increases in strength have also been recorded when each contraction is held for longer (say 60 s). This may be because the higher-threshold units can be recruited as the lower-threshold units become fatigued (for reviews see Edström and Grimby, 1986; Jones, Rutherford and Parker, 1989; Lieber, 1986).

It has been claimed that, prior to training, muscle cannot be maximally activated by voluntary activity and that large, fast motor units are recruited only when higher forces are applied. It is possible that some of these fast units are never recruited in the untrained state and there is evidence to show that in trained muscle there is increased synchronisation (see Komi, 1986).

In the first 6–8 weeks before changes in muscle size become apparent, activation and therefore strength increases as a result of establishing appropriate motor patterns of control of the muscles and of increased neural drive. If training is continued beyond about 12 weeks, a steady and slow increase occurs in both size and strength of the exercised muscles (for a review see Jones, Rutherford and Parker, 1989).

A recent study (Hortobágyi et al., 2000) of the rate of muscle strength recovery after immobilisation and retraining showed that in those individuals whose retraining was eccentric and mixed, compared with concentric training, the rate of strength recovery was faster and the eccentric and isometric strength gains were greater. They suggested that the faster rate of strength recovery and the greater strength gains after eccentric training were due to the unique aspects of the muscle lengthening. Immobilisation reduces type I, IIa and IIx muscle fibre areas and significantly greater hypertrophy of the muscle fibres was found after eccentric training, and upregulation of type IIx myosin heavy-chain messenger RNA.

Training studies tend to be of short duration (less than 5 weeks) and confined to a period when neural adaptations are thought to underlie the increases in strength, so at present it is still unclear whether the gains in strength with short-term electromyostimulation are superior to voluntary training.

Effects of electrical stimulation

The order of motor unit activation by electrical stimulation depends on at least three factors:

- the diameter of the motor axon
- the distance between the axon and the active electrode
- the effect of input from cutaneous afferents that have been activated by the artificial stimulus.

The hierarchical order of recruitment of the motor units in electrical stimulation is the reverse of the natural sequence (Trimble and Enoka, 1991; also see section Recruitment of motor units in voluntary contractions in Ch. 4). Because of their large diameter axons and low activation threshold, the larger normally inactive motor units are recruited first and may experience the most profound change in their use. These fast-contracting, high-tension generating, easily fatigable motor units are often found in the superficial layers of a muscle and are closer to the stimulating electrodes. The stimulation will also be conducted antidromically, that is, going towards the spinal cord, along the motor nerve and by the afferent sensory nerves. This too has been shown to cause a reversal of the normal order of motor unit recruitment (see Ch. 4) (Garnett *et al.*, 1978).

Imposed electrical stimulation is seen to have certain advantages in increasing muscle activity compared with exercise:

- the rigid hierarchical order of recruitment is bypassed
- electrical stimulation can attain higher levels of activity than any exercise regimen and therefore the adaptive potential of the system is challenged to its limits
- enhanced activity is restricted to the target muscle with few if any secondary systemic effects.

LOW-FREQUENCY ELECTRICAL STIMULATION

As already stated, low-frequency electrical stimulation in human studies where the impulses are no faster than 1000 Hz and usually lower than 100 Hz has traditionally been used to facilitate or to mimic voluntary contractions of skeletal muscle and as a supplement to normal training procedures. Hardly surprisingly, the focus in animal studies has been on the effect of long-term, low-frequency electrical stimulation where there is no need for active cooperation. More surprising is the paucity of human studies that evaluate any physiological changes which may occur, or that identify and monitor aspects of motor performance, such as skill and the restoration of functional performance in response to either short- or long-term electrical stimulation.

Short-term electrical stimulation

This form of electrical stimulation is sometimes known as electromyostimulation or faradic-type (i.e. shorter pulses usually between 0.1 and 1 ms duration and applied at between 30 and 100 Hz) stimulation. The therapeutic rationale is based on the assumption that the output of the motor system is insufficient and needs to be supplemented by artificial means. This seems reasonable, particularly where the function of the nervous system may have been compromised by a traumatic event or by some disease process.

Clinically, electrical stimulation is used for strengthening in cases involving immobilisation or where there is contraindication to dynamic exercise. In the early stages of rehabilitation after injury or surgery, there can be diminished voluntary control and an inability to exert muscular force. In athletic and sports training regimens, electrical stimulation may be used as an adjunct to voluntary exercise, especially at the end of a session when the motivation to continue exercising may begin to decline.

It is sometimes suggested that it is difficult to evaluate the relative effectiveness of various protocols because sufficient details have not been provided of the parameters that have been used. Most, although not all, studies have shown that it is possible to induce strength gains in both healthy and weakened skeletal muscles with short-term, low-frequency electrical stimulation. The general conclusion to emerge is that strength gains are similar to, but not greater than, those that can be achieved with normal voluntary training.

Gains in strength have been attained with a variety of stimulus parameters ranging from low frequencies (25–200 Hz) to trains of high-frequency sinusoidal pulses that are modulated at low frequencies. Enoka (1988), reviewing the training effects underlying neuromuscular stimulation, suggested that an optimum protocol used interferential stimulation (see section on Interferential therapy in Ch. 18). A disadvantage of this form of regimen is that it requires sophisticated equipment; the advantage of low-frequency stimulation is that it is usually self- applied using a battery-driven stimulator. Selkowitz (1989) identified two major categories of electrical stimulation: low-frequency, endurance-training programmes, and strength training using interferential stimulation. He suggested that low-frequency, muscle endurance regimens have relatively short intervals between contractions, with the contraction durations approximately equal to the rest periods (usually 4/15 seconds on/off) and lasting for a total of 6–15 minutes for each treatment session.

Snyder-Mackler and her colleagues (1994), in a study of two groups of patients recovering from anterior cruciate ligament reconstruction, investigated the use of electrical stimulation together with a rigorous exercise programme. Both groups of patients received electrical stimulation for 15 minutes four times a day, for 5 days a week. Those patients training with an interferential stimulator (2500 Hz triangular alternating current at a burst rate of 75 Hz) trained at higher intensities (i.e. percentage of the uninvolved MVC) than those training with portable battery-operated stimulators (pulse duration of 300 μs at 55 Hz, on/off time = 15/50 seconds). Their findings showed a dose-related response and a linear correlation between the training intensity and the strength of the quadriceps femoris muscle.

Long-term (chronic) electrical stimulation of skeletal muscle

Investigations in animals and recent studies in human muscle have confirmed that it is possible to modify the properties of mammalian skeletal muscle by long-term electrical stimulation. Skeletal muscle has a remarkable ability to change its properties in response to demand, so much so that it is now recognised that appropriate use of chronic low-frequency stimulation can change most cellular elements of a muscle in an orderly sequence. This model has provided a means for researchers to correlate functional changes with changes at the molecular level and has enabled investigations to be undertaken that explore the extent of muscle plasticity. Observation of the time course of changes has led to the study of gene expression of different functional elements in muscle fibres and transformation of their phenotype (Pette and Vrbová, 1999).

The ability to change properties of skeletal muscles by chronic, low-frequency stimulation is now well established in both animal and human muscles and a number of reviews have

summarised the major effects (Enoka, 1988; Lieber, 1986; Pette and Vrbová, 1992; Salmons and Henriksson, 1981). Variation in the parameters used in animal studies, inherent differences between species, and the varying condition of animals prior to stimulation have made it difficult to compare results from different studies. Nevertheless, the findings are largely complementary and an overall pattern of transformation has been established.

Although we know that the neuronal control and patterns of activation are different for each activity and for each muscle, and even for the constituent motor units, we do not yet know how best to exploit this ability to change muscle properties. The time course of reversal of induced changes when stimulation is discontinued appears to be different for each muscle property but, in general terms, it is comparable to the time course of transformation.

Changes in contractile properties

In response to chronic, low-frequency stimulation in both rabbit and cat fast-contracting muscles, the first effect noted was an increase in both contraction and relaxation times of stimulated muscles when compared with those of control muscles (Pette *et al.*, 1973; Salmons and Vrbová, 1969; Vrbová, 1966). There was also an alteration in the ratio of twitch to tetanic force, in that the twitch tension was very similar to that of the control muscle but the maximal tetanic tension was considerably reduced. The slowing effect became apparent after 9–12 days of stimulation.

Similar changes within 3 weeks of superimposed stimulation have been reported in chronically stimulated tibialis anterior muscle, adductor pollicis human adult muscles (Rutherford and Jones, 1988; Scott *et al.*, 1985b) and more recently in quadriceps femoris muscle (Cramp, Manuel and Scott, 1995). A consistent finding in both animal and human studies in response to long-term stimulation has been an increased resistance to fatigue. Having been described in a large number of animal studies, this was first demonstrated in adult human muscle in a study of tibialis anterior muscle by Scott *et al.* (1985b), then in adductor pollicis by Rutherford and Jones (1988), and latterly in quadriceps femoris muscle by Cramp, Manuel and Scott (1995).

Metabolic changes

In animal muscles, the increased resistance to fatigue has been associated with increases in aerobic–oxidative capacity and with a marked decrease in glycolytic enzyme activities. Transformation of fast-twitch muscle fibres into slow ones (see section Classification—matching motoneurons to the muscle fibres in Ch. 4) by chronic stimulation at 10 Hz is well documented. It is associated with changes of contractile characteristics, shifts of metabolic enzyme patterns, Ca^{2+} uptake by the sarcoplasmic reticulum, and eventual changes in myosin heavy and light chains. These changes of metabolic, histochemical and structural properties have been extensively reviewed (Enoka, 1988; Pette and Vrbová, 1992, 1999; Salmons and Henrikson, 1981) and are shown schematically in Figure 8.1.

Circulatory changes

The earliest changes recorded in animal muscles can be identified as changes in the sarcoplasmic reticulum, an increase in blood supply followed by an increase in capillary density surrounding the stimulated muscle fibres, and a decrease in muscle fibre diameter (Cotter, Hudlická and Vibová, 1973). It was found (Hudlická et al., 1977) that, after 4 days, the stimulated muscles fatigued less than the control muscles, suggesting that increased capillary density provided a more homogeneous distribution of blood and better diffusion of oxygen. It was suggested that this might be because a greater number of muscle fibres would have access to oxygen, which would facilitate rephosphorylation of ATP and creative phosphate (see section The sliding-filament hypothesis in Ch. 4).

Structural changes

Heilmann and Pette (1979), investigating effects of continuous 10 Hz stimulation on rabbit fast-twitch muscles, found that one of the earliest changes was a reduction in both the initial and total Ca^{2+} uptake, accompanied by a change in the polypeptide patterns of the sarcoplasmic reticulum. Stimulation-induced changes in muscle fibres include a more homogeneous population of fibres with a smaller cross-sectional area, but no loss of muscle fibres.

Myofibrillar ATPase histochemistry has shown a stimulation-induced increase in the number of type I muscle fibres in many species, and detailed analysis of chronically stimulated extensor digitorum longus and tibialis anterior in rabbit muscles has shown an overall transition of fast-type muscle to slow, including changes in the myosin molecule.

Particular attention has been paid to changes in the myofibrillar protein myosin, and to the regulatory proteins tropomyosin and troponin, which are associated with actin. Changes in the myosin molecule were first observed after 2–4 weeks, but the complete fast-to-slow transition of the myosin light chains appears to take several months (for further details see Pette and Vrbová, 1992, 1999).

Different patterns of stimulation

Much less research has been carried out into the transformation of slow muscle to fast (apart from early work on the soleus muscle—Vrbová, 1963), but in recent years more work has been done on the effect of different patterns of stimulation in human muscle.

Throughout many of the studies, investigators have been concerned to consider the effect of external factors on the changes that have been observed in response to stimulation. Such external factors may be of importance when considering the possible effect of long-term stimulation in human muscles. In animal studies, it is usual for the entire muscle to be stimulated using implanted electrodes. In human studies, in contrast, muscles are generally stimulated using surface electrodes (rather than through implants) and so it is important to be aware of the percentage of a muscle that is being stimulated.

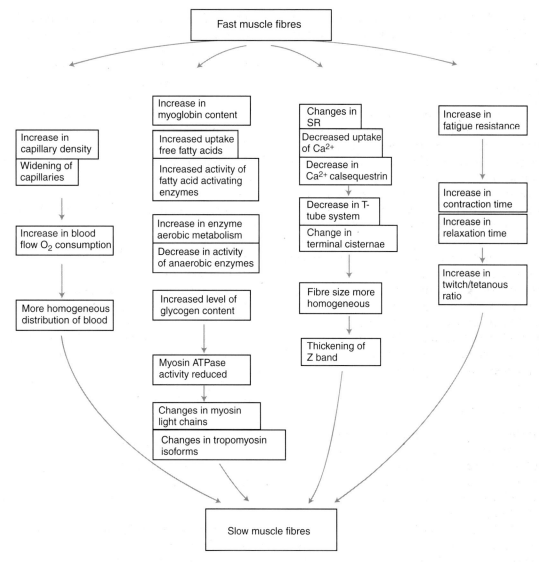

Figure 8.1 Schematic representation of effects of chronic low-frequency stimulation on fast muscle fibres.

As already observed, the position and loading of the muscle during stimulation are likely to affect the changes that occur. Studies on muscle protein metabolism by Williams and Goldspink (1986 and 1988) showed the importance of stretch on muscle proteins. Cotter and Phillips (1986) showed that the transition from fast to slow muscle was accelerated in rabbit tibialis anterior muscle with immobilisation in the neutral position; Williams *et al.* (1986) found greater increases in type I and type IIa fibres when a muscle was immobilised in a stretched position.

Studies on healthy human muscles

In 1985, Scott *et al.* investigated the effect on contractile properties of tibialis anterior by stimulating the intramuscular branches of the lateral popliteal nerve at 10 Hz for an hour, three times a day for 6 weeks. Using an asymmetrical biphasic waveform of sufficient intensity to give a visible contraction of the tibialis anterior accompanied by movement of the foot, they monitored the effect of chronic low-frequency stimulation and showed that it was possible to change the contractile characteristics of this muscle in human subjects. As in animal studies, long-term low-frequency stimulation induced a significant increase in resistance to fatigue in the stimulated muscles compared with unstimulated controls, suggesting a change in properties of the type II, fast-contracting, easily fatigable, glycolytic fibres.

Comparing the effect of long-term, low-frequency stimulation with a non-uniform pattern of stimulation incorporating a range of low through to high frequencies (5–40 Hz), Rutherford and Jones (1988) found there were similar changes in the fatigue characteristics in response to both patterns of stimulation. However, those subjects whose muscles were stimulated with a low-frequency pattern lost muscle strength, whereas those subjects whose muscles were stimulated using a mixed pattern of stimulation became stronger. The reduction in muscle bulk as well as strength that was reported may have been due to reduction of fibre diameter of the largest and most fatigable muscle fibres being exposed to sudden excessive activity.

More recently Cramp *et al.* (1995) explored the effects of selected patterns of long-term electrical stimulation on quadriceps femoris muscle of 21 healthy subjects. Stimulated muscles showed significant increases in strength, fatigue resistance and relaxation times after 3 weeks and in force–frequency output after 6 weeks. Significant changes were observed in those muscles stimulated with a mixed or random pattern of activation, indicating that a mixed or random pattern of activation induced greater changes than a uniform 8 Hz pattern.

Clinical studies

Facial paralysis (Bell's palsy). In some studies, attempts were made to simulate motoneuron discharge patterns on the basis that the natural pattern of discharge of a single, slow motor unit is not a uniform one. Farraher, Kidd and Tallis (1987) described this form of stimulation as 'eutrophic stimulation', identifying a 'neurotrophic effect' of the simulated pattern, and reporting considerable clinical merit for patients suffering from intractable Bell's palsy.

Rheumatoid arthritis. Kidd and Oldham in 1988, and then Oldham and Stanley in 1989, gave accounts of the benefits of using eutrophic stimulation on the small muscles of the hand in patients with rheumatoid arthritis and reported significant improvement in functional ability and voluntary fatigue in the hand muscles of these patients. Their pattern of stimulation was derived from a fatigued motor unit from the first dorsal interosseus muscle in a normal hand.

Duchenne muscular dystrophy. Studies using different patterns of long-term electrical stimulation on the muscles of boys with Duchenne muscular dystrophy identified the importance of the pattern of stimulation (Scott *et al.*, 1986, 1990). The application of a uniform 8 Hz pattern to stimulate the tibialis anterior and quadriceps femoris of young boys with DMD resulted in improvements in maximum voluntary contraction of stimulated muscles in comparison with unstimulated controls. In contrast, use of a 30 Hz pattern of stimulation on a group of six boys with DMD resulted in a decrease in maximum voluntary contraction. Three of the latter group subsequently stimulated their muscles with the uniform 8 Hz pattern and gained voluntary strength.

Functional electrical stimulation (FES). Functional electrical stimulation is electrical stimulation of muscle deprived of normal control to produce a functionally useful contraction (see Singer, 1987). The first portable stimulator was developed in 1960 by Wladimir Liberson to provide a foot assistance in hemiplegic patients. It was triggered with a foot switch in the shoe of the affected leg.

FES serves to provoke contraction of a paralysed muscle and to affect the sensory pathways, contributing to the normalisation of basic reflex motor activities. It has been used primarily in the rehabilitation of:

- hemiplegics
- paraplegics and quadriplegics

- children with cerebral palsy
- other patients suffering from impairment or disease of the central nervous system (multiple sclerosis, head injuries etc.) (Vodovnik, 1981).

PATIENT TOLERANCE

Comparative comfort is a key issue and tends to limit widespread application of electrical stimulation (Baker, Bowman and McNeal, 1988; Delitto et al., 1992). Surface stimulation activates sensory receptors on the surface of the skin (see sensory-motoneuron activation in Ch. 4, p. 71). The resulting discomfort and pain can often limit application of effectiveness of stimulation. However subjects adapt to this sensory experience relatively quickly, developing an increased tolerance to all types of stimulation over a number of sessions. The sensation of stimulated muscle contraction can be disconcerting and subjects often comment that a relatively low percentage of their MVC feels like a very strong contraction.

Stimulus waveform and pulse duration play a major role in subject comfort. It is often stated that levels of pain and of unpleasant sensation are minimised by the use of short pulse widths (50 µs is often chosen) and high frequencies (40–50 Hz or higher). There is a need for continual reassessment of the therapeutic level of contraction for each muscle that is stimulated to ensure that optimal effects are being obtained.

MONITORING AND MEASUREMENT

Singer (1987) recommended minimum requirements when reporting muscle strength testing, the stimulus parameters and the design of training programmes. Their objective was to provide a guide toward more appropriate protocols for further research and clinical practice. More than 10 years later, these criteria are as relevant to the clinician recording details of patient progress and requiring a sound basis for therapeutic evaluation as they are to the researchers in their investigative studies and to individuals concerned with their own well being.

Summary

There is still uncertainty concerning optimum patterns of stimulation and increasingly studies in both animals and human subjects have highlighted the need to consider the effect of loading and normal use of the muscle during periods of stimulation. A concern that has not yet been resolved has been the possible damaging effect of high frequencies of stimulation on young developing muscles. The effect of different patterns of stimulation may, of course, be a key factor, but there are additional considerations of patient compliance and acceptability that need to be considered (Baker, Bowman and McNeal, 1988).

REFERENCES

Andersen, JL, Cruschy-Knudsen, T, Sandri, C, Larsson, L, Schiaffino, S (1999) Bed rest increases the amount of mismatched fibres in human skeletal muscle. *Journal of Applied Physiology* **86**(2): 455–460.

Baker, L, Bowman, BR, McNeal, DR (1988) Effects of waveform on comfort during neuromuscular electrical stimulation. *Clinical Orthopaedics and Related Research* **233**: 75–85.

Bateman, A, Greenwood, RJ, Scott, OM (1988) Quadriceps femoris strength and fatiguability in patients after recent head injury. *Journal of Physiology* **509**: 44P.

Cotter, M, Phillips, P (1986) Rapid fast to slow fiber transformation in response to chronic stimulation of immobilized muscles of the rabbit. *Experimental Neurology* **93**: 531–545.

Cotter, M, Hudlická, O, Vrbová, G (1973) Growth of capillaries during long-term activity in skeletal muscle. *Bibliography of Anatomy* **11**: 395–398.

Cramp, MC (1998) *Alterations in Human Muscle and Central Control Mechanisms*. PhD thesis, University of East London.

Cramp, MC, Manuel, JA, Scott, OM (1995) Effects of different patterns of long-term electrical stimulation on human quadriceps femoris muscle. *Journal of Physiology (Lond)* **483**: 82P.

Delitto, A, Strube, MJ, Shulman, AD, Minor, SD (1992) A study of discomfort with electrical stimulation. *Physical Therapy* **72**: 410–424.

Dietz, V, Ketelsen, UP, Berger, W, Quintern, J (1986) Motor unit involvement in spastic paresis: relationship between leg activation and histochemistry. *Journal of the Neurological Sciences* **75**: 89–103.

Duchateau, J, Hainaut, K (1990) Effects of immobilisation on contractile properties, recruitment and firing rates of human motor units. *Journal of Physiology* **422**: 55–65.

Edwards, RHT, Young, A, Hoskings, GP, Jones, DA (1977) Human skeletal muscle function: Description of tests and normal values. *Scientific Molecular Medicine* **52**: 283–290.

Edström, L, Grimby, L (1986) Effect of exercise on the motor unit. *Muscle and Nerve* **9**: 104–126.

Enoka, RM (1997) Neural adaptations with chronic physical activity. *Journal of Biomechanics* **30**(5): 447–455.

Enoka, RM (1988) Muscle strength and its development: new perspectives. *Sports Medicine* **6**: 146–168.

Farraher, D, Kidd, GL, Tallis, RC (1987) Eutrophic electrical stimulation for Bellís palsy. *Clinical Rehabilitation* **1**: 265–271.

Garnett, RAF, O'Donnovan, MJ, Stephens, JA, Taylor, A (1978) Motor unit organisation of human medial gastrocnemius. *Journal of Physiology (Lond)* **287**: 33–43.

Gerrits, HL, de Hann, A, Hopman, MTE, van der Woude, LHV, Jones, DA, Sargeant, AJ (1999) Contractile properties of the quadriceps muscle in individuals with spinal cord injury. *Muscle & Nerve* **22**: 1249–1253.

Harridge, SDR, Kryger, A, Stensgaard, A (1999) Knee extensor strength, activation and size in very elderly people following strength training. *Muscle & Nerve* **22**: 831–839.

Heilmann, C, Pette, D (1979) Molecular transformations in sarcoplasmic reticulum of fast twitch muscle by electrostimulation. *European Journal of Biochemistry* **93**: 437–446.

Hortobágyi, T, Dempsey, D, Fraser, D, *et al.* (2000) Changes in muscle strength, muscle fibre size and myofibrillar gene expression after immobilisation and retraining in humans. *Journal of Physiology* **524**(1): 293–304.

Hudlická, O, Brown, M, Cotter, M, Smith, M, Vrbová, G (1977) The effect of long-term stimulation on fast muscles on their blood flow, metabolism and ability to withstand fatigue. *Pflugers Archives* **369**: 141–149.

Jones, DA, Rutherford, OM, Parker, DF (1989) Physiological changes in skeletal muscle as a result of strength training. *Quarterly Journal of Experimental Physiology* **74**: 233–256.

Kidd, GL, Oldham, JA (1988) Eutrophic electrotherapy and atrophied muscle: a pilot clinical study. *Clinical Rehabilitation* **2**: 219–230.

Komi, PV (1986) Training of muscle strength and power: Interaction of neuromotoric, hypertrophic and mechanical factors. *International Journal of Sports Medicine* **7**: 10–15.

Lenman, AJR, Tulley, FM, Vrbová, G (1989) Muscle fatigue in some neurological disorders. *Muscle and Nerve* **12**: 938–942.

Lieber, RL (1986) Skeletal muscle adaptability: Muscle properties following chronic electrical stimulation. *Developmental Medicine and Child Neurology* **28**: 662–670.

Low, J, Reed, A (2000) *Electrotherapy Explained*, 3rd edn. Butterworth-Heinemann, Oxford.

O'Connor, MC, Carnell, P, Manuel, JM, Scott, OM (1993) Characteristics of human quadriceps femoris muscle during voluntary and electrically induced fatigue. *Journal of Physiology* **473**: 71P.

O'Dwyer, NJ, Ada, L, Neilson, PD (1996) Spasticity and muscle contracture in relation to spastic hypertonia. *Current Opinion in Neurology* **9**: 451–455.

Oldham, JA, Stanley, JK (1989) Rehabilitation of atrophied muscle in the rheumatoid arthritic hand: a comparison of two methods of electrical stimulation. *Journal of Hand Surgery (British volume)* **14B**: 294–297.

Pette, D, Vrbová, G (1992) Adaptation of mammalian skeletal muscle fibres to chronic electrical stimulation. *Review of Physiological Biochemistry* **120**: 116–202.

Pette, D, Vrbová, G (1999) What does chronic electrical stimulation teach us about muscle plasticity? *Muscle and Nerve* **22**: 666–677.

Pette, D, Smith, ME, Staudte, HW, Vrbová, G (1973) Effects of long-term electrical stimulation on some contractile and metabolic characteristics of fast rabbit muscles. *Pflugers Archives* **338**: 257–272.

Roos, MR, Rice, CL, Connelly, DM, Vandervoot, AA (1999) Quadriceps muscle strength, contractile properties, and motor unit firing rates in young and old men. *Muscle & Nerve* **22**: 1094–1103.

Rutherford, OM, Jones, DA (1988) Contractile properties and fatigability of the human adductor muscle and first dorsal interosseus: a comparison of the effects of two chronic stimulation patterns. *Journal of Neurological Science* **85**: 319–331.

Salmons, S, Henriksson, J (1981) The adaptive response of skeletal muscle to increased use. *Muscle and Nerve* **4**: 94–105.

Salmons, S, Vrbová, V (1969) The influence of activity on some contractile characteristics of mammalian fast and slow muscles. *Journal of Physiology* **201**: 535–549.

Scott, OM, Vrbová, G, Hyde, SA, Dubowitz, D (1986) Responses of muscles of patients with Duchenne muscular dystrophy to chronic electrical stimulation. *Journal of Neurology, Neurosurgery and Psychiatry* **49**: 1427–1434.

Scott, OM, Vrbová, G, Hyde, SA, Dubowitz, D (1985) Effects of chronic, low-frequency electrical stimulation on normal tibialis anterior muscle. *Journal of Neurology, Neurosurgery and Psychiatry* **48**: 774–781.

Scott, OM, Hyde, SA, Vrbová, G, Dubowitz, V (1990) Therapeutic possibilities of chronic low frequency electrical stimulation in children with Duchenne muscular dystrophy. *Journal of Neurological Sciences* **95**: 171–182.

Selkowitz, DM (1989) High frequency electrical stimulation in muscle strengthening: A review and discussion. *American Journal of Sports Medicine* **17**(1): 103–111.

Singer, B (1987) Functional electrical stimulation of the extremities in the neurological patient: A review. *Australian Journal of Physiotherapy* **33**(1): 33–42.

Snyder-Mackler, L, Binder-Macleod, SA, Williams, PR (1993) Fatigability of human quadriceps femoris muscle following anterior cruciate ligament reconstruction. *Medicine and Science in Sports and Exercise* **25**(7): 783–789.

Snyder-Mackler, L, Delitto, A, Stralka, SW, Bailey, SL (1994) Use of electrical stimulation to enhance recovery of quadriceps femoris muscle force production in patients following anterior cruciate ligament reconstruction. *Physical Therapy* **74**(10): 901–907.

Thomson, LV (1994) Effects of age and training on skeletal muscle physiology and performance. *Physical Therapy* **74**: 71–81.

Trimble, MH, Enoka, RM (1991) Mechanisms underlying the training effects associated with neuromuscular electrical stimulation. *Physical Therapy* **71**(4): 273–282.

Vodovnik, L (1981) Functional electrical stimulation of extremities. In: *Advances in Electronics and Electron Physics*. Academic Press, New York.

Vrbová, G (1963) The effect of motoneurone activity on the speed of contraction of striated muscle. *Journal of Physiology (Lond)* **169**: 513–526.

Vrbová, G (1966) Factors determining the speed of contraction of striated muscle. *Journal of Physiology (Lond)* **185**: 17P–18P.

Williams, PE (1988) Effect of intermittent stretch on immobilised muscle. *Annals of Rheumatic Diseases* **47**: 1014–1016.

Williams, PE, Goldspink, G (1973) The effect of immobilization on the longitudinal growth of striated muscle fibres. *Journal of Anatomy* **116**: 45–55.

Williams, PE, Goldspink, G (1984) Connective tissue changes in immobilized muscle. *Journal of Anatomy* **138**(2): 343–350.

Williams, PE, Watt, P, Bicik, V, Goldspink, G (1986) Effects of stretch combined with electrical stimulation on the type of sarcomeres produced at the ends of muscle fibres. *Experimental Neurology* **93**: 500–509.

Yue, GH, Bilodeau, M, Enoka, RN (1994) Elbow joint immobilization decreases fatiguability and alters the pattern of activation in humans. *Society of Neurosciences Abstracts* **20**: 1205.

Conductive agents

9

Heat and cold: conduction methods

Sheila Kitchen

INTRODUCTION

Both heat and cold can be effective forms of treatment for conditions, such as musculoskeletal lesions, pain and spasticity. Chapter 6 has described in some detail the nature of the physical and physiological changes which can arise in the human body due to thermal variation. This chapter will discuss the use of agents which effect temperature changes through direct physical contact with tissue.

Heat or cold?

Many, though not all, of the clinical benefits produced by heat and cold are similar. Selection is therefore based on a number of factors which may, on occasion, be empirical but are nevertheless of importance.

• **Stage of inflammation.** Generally, cold is preferable during the acute stage of inflammation to relieve pain, reduce bleeding and possibly reduce swelling. Heat, in contrast, can exacerbate the early inflammatory process. However, it should be remembered that cold can retard the basic healing process.
• **Oedema.** Heat tends to increase this, especially in the early stages of inflammation and injury. Cold can help to limit oedema.
• **Collagen extensibility.** This is more likely to be affected beneficially by a rise in temperature; collagen becomes stiffer with cold.

- **Pain.** Both heat and cold may be used to relieve pain. The effect of cold may be more prolonged but can increase pain in certain situations.
- **Spasm.** Both heat and cold can decrease muscle spasm associated with musculoskeletal injuries and nerve root irritation. Similarly, both will reduce spasticity due to upper motor neuron dysfunction, though heat will do so for only a short period of time; cold is more effective under these circumstances as the return to normal temperatures takes longer.
- **Muscle contraction.** Moderate cooling to approximately 27°C leads to an increase in the ability of a muscle to sustain a contraction. There appears to be a slight increase in the strength of contraction with a rise in temperature.
- **Area to be treated.** In some subjects the application of cold to the hands and feet leads to considerable discomfort and this may therefore be an indication for heat therapy.
- **Ease of use.** This can be especially important when considering home therapy administered by the patient.
- **Patient preference.** Some subjects find cold intolerable; the use of heat to relieve both pain and muscle spasm may be more acceptable and lead to greater compliance with treatment.

Wet or dry?

A second important factor to be considered when selecting contact treatment is that of choosing between wet and dry contact techniques. Little is known about the relative efficacy of one compared with the other; however, Abramson (1967) has suggested that dry heat can elevate surface temperature to a slightly greater degree, whilst wet heat can lead to rises in temperature at slightly deeper levels.

Heat *and* cold

The effects of heat and cold are described separately in the following sections. Occasionally the two are used alternatively, most commonly in contrast baths.

Contrast baths. Most commonly, contrast baths comprise two water baths at different temperatures: a hotter bath at 40–42°C (immersion for 3–4 minutes) and a colder one at 15–20°C (for about 1 minute). The body part is immersed in each of the baths alternatively, and it is normal practice to begin and end with the hotter bath. Lehmann and de Lateur (1990) have suggested that a 10 minute immersion in the warmer bath prior to the use of the colder contrasting temperatures may be useful in producing an initial hyperaemia.

Few studies have examined the efficacy of this treatment but it is suggested that hyperaemia, reduced oedema due to vasodilation (Woodmansey, Collins and Ernst, 1938) and pain relief, possibly through the pain gate mechanism, may be implicated (Lehmann and de Lateur, 1999). Myrer, Draper and Durrant (1994) demonstrated that contrast baths are unlikely to result in an increase in intramuscular temperature.

HEAT: CONTACT TECHNIQUES

Contact methods of heating require, by definition, physical contact between the therapeutic agent and the tissues. Changes in temperature are the result of heat transfer through conduction (see Ch. 6 for details); the resulting oscillation or vibration of ions and molecules, or both, give rise to the heating. Heating of deeper tissues is due to conduction within the tissues themselves, as well as convection through fluids (e.g. blood).

When superficial contact heat is applied, the surface tissue temperature change will depend on:

- the intensity of the heat (watts/cm^2)
- the length of exposure to the heat (minutes)
- size of area exposed (cm^2)
- the thermal medium; this is a product of the thermal conductivity, density and specific heat characteristics of the tissue (Hendler, Crosby and Hardy, 1958).

In order to achieve therapeutic levels of heating, the temperature obtained in the tissues should be between 40 and 45°C (Lehman and de Lateur, 1990). Burning is likely to occur above this level, and below 40°C the effects of heating are considered too mild to be of therapeutic use.

Maximal elevation of the temperature of the skin and very superficial tissue will occur within 6–8 minutes. The underlying muscle will respond to a lesser extent and more slowly, and, at tolerable temperatures, muscle temperature can be expected to be raised by about 1°C at a depth of 3 cm. However, where subcutaneous fat is present, heating of deeper tissues is reduced because of insulation. Where a greater depth of penetration is required, deep-heat modalities such as short-wave diathermy, should be considered.

Physiological effects

These are described in detail in Chapter 6; they include effects on cell function in general, on circulation (blood flow, oedema, haemorrhaging), on collagen, on neurological tissue (pain, spasm), on muscle (contraction rates and intensity, agility) and on tissue repair. It is important to remember that contact methods produce only relatively superficial thermal changes; thus effects will be limited in the deeper tissues of the body.

Clinical efficacy

Much of the work to examine the clinical efficacy of heat was conducted using contact methods such as water baths. Lehmann and de Lateur (1990) and Chapman (1991) review this literature in some detail, and it forms the basis of the discussion in Chapter 6. Relatively few recent articles have been published in this area.

Methods of application

Surface heat may be applied in a number of ways. All methods raise superficial tissue temperatures; however, some may be more suitable in given situations owing to the material used (e.g. wet or dry heat) and the practicalities of application.

Wax

Paraffin wax, with a melting point of approximately 54°C, is combined with a mineral oil such as liquid paraffin to produce a temperature-controlled bath at a temperature between 42°C and 50°C. These temperatures are slightly higher than would be tolerated if the body part were placed in hot water. This is because the specific heat of paraffin wax is less than that of water (2.72 kJ/kg per degree centigrade for wax and 4.2 kJ/kg per degree centigrade for water). Wax therefore releases less energy than water when cooling. Selkins and Emery (1990) note that the amount of heat imparted to the tissue due the solidification of the wax—the latent heat of fusion—is small. At the same time, heat loss is prevented owing to the insulating nature of the material. The net result is a well-insulated, low-temperature method of heating tissue.

Slightly higher temperatures may be used for the upper extremities and lower temperatures for the lower extremities and newly healed tissue (Burns and Conin, 1987; Head and Helms, 1977).

Application: the body part is inspected for any contraindications (see the following section), and washed. In the *dip and wrap method*, the part is first immersed in the warm wax. It is then withdrawn and the wax allowed to set. The procedure is repeated, normally 6 to 12 times, to develop a 'wax glove'. The whole is then wrapped in plastic or waxed paper and an insulating layer of material such as a towel.

Alternatively, the part may be retained in the bath following the development of the wax glove—the *dip and reimmerse method*. This technique results in a greater increase in temperature (Abramson *et al.*, 1964; Abramson, Chu and Tuck, 1965).

Heated pads and packs

A variety of heated pads may be used to provide heat to small areas.

Hydrocollated pads. These consist of hydrophilic silicate gel (which absorbs water) within a cotton wrapping. The temperature of the pack is raised in a hot water bath of approximately 75°C, wrapped in a material such as towelling and then applied to the part. The temperature of the final pack should be around 40–42°C. Gradual cooling will occur. Replacement of the packs during treatment can result in prolonged heating, though no significant differences in subcutaneous temperatures result (Lehmann *et al.*, 1966).

Moist pads. These are immersed in hot water (at approximately 36–41°C) and perform a similar function to those above but tend to cool more quickly as it is not practical to provide an insulation layer. Such pads need to be replaced after approximately 5 minutes.

Electrically heated pads. These vary in size greatly. Electrical resistance wire lies within the structure and the design allows the temperature (40–42°C) to be controlled thermostatically. These pads can be used at lower temperatures, some having a range of 1–42°C.

Hydrotherapy

The use of hot water to heat tissue is an effective way of increasing temperature, and both whirlpools and still water baths may be used for local treatment. Temperatures are usually between 36 and 41°C (lower than wax temperatures for the reasons discussed above). Borell *et al.* (1980) confirmed that treatment at these temperatures results in an increase in subcutaneous temperature. The motion of the water in whirlpool baths may, in addition, stimulate receptors in the skin surface, giving rise to pain relief through the pain gate mechanism.

Other methods

Hot air (at about 70°C), both dry and moist, can be used to warm the tissues. Due to the low conductivity of air, the tissue temperature remains lower than 70°C, again at around 35–40°C. Fluidotherapy is a form of dry heating (38–45°C), and involves a suspension of cellulose particles which are kept in motion by air movement. It makes use of convection forces to transfer energy. Neither form of heating is commonly used in clinical practice, probably because of the need for special cabinets for the treatment.

Hazards

These include the following.

• **Burns.** Burns are the main hazard associated with contact-heating methods. They can arise if there is inadequate testing of materials and equipment, the patient has severely impaired circulation, or the tissue is devitalised.

• **Foreign material.** This may be introduced into open wounds. Particles of wax may remain in lesions, and water and wet materials may carry infection if not carefully controlled. Patients with any kind of open wound or infection should not use communal baths (e.g. wax baths).

Contraindications

The presence of the following may either fully contraindicate this type of treatment or may indicate that extra care is needed in its application:

• lack of local thermal sensitivity on the part of the patient
• impaired circulation
• areas of recent bleeding or haemorrhaging
• devitalised skin, e.g. after deep X-ray treatment
• open wounds
• certain skin conditions, e.g. skin carcinomas, acute dermatitis (especially with wax)
• cardiovascular impairment—in some individuals immersion in warm liquids may be inappropriate if a large body area part is to be treated
• damaged or infected tissues, as moisture may encourage these to break down.

COLD: CONTACT TECHNIQUES (CRYOTHERAPY)

Contact techniques may be used to cool tissue for therapeutic reasons. The changes in temperature that can be achieved have been reported in many studies and vary enormously. This variation can be attributed to:

• different methods of application
• the length of time over which cooling has been applied

- the initial temperature of the technique used, e.g. water temperature.

Skin temperatures. The greatest changes in temperature reported in a variety of studies for the different methods of application are as follows:

- immersion in water: a drop of 29.5°C at a water temperature of 4°C after 193 minutes
- ice massage: a drop of 26.6°C at an ice temperature of 2°C after 10 minutes' application
- evaporation sprays: a drop of 2°C with spraying for 15–30 seconds
- ice packs: a drop of 20.3°C at a contact temperature of 0–3°C after 10 minutes
- ice towels: a drop of 13°C after a 7 minute period.

Intramuscular temperature. The associated drop in temperature depends on the duration of the treatment, the depth of the muscle from the surface and the initial temperature of the treatment agent; cooling persists for several hours (Meussen and Lievens, 1986).

Joint temperature. This appears to remain low after the application of cold, although some investigators have reported an initial brief rise in temperature (Kern *et al.*, 1984).

Physiological effects

These are described in detail in Chapter 6 and include effects on cell function in general, circulation (blood flow, oedema, haemorrhaging), collagen, neurological tissue (pain, spasm), muscle (contraction rates and intensity, agility) and tissue repair. It is important to remember that contact methods of cooling produce only relatively superficial changes, so effects will be limited in the deeper tissues of the body.

Clinical efficacy

Studies examining clinical efficacy support the empirical evidence for the use of ice for a number of symptoms.

Cooling can reduce swelling (e.g. Basur, Shephard and Mouzos, 1976). However, in clinical practice cooling is often accompanied by compression, which means that it is difficult to ascribe the benefits to cooling alone. The treatment may lead to a reduction in bleeding; again, however, this may be due to a reduction in blood flow and is most likely to occur during the early phase of treatment. Elevation of the pain threshold has been demonstrated in patients with rheumatoid arthritis (Curkovic *et al.*, 1993) immediately following treatment but declines within 30 minutes. Pain may sometimes be due to particular tissue irritants. For example, a number of studies have suggested that patients with arthritis may experience pain relief owing to the adverse effects of cooling on the activity of destructive enzymes within the joints (Harris and McCroskery, 1974; Pegg, Littler and Littler, 1969). A report was published in 1997 by Lessard *et al.* evaluating the effect of cold on recovery from minor arthroscopic knee surgery. A significant difference was found between the groups (exercise regimen plus cold, or exercise regimen only) in terms of increased compliance and weight bearing, and of reduced drug consumption.

Effects on muscle strength are described in Chapter 6, and clinical studies lend some support to these findings (e.g. Oliver *et al.*, 1979); there is some evidence that muscle performance improves above pretreatment levels during the hours following cooling.

A number of recent reviewers have examined the evidence for efficacy of cooling. Sauls (1999) undertook a review of the effects of cold for pain relief by the nursing profession. Some benefits were noted for certain orthopaedic procedures and for injections in adults; in contrast, pain relief was not recorded during abdominal procedures or injections in children. She noted, however, along with other researchers, that the quality of many reports is questionable and that care should be taken when evaluating and implementing their results.

Detrimental effects of cooling. When considering the beneficial effects of cooling it is important that other, less therapeutically useful effects are not underestimated. For instance, the immediate increase in peripheral vascular resistance associated with vasoconstriction that occurs with cooling causes an increase in blood pressure. This may preclude the safe use of this modality in patients who have a history of hypertension. Ice should not be applied to areas affected by peripheral vascular disease as vasoconstriction will further impair the blood supply to an area which is already compromised. The later vasodilation, which occurs as part of the 'hunting reaction', is also of limited value as the shift to the left of the O_2-dissociation curve which also occurs with cooling means that O_2 is not readily available to the tissues.

Therapeutic effects may not occur in patients with sympathetic dysfunction, as some circulatory responses are mediated by the sympathetic nervous system.

The effects on muscle strength discussed above should be considered when making objective measures of muscle strength, as such measures may be unreliable if made after cooling.

The effects of temperature on collagen have been discussed in the section on collagen heating. It is important to note, however, that a reduction in temperature is likely to increase the mechanical stiffness of collagenous tissue and therefore also increase joint stiffness (Hunter, Kerr and Whillans, 1952).

Methods of application

Cold may be applied in a number of ways, including wet and dry packs and the use of evaporating sprays. During the application of cold therapy, the subject will experience a number of sensations; these may include:

- intense cold
- burning
- aching
- analgesia.

Cold packs

Cold packs may be either 'homemade' by the clinician or purchased. Satisfactory packs may be made by wrapping flaked ice in damp terry towels. These can be applied to the body part to be treated for anything up to 20 minutes. The rate of initial cooling is rapid but decreases as a film of water forms between the pack and the skin; this means that the temperature of the skin is usually above that of the melting ice and is generally in the region of 5–10°C.

Ice packs produced commercially are of two types. First, bags which contain a mixture of water and an antifreeze substance are available. These may be cooled in a freezer and then molded to the body part. Care should be taken on initial application as the temperature of the pack can be below 0°C and therefore lead to very rapid cooling of the surface tissue. A damp towel placed between the skin and the pack can ensure that the contact temperature remains at about 0°C. Secondly, packs are available that rely on a chemical reaction for their cooling properties. Such packs may be used only once. Though both types of pack are effective in reducing tissue temperatures, McMaster, Liddle and Waugh (1978) demonstrated that chemical packs are more effective in lowering subcutaneous temperatures. However, as suggested earlier in this section, the final temperature developed depends on a variety of factors.

Ice towels

Very superficial cooling may be achieved through the use of ice towels. Towelling is placed in a mush of flaked ice and water, wrung out and applied to the part. Large areas may be covered but the towel will need to be replaced frequently as it warms up rapidly. Treatment may be given for up to 20 minutes.

Cold baths

One of the simplest methods of cooling tissue is to place the body part in cold water or a mixture of ice and water. The temperature can be controlled by varying the ratio of ice to water. Lee, Warren and Mason (1978) suggest that a temperature of 16–18°C may be tolerated for 15–20 minutes. Lower temperatures may be used, but will require intermittent immersion of the part.

Vaporising sprays

Chapter 1 discussed the role of evaporation in producing cooling of the skin. Techniques which use this method of reducing skin temperature result in effective but short-lived tissue cooling. A volatile liquid is sprayed directly on to the area to be treated. It is important that the spray should be both non-flammable and non-toxic for safety reasons. It should be applied over the area in a number of short bursts (of approximately 5 seconds each). Generally, three to five bursts are adequate. Unpublished work suggests that rewarming begins about 20 seconds after the preceding application, and that statistically significant decreases in temperature can be produced with repeated applications (Griffin, 1997).

Ice massage

Ice 'lollipops' or blocks may be used for this technique. First, ice message may be used to produce analgesia. It is normally performed over a small area such as a muscle belly or trigger point and may be used prior to other techniques such as deep massage. Waylonis (1967) discusses the physiological effects of ice massage and suggests that an area of $10 \times 15\,cm$ should be treated for up to 10 minutes or until analgesia occurs. A slow, circular motion over a small area is used. Temperatures do not drop to levels below 15°C with this method. Secondly, ice massage may be used to facilitate muscle activity. In this case, ice is applied briskly and briefly over the skin dermatome of the same nerve root as the muscle in question.

Hazards

Damage due to the therapeutic use of cold therapy is rare. However, *ice burns* can arise if the use of cold is excessive or the pathology of the patient is such as to predispose to damage at temperatures which are normally acceptable. Damage appears, a few hours after the application of cold, in the form of erythema and tenderness. More severe damage can lead to fatty necrosis and the appearance of bruising; ultimately, severe

cooling can lead to frost bite. The last two are very unlikely to occur, however, if the methods described above are used.

Contraindications

The following conditions contraindicate the use of cryotherapy:

* arteriosclerosis
* peripheral vascular disease—cold will compromise the already inadequate blood supply in the area
* vasospasm—e.g. conditions such as Raynaud's disease, which is associated with excessive vasospasm
* cryoglobinaemia—abnormal blood proteins can precipitate at low temperatures, and this can lead to vessel blockage; the condition may be associated with rheumatoid arthritis and systemic lupus erythematosus
* cold urticaria—histamine, released by mast cells, leads to local weal formation, itching and the development of an erythema; changes in blood pressure (lowered) and pulse rate (raised) occur occasionally.

Caution should also be exercised when treating patients with the following problems:

* cardiac disease and altered arterial blood pressure—these may be important factors if a large area of tissue is to be cooled
* defective skin sensation—although most ice therapy leads to analgesia and it is therefore unnecessary for patient to be sensorily aware during treatment, loss of sensory awareness may indicate other neuromuscular and autonomic problems which may preclude the use of cold therapy
* skin hypersensitivity
* adverse psychological factors—some subjects have a strong dislike of cold and it should therefore not be used in these cases.

In addition, care should be taken when applying cooling agents to areas in which nervous tissue is very superficial. A number of authors have reported neural damage, including confirmed axonotmesis, following cooling of the peroneal nerve, the lateral cutaneous femoral nerve and the cutaneous femoral nerve (Covington and Bassett, 1993; Green, Zachazewski and Jordan, 1989; Parker, Small and Davis, 1983).

REFERENCES

Abramson, DI (1967) Comparison of wet and dry heat in raising temperature of tissue. *Archives of Physical Medicine in Rehabilitation* **48**: 654.

Abramson, DI, Tuck, S, Chu, L *et al.* (1964) Effect of paraffin bath and hot fomentations on local tissue temperature. *Archives of Physical Medicine in Rehabilitation* **45**: 87–94.

Abramson, DI, Chu, LSW, Tuck, S (1965) Indirect vasodilation in thermotherapy. *Archives of Physical Medicine in Rehabilitation* **46**: 412.

Basur, R, Shephard, E, Mouzos, G (1976) A cooling method in the treatment of ankle sprains. *Practitioner* **216**: 708.

Borell, PM, Parker, R, Henley, EJ *et al.* (1980) Comparison of *in vivo* temperatures produced by hydrotherapy, paraffin wax treatment and fluidotherapy. *Physical Therapy* **60**: 1273–1276.

Burns, SP, Conin, TA (1987) The use of paraffin wax in the treatment of burns. *Physiotherapy Canada* **39**: 258.

Chapman, CE (1991) Can the use of physical modalities for pain control be rationalized by the research evidence? *Canadian Journal of Physiology and Pharmacology* **69**: 704–712.

Covington, DB, Bassett, FH (1993) When cryotherapy injures. *Physician and Sports Medicine* **21**(3): 78–93.

Curkovic, B, Vitulic, V, Babic-Naglic, D, Durrigl, T (1993) The influence of heat and cold on the pain threshold in rheumatoid arthritis. *Zeitschrift für Rheumatologie* **52**: 289–291.

Green, GA, Zachazewski, JE, Jordan, SE (1989) Peroneal nerve palsy induced by cryotherapy. *The Physician and Sports Medicine* **17**(9): 63–70.

Griffin, S (1997) Study to examine the change in skin temperature produced by the application of ice spray on the ankle. BSc dissertation, King's College London.

Harris, ED, McCroskery, PA (1974) The influence of temperature and fibril stability on degradation of cartilage collagen by rheumatoid synovial collegenase. *New England Journal of Medicine* **290**: 1–6.

Head, MD, Helms, PS (1977) Paraffin and sustained stretching in the treatment of burns contracture. *Burns* **4**: 136.

Hendler, E, Crosby, R, Hardy, JD (1958) Measurement of heating of the skin during exposure to infrared radiation. *Journal of Applied Physiology* **12**: 177.

Hunter, J, Kerr, EH, Whillans, MG (1952) The relation between joint stiffness upon exposure to cold and the characteristics of synovial fluid. *Canadian Journal of Medical Science* **30**: 367–377.

Kern, H, Fessl, L, Trnavsky, G, Hertz, H (1984) Das Verhalten der Gelenkstemperatur unter Eisapplikation—Grundlage

für die praktische Anwendung. *Wiener Klinische Wochenschrift* **96**: 832–837.

Lee, JM, Warren, MP, Mason, SM (1978) Effects of ice on nerve conduction velocity. *Physiotherapy* **64**: 2–6.

Lehmann, JF, de Lateur, JB (1990) Therapeutic heat. In: Lehman JF (ed) *Therapeutic Heat and Cold*, 4th edn. Williams and Wilkins, Baltimore, pp 417–581.

Lehmann, JF, de Lateur, JB (1999) Ultrasound, shortwave, microwave, laser, superficial heat and cold in the treatment of pain. In: Wall, PD, Melzack, R (eds) *Textbook of Pain*, 4th edn. Churchill Livingstone, New York, pp 1383–1397.

Lehmann, JF, Silvermann, DR, Baum, B *et al.* (1966) Temperature distribution in the human thigh produced by infrared, hot pack and microwave applications. *Archives of Physical Medicine in Rehabilitation* **47**: 291–299.

Lessard, LA, Scudds, RA, Amendola, A, Vaz, MD (1997) The effect of cryotherapy following arthroscopic knee surgery. *Journal of Orthopaedic and Sports Physical Therapy* **26**(1): 14–22.

McMaster, WC, Liddle, S, Waugh, TR (1978) Laboratory evaluation of various cold therapy modalities. *American Journal of Sports Medicine* **6**(5): 291–294.

Meussen, R, Lievens, P (1986) The use of cryotherapy in sports injuries. *Sports Medicine* **3**: 398–414.

Myrer, JW, Draper, DO, Durrant, E (1994) Contrast therapy and intramuscular temperature in the human leg. *Journal of Athletic Training* **29**(4): 318–322.

Oliver, RA, Johnson, DJ, Wheelhouse, WW *et al.* (1979) Isometric muscle contraction response during recovery from reduced intramuscular temperature. *Archives of Physical Medicine in Rehabilitation* **60**: 126.

Parker, JT, Small, NC, Davis, DG (1983) Cold induced nerve palsy. *Athletic Training* **18**: 76.

Pegg, SMH, Littler, TR, Littler, EN (1969) A trial of ice therapy and exercise in chronic arthritis. *Physiotherapy* **55**: 51–56.

Sauls, J (1999) Efficacy of cold for pain: fact or fallacy? *Online Journal of Knowledge Synthesis for Nursing* **6**(8).

Selkins, KM, Emery, AF (1990) Thermal science for physical medicine. In: Lehmann, JF (ed) *Therapeutic Heat and Cold*, 4th edn. Williams and Wilkins, Baltimore, pp 62–112.

Waylonis, GW (1967) The physiological effect of ice massage. *Archives of Physical Medicine in Rehabilitation* **48**: 37–41.

Woodmansey, A, Collins, DH, Ernst, MM (1938) Vascular reactions to the contrast bath in health and in rheumatoid arthritis. *Lancet* **2**: 1350–1353.

Electromagnetic agents

SECTION CONTENTS

10

Infrared irradiation

Sheila Kitchen

INTRODUCTION

Infrared irradiation is a superficial, thermal agent used for the relief of pain and stiffness, to increase joint motion and to enhance the healing of soft tissue lesions and skin conditions (Kitchen and Partridge, 1991; Lehmann and de Lateur, 1999; Michlovitz, 1986).

Physical characteristics

Infrared (IR) radiations lie within that part of the electromagnetic spectrum which gives rise to heating when absorbed by matter (see Fig. 1.20). The radiations are characterised by wavelengths of 0.78–1000 μm, which are between those of microwaves and visible light. Many sources which emit visible light or ultraviolet (UV) radiation also emit IR. The International Commission on Illumination (CIE) describes infrared irradiation in terms of three biologically significant bands, which differ in the degree to which they are absorbed by biological tissues and therefore their effect upon those tissues:

- IRA: spectral values of 0.78–1.4 μm
- IRB: spectral values of 1.4–3.0 μm
- IRC: spectral values of 3.0–1.0 mm.

The wavelengths mainly used in clinical practice are those between 0.7 μm and 1.5 μm, and are therefore concentrated in the IRA band.

Production of infrared irradiation by bodies

Infrared irradiation is produced as a result of molecular motion within materials. An increase in temperature above absolute zero results in the vibration or rotation of molecules within matter, which leads to the emission of infrared irradiation. The temperature of the body affects the wavelength of the radiation emitted, with the mean frequency of emitted radiation rising with an increase in temperature. Thus, the higher the temperature of the body the higher is the mean frequency output and, consequently, the shorter the wavelength. Most bodies do not, however, emit IR of a single wave band. A number of different wavelengths may be emitted owing to interplay between the emission and absorption of radiations affecting the behaviour of molecules.

Sources of infrared irradiation

Infrared sources can be either natural (for example, the sun) or artificial. Artificial IR is normally produced by passing an electrical current through a coiled resistance wire. Luminous generators (or radiant heaters) consist of a tungsten filament within a glass bulb which contains an inert gas at low pressure (Fig. 10.2); they emit both infrared and visible radiations with a peak wavelength of around 1 μm. Filters may be used to limit the output to particular wave bands, such as when a red filter is used to filter out blue and green light waves.

Non-luminous generators (Fig. 10.1) most commonly consist of a coiled resistance wire which is wound around or embedded in a ceramic insulating material. Infrared irradiation will therefore be emitted by both the wire and the heated materials surrounding it, resulting in the emission of radiations of a number of different frequencies. Non-luminous generators produce radiations which peak at a wavelength of around 4 μm.

Luminous lamps (Fig. 10.2) are generally available with power levels of between 250 and 1500 W, and non-luminous lamps with levels between 250 and 1000 W. Both require a 'warm-up' period, as the energy emitted increases over a period of time (Orenberg *et al.*, 1986; Ward, 1986).

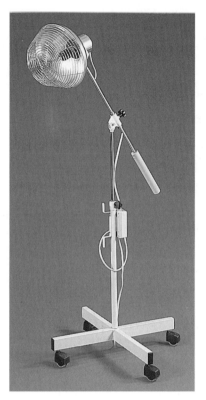

Figure 10.1 A non-luminous infrared unit. (Photograph courtesy of Chatanooga Group Ltd, Bicester.)

Non-luminous lamps take longer than luminous lamps to reach a stable, peak level of heat emission as the molecular oscillation causing heating spreads through the body of the heater.

PHYSICAL BEHAVIOUR OF INFRARED RADIATION

Infrared radiations can be reflected, absorbed, transmitted, refracted and diffracted by matter (see Ch. 1 for details), the reflection and absorption being of most biological and clinical significance. These effects moderate the penetration of energy into the tissues and thus the biological changes which take place.

Absorption, penetration and reflection

Skin is a complex material and consequently its reflective and absorptive characteristics are not

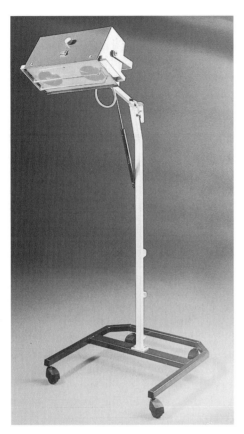

Figure 10.2 A luminous infrared unit. (Photograph courtesy of Electro-Medical Supplies (Greenham) Ltd, Wantage.)

uniform (Moss *et al.*, 1989). Radiation must be absorbed in order to facilitate changes within the body tissues, and the absorption is dependent on: structure and type of tissue, vascularity, pigmentation and wavelength. Penetration of energy into a medium is dependent upon the intensity of the source of infrared, the wavelength (and consequent frequency of the radiation), the angle at which the radiation hits the surface and the coefficient of absorption of the material.

Hardy (1956) pointed out that short wavelengths are scattered more than long wavelengths but that the differences are minimised as the thickness of the skin increases. Penetration therefore depends both on the absorptive properties of the constituents of the skin and on the degree of scattering brought about by the skin microstructure. Jacques and Kuppenheim (1955)

examined the reflection characteristics of human skin and noted that maximum reflectivity occurs at IR wavelengths of between 0.7 and 1.2 μm— the range of many therapeutic lamps.

Maximum penetration occurs with wavelengths of 1.2 μm, whereas the skin is virtually opaque to wavelengths of 2 μm and more (Moss *et al.*, 1989). Hardy (1956) showed that at least 50% of radiations of 1.2 μm penetrated to a depth of 0.8 mm, allowing interaction with capillaries and nerve endings. Because the energy penetration decreases exponentially with depth, most heating due to IR will occur superficially. Selkins and Emery (1990) demonstrated that almost all energy was absorbed at a depth of 2.5 mm and Harlen (1980) noted penetration depths of 0.1 mm for long IR wavelengths and up to 3 mm for the shorter wavelengths.

Heating of body tissue

Infrared radiations produce thermal changes owing to the absorption of radiation, which leads to molecular vibration, and this motion in turn leads to the thermal changes. Some heating may occur at a greater depth owing to the transfer of heat from the superficial tissue both by direct conduction and by convection, largely through the increased local circulation. Infrared should, however, be regarded as a surface heating modality. (Further details about the transfer of heat by conduction are given in Chapter 1.)

BIOLOGICAL EFFECTS

It is generally assumed by most specialists that IR photons do not give rise to photochemical effects. The main physiological effects claimed for IR are, therefore, the result of local tissue heating, as discussed in detail in Chapter 6. These effects include alterations in metabolic and circulatory behaviour, in neural function and in cellular activity.

Evidence for clinical efficacy

There is limited evidence of efficacy directly related to the use of IR; nevertheless, evidence from the use of other forms of superficial heating that give rise to superficial thermal changes only (e.g. conduction heating) is also applicable.

Pain

Lehmann, Brunner and Stow (1958) demonstrated that when IR was applied to the ulnar nerve region at the elbow, an analgesic effect was noted distal to the point of application. Kramer (1984) utilised IR as a control when evaluating the heating effect of ultrasound in nerve conduction tests on normal subjects. IR and ultrasound were applied separately to the distal humeral segment of the ulnar nerve in dosages that generated a rise in tissue temperature of 0.8°C; an increase in the post-treatment ulnar nerve conduction velocity was found in both cases. The studies of Halle, Scoville and Greathouse (1981) and Currier and Kramer (1982), also indicate that IR can cause an increase in the conduction velocity of normal nerves in humans.

Joint stiffness

Joint stiffness encompasses a number of parameters such as the behaviour of ligaments, joint capsule and periarticular structures, and alterations in fluid pressure. Wright and Johns (1961) applied IR to a normal hand joint in vivo, producing a surface temperature of 45°C. They measured a 20% drop in joint stiffness at 45°C when compared with the stiffness at a temperature of 33°C. However, this work was performed with two subjects only, and no replication studies have been identified.

Oedema

Wadsworth and Chanmugan (1980) advocate the use of IR irradiation in the management of oedema of the extremities. They claim that the use of IR will cause vasodilation of the vessels and encourage increased rates of tissue fluid exchange. No studies have been found to substantiate these claims or to indicate that the addition of IR to other treatments actually facilitates the reduction of oedema.

Skin lesions

Some skin lesions may benefit from a drying heat. Fungal infections, such as paronychia, and psoriasis may be managed with IR treatment. Westerhof et al. (1987) exposed patients with psoriasis to IR for one month, with a skin temperature of 42°C. Eighty per cent of these patients experienced remission, with 30% experiencing a dramatic improvement. Orenberg et al. (1986) confirmed these results. Infrared irradiation should not be used to treat open wounds, however, as evidence indicates that its tendency to dehydrate the tissue causes further damage and inhibits healing.

Dosage

Whilst the level of heating produced in the tissue may be calculated mathematically (e.g. Orenberg et al., 1986) or may be recorded by heat sensors (e.g. Westerhof et al., 1987), it is normal clinical practice to gauge the level of heating developed in the surface tissues by the sensory report of the patient. The amount of energy received by the patient will be governed by:

- the intensity of the output of the lamp (in watts)
- the distance of the lamp from the patient
- the duration of the treatment.

In order for therapeutic effects to occur it has been suggested that there is a need for a temperature of between 40 and 45°C to be maintained for at least 5 minutes (Lehmann and de Lateur, 1990). Crockford and Hellon (1959) demonstrated a gradual rise in temperature during the first 10 minutes of irradiation, with the return to normal taking an average of 35 minutes.

The intensity is altered either by changing the distance of the lamp from the body part or by altering the output of the generator. By the end of a treatment, a mild dose should generate skin temperatures in the region of 36–38°C, and a moderate dose should produce temperatures of between 38–40°C. Infrared treatment is normally continued for a period of between 10 and 20 minutes, depending on the size and vascularity of the body part, the chronicity of the lesion and the nature of the lesion. Small avascular parts, acute conditions, and skin lesions tend to be treated for shorter periods of time.

CLINICAL APPLICATION

The following procedure should be used when giving infrared therapy to a patient.

- **Select equipment.** Luminous (radiant) or non-luminous lamp.
- **Warm-up.** This maximises the output. Non-luminous lamp: approximately 15 minutes; luminous lamp: a few minutes only.
- **The subject.** A comfortable, supported position is used to allow the subject to remain still for the treatment. The skin should be uncovered, clean and dry, all liniments and creams being removed.
- **Safety precautions.** The nature, effects and dangers of the treatment should be explained, contraindications checked and the thermal sensitivity of the skin examined. Eyes should be shielded if they are likely to be irradiated in order to prevent drying of the surface. The patient should be warned of any dangers, including burns.
- **Lamp positioning.** The lamp is positioned to allow the radiations to strike the skin at a right angle, to facilitate maximum absorption of energy. The distance of the lamp from the part will vary according to the output of the lamp, but is usually between 50 and 75 cm.
- **Dosage (see p. 142).** This is determined by the response of the subject. It is essential, therefore, that the patient is advised of the appropriate level of heating and understands the importance of reporting any changes from this.
- **Follow-up.** Following the cessation of treatment, the temperature of the skin should feel mildly or moderately warm to touch. The degree of erythema induced should be noted and any unexpected changes evaluated. Records should be kept of each treatment, and the changes induced by the radiation.

HAZARDS

- **Skin.** Acute burns may follow a single, excessive exposure to IR at temperatures of 46–47°C and above. Pain, however, occurs at 44.5 ± 1.3°C and should, therefore, provide protection by evoking a withdrawal response (Hardy, 1951; Stevens, 1983). Chronic damage may follow prolonged exposure at tolerable temperatures (Kligman, 1982); epidermal hyperplasia and a large increase in ground substance occurred in guinea pigs.
- **Subdermal tissues.** Tissues exposed to IR during surgical procedures show an increased tendency to develop adhesions.
- **Testicles.** There is a temporary lowering of sperm count.
- **Respiratory system.** Infants exposed to radiant warmers may be subject to periods of apnoea.
- **Susceptible subjects.** For instance, elderly people may suffer dehydration and temporary lowering of the blood pressure, or symptoms including dizziness and headaches following treatment, especially to large areas such as the back or neck/shoulders.
- **Optical damage.** Corneal burns, retinal and lenticular injury may occur. This type of injury is normally associated with industrial environments (Moss et al., 1989).

SAFETY PRECAUTIONS AND CONTRAINDICATIONS

The electrical safety of the equipment should be checked regularly (see Appendix). The output of the lamp should be checked, and the mechanical stability, alignment and security of all parts of the lamp should be examined.

Contraindications

Whilst not all factors listed have been substantiated fully through research, the following have resulted in minimal reporting of damage in patients:

- areas with poor or deficient cutaneous thermal sensitivity
- subjects with advanced cardiovascular disease

- local areas of impaired peripheral circulation
- scar tissue or tissue devitalised by deep X-ray treatment or other ionising radiations (which may be more subject to burning)
- malignant tissue of the skin (though such tissue may occasionally be treated through the use of infrared irradiation)

- subjects with a reduced level of consciousness or understanding of the dangers of treatment
- subjects with acute febrile illness
- some acute skin diseases such as dermatitis or eczema
- the testes.

REFERENCES

Crockford, GW, Hellon, RF (1959) Vascular responses of human skin to infrared radiation. *Journal of Physiology* **149**: 424–432.

Currier, DP, Kramer, JF (1982) Sensory nerve conduction: heating effects of ultrasound and infrared. *Physiotherapy Canada* **34**: 241–246.

Halle, JS, Scoville, CR, Greathouse, DG (1981) Ultrasound's effect on the conduction latency of the superficial radial nerve in man. *Physical Therapy* **61**: 345–350.

Hardy, JD (1951) Influence of skin temperature upon pain threshold as evoked by thermal irradiation. *Science* **114**: 149–150.

Hardy, JD (1956) Spectral transmittance and reflectance of excised human skin. *Journal of Applied Physiology* **9**: 257–264.

Harlen, F (1980) In: Docker, MF (ed) *Physics in Physiotherapy, Conference Report Series—35.* Hospital Physicists Association, London, p 180.

Jacques, JA, Kuppenheim, HF (1955) Spectral reflectance of human skin in the region of 0.7–2.6 μm. *Journal of Applied Physiology* **8**: 297–299.

Kitchen, SS, Partridge, CJ (1991) Infrared therapy. *Physiotherapy* **77**(4): 249–254.

Kligman, LH (1982) Intensification of ultraviolet-induced dermal damage by infrared radiation. *Archives of Dermatological Research* **272**: 229–238.

Kramer, JF (1984) Ultrasound: evaluation of its mechanical and thermal effects. *Archives of Physical Medicine and Rehabilitation* **65**: 223–227.

Lehmann, JF, de Lateur, BJ (1990) Therapeutic heat. In: Lehmann, JF (ed) *Therapeutic Heat and Cold*, 4th edn. Williams and Wilkins, Baltimore, MD, pp 417–581.

Lehmann, JF, de Lateur, BJ (1999) Ultraosund, shortwave, microwave, laser, superficial heat and cold in the treatment of pain. In: Melzack, PD, Wall, R (1999) *Textbook of Pain*, 4th edn. Churchill Livingstone, New York, pp 1383–1397.

Lehmann, JF, Brunner, GD, Stow, RW (1958) Pain threshold measurements after therapeutic application of ultrasound, microwaves and infrared. *Archives of Physical Medicine and Rehabilitation* 39, 560–565.

Michlovitz, SL (1986) *Thermal Agents in Rehabilitation, Contemporary Perspectives in Rehabilitation*, Vol 1. F A Davies, Philadelphia.

Moss, C, Ellis, R, Murray, W, Parr, W (1989) *Infrared Radiation, Nonionising Radiation Protection*, 2nd edn, WHO Regional Publications, European Series, no. 25.

Orenberg, EK, Noodleman, FR, Koperski, JA, Pounds, D, Farber, EM (1986) Comparison of heat delivery systems for hyperthermia treatment of psoriasis. *International Journal Hyperthermia* **2**(3): 231–241.

Selkins, KM, Emery, AF (1990) Thermal science for physical medicine. In: Lehmann, JF (ed) *Therapeutic Heat and Cold*, 3rd edn. Williams and Wilkins, Baltimore, MD, pp 62–112.

Stevens, J (1983) Thermal sensation: infrared and microwaves. In: Adair, E (ed) *Microwaves and Thermal Regulation*. Academic Press, London, pp 134–176.

Wadsworth, H, Chanmugan, APP (1980) *Electrophysical Agents in Physiotherapy: Therapeutic and Diagnostic Use*. Science Press, Mackerville, NSW, Australia.

Ward, AR (1986) *Electricity Fields and Waves in Therapy*. Science Press, Mackerville, NSW, Australia.

Westerhof, W, Siddiqui, AH, Cormane, RH, Scholten, A (1987) Infrared hyperthermia and psoriasis. *Archives of Dermatological Research* **279**: 209–210.

Wright, V, Johns, RJ (1961) Quantitative and qualitative analysis of joint stiffness in normal subjects and in patients with connective tissue disease. *Annals of Rheumatological Disease* **20**: 26–36.

11

Diathermy

Shona Scott
(Part 1 Short-wave diathermy)
Joan McMeeken
Barry Stillman
(Part 2 Microwave diathermy)

PART 1
SHORT-WAVE DIATHERMY

BRIEF HISTORY

Short-wave diathermy (SWD) is non-ionising radiation from the radio frequency portion of the electromagnetic (EM) spectrum. It is used by physiotherapists to deliver heat and 'energy' to deeply situated tissues.

Reference to the medical use of high-frequency electrical currents can be traced as far back as the 1890s when d'Arsonval passed a 1 ampere current at high frequency through himself and an assistant. Although similar amounts of electricity at low frequencies were known to be potentially fatal, he reported feeling only a sensation of warmth (Guy, Chou, and Neuhaus, 1984). Subsequent work led to the development of inductive and capacitive methods of applying high-frequency currents to the body to produce what was claimed to be non-superficial heating (Guy, Chou and Neuhaus, 1984). These methods became known as 'diathermy'.

High-frequency currents became popular therapies in Europe from the 1920s onwards. During this time, interest in the non-thermal properties of electromagnetic fields was also developing and by the 1950s a method of rapidly switching on and off the field and producing pulsed short-wave diathermy (PSWD) had been developed. In the early years of its development PSWD in particular was hailed as the cure for many ailments.

Today, PSWD is still a very popular modality. A survey of physiotherapists working in England in 1995 indicated that 75% of the sample used PSWD, with approximately 50% using the modality two to three times a day. SWD was a less popular modality, with about 8% using it two to three times per day (Pope, Mockett and Wright, 1995). Despite this obvious popularity many questions remain regarding the application of PSWD and SWD, for example it is still not possible to answer conclusively in which circumstances PSWD or SWD respectively should be used or what the treatment doses should be. Similar criticism can be levelled at many other areas of physiotherapy practice, however. For example, the Cochrane Library Review of Physical Medicine Modalities for Mechanical Neck Disorders concluded: 'There is little information available from trials to support the use of physical medicine modalities for mechanical neck pain.' (Gross *et al.*, 1999).

Nevertheless, physiotherapists do find PSWD and SWD to be useful adjuncts in the management of a variety of conditions, so this chapter aims to establish best practice guidelines and to highlight where more research is required. As Pope (1999) aptly pointed out, we should not simply discard PSWD and SWD from our list of modalities just because it is an underresearched area of practice or is becoming unfashionable. What is needed is that the established areas in which PSWD and SWD are currently used are subjected to evaluation so that informed decisions can be made as to if, when and how this modality can be most usefully employed. It is not simply enough to say, 'we can't prove its value, so let's not use it' and immediately replace it with some other underresearched treatment approach. Physiotherapists need to be more critical in their thinking and not just follow the latest fashion (Kitchen and Partridge, 1992).

PHYSICAL CHARACTERISTICS

Short-wavelength radio waves lie between microwaves and medium-wavelength radio waves on the electromagnetic spectrum, as shown in Figure 1.20, and have a frequency range of 10–100 MHz. Therapeutic diathermy uses the radiofrequency wave bands of 27.12 MHz. This 27.12 MHz frequency is used to prevent interference with other frequency bands that are used in communications. Historically, three high-frequency bands were allocated for medical use and SWD makes use of one of these frequency bands (27.12 MHz ± 160 kHz, with a corresponding wavelength of around 11.062 m). Radio waves have the longest wavelength of any region of the electromagnetic spectrum and therefore the lowest frequency, so they also have the lowest energy per quantum.

Short-wave electromagnetic energy has very little effect on living tissues itself. However, the presence of an electromagnetic field (such as in SWD) creates tiny electric currents and a magnetic field within the tissues. It is these that are responsible for any physiological effects, such as a rise in tissue temperature.

An electric field (E) is set up in the presence of electrical charges; this field is characterised by both its direction and magnitude. An electrically charged particle, such as an electron or proton, placed within this field will experience a force (F). E and F are related as follows:

$$F = qE \qquad [1]$$

where q is the strength of the charge placed in the field. In electrically conductive materials, such as living tissues, these forces will result in the production of electrical currents.

A magnetic field is produced by a moving electrical charge and, since magnetic fields exert forces on other charges in motion, an alternating electrical current (i.e. a moving charge) will initiate the production of a magnetic field, which in turn may initiate the production of an *induced* current. Magnetic fields are specified by two quantities: the magnetic flux density (B) and magnetic field strength (H), which are measured in units of tesla (T) and amperes per metre (A/m) respectively.

Both electric and magnetic fields are set up in human tissues which are subjected to SWD. During SWD application, the patient is made part of the electrical circuit by the use of an inductive coil or capacitive type electrodes; this is shown in Figure 11.1. The resonator (or patient circuit) and generator circuit are tuned by use of

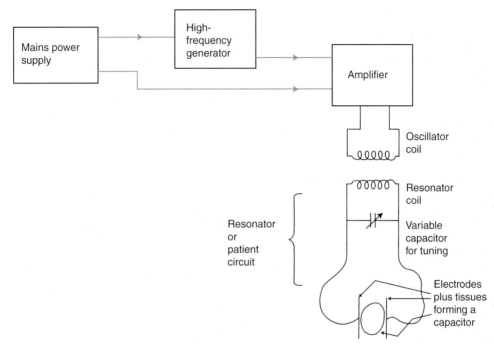

Figure 11.1 Block diagram to show short-wave diathermy generation. (After Low and Reed, 2000, with permission of Butterworth-Heinemann.)

a variable capacitor in order to match the parameters of each circuit and thus generate maximum power transfer.

The interaction between the field and the tissues is affected by a macroscopic property of the tissue called the 'complex permittivity'; this is related to the dielectric constant and the loss factor of the tissue (Delpizzo and Joyner, 1987). The dielectric constant represents the depolarisation characteristics of a tissue, and is primarily dependent upon the water content. Complex permittivity is also a function of the field frequency and, therefore, the propagation and attenuation of the electromagnetic waves are dependent upon frequency.

Absorption of radiofrequency energy

Using a *capacitive circuit* to treat tissues requires that they lie within the oscillating electrical field; this causes vibration of tissue molecules and thus heating within the tissues. High-frequency alternating voltage applied to tissues gives rise to two types of current: conduction current and displacement current.

1. Conduction current (I_R)

Heat develops in relation to the following equation:

$$Q = I^2 Rt \qquad [2]$$

where Q = heat in joules, I_R = the amplitude of the current in amperes, R = ohmic resistance, and t = time.

2. Displacement current (I_C)

A displacement of electrical energy occurs as the result of polarisation of the tissue, and its magnitude depends upon the capacitance of the tissue and the frequency of the alternating current.

The use of an *inductive applicator* relies on the tissue being placed within a rapidly alternating magnetic field which is generated by passing the high-frequency current through a coil; this results in the creation of eddy currents within the tissue, induced by the oscillating electromagnetic field.

The rise in tissue temperature during the application of SWD depends on a factor known as the specific absorption rate (SAR). The SAR is the rate at which energy is absorbed by a known mass of tissue, and is calculated in units of watts per kilogram (W/kg). SAR is a function of tissue conductivity and the electrical field magnitude in tissue. *Tissue conductivity* reflects the ease in which an electric field can be set up in the tissue. The SAR, and therefore the heating produced by SWD, is dependent upon the electrical properties of tissue within the electromagnetic field (Kloth and Ziskin, 1990). The concentration of the electric field will be highest in the tissues with the greatest conductivity. Living tissues can be considered to consist of three molecular types: charged molecules, dipolar molecules and non-polar molecules (Ward, 1980). Different tissues contain varying proportions of these molecules, influencing the conductivity and hence the SAR and heating pattern when irradiated by SWD.

Heat production in tissues

Charged molecules

Within living tissue there is an abundance of charged molecules—mainly ions and certain proteins. In response to the forces of repulsion and attraction that occur between charged molecules, exposure to a SWD field causes the charged molecules to be accelerated along the lines of electric force. The high-frequency field causes charged molecules to oscillate about a mean position (Fig. 11.2), converting kinetic energy into heat (Ward, 1980). Oscillation of charged molecules is an efficient means of heat production (Ward, 1980). Tissue containing high proportions of charged molecules will in theory be heated most during SWD treatment.

Dipolar molecules

The dipolar molecules found in living tissues consist principally of water and some proteins.

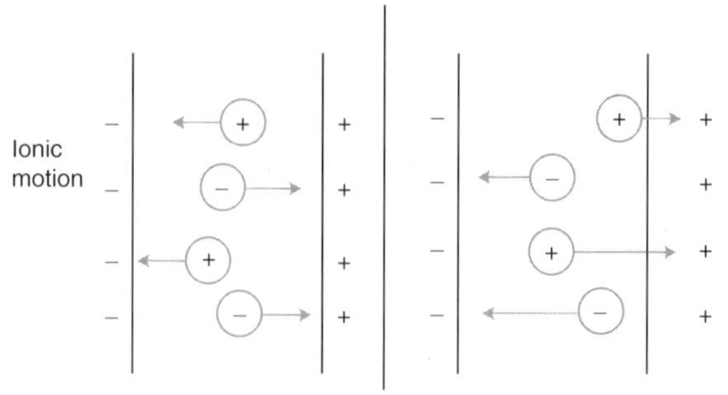

Figure 11.2   Charged ions move to and fro in response to an oscillating electric field.

They can also be affected by electric fields—for example, since the positive pole of the molecule aligns itself towards the negative pole of the electric field, the alternating SWD field causes rotation of these molecules as the charge of the plates alters rapidly (Fig. 11.3). Heating results from the frictional drag between adjacent molecules. Ward (1980) describes this process as a moderately efficient means of heating.

Non-polar molecules

Fat cells are an example of non-polar molecules. Although non-polar molecules do not have free ions or charged poles, they still respond to the influence of the SWD field. During exposure to SWD the electron cloud becomes distorted, but negligible heat is produced (Fig. 11.4).

Tissues that have a high ionic content in solution or a large number of free ions (an example of which is blood) are the best conductors and therefore any highly vascular tissue is a good

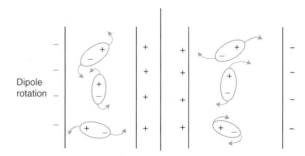

Figure 11.3   Dipolar molecules rotate as the electric field oscillates.

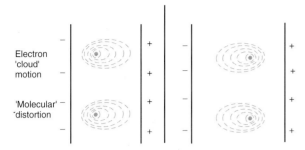

Electron
'cloud'
motion

'Molecular'
distortion

Figure 11.4   The paths of orbiting electrons are distorted in alternate directions as the electric field oscillates. (After Low and Reed, 2000, with permission of Butterworth-Heinemann.)

conductor. Similarly, both metal and sweat are good conductors. This means if a metal implant or drop of sweat are within the electric field they will create an area of high field density and adjacent tissues may be exposed to a large thermal load, which may be sufficient to cause a burn. Adipose tissue, on the other hand, is a poor conductor and, therefore, the magnitude of current set up in fat will be minimal.

Pulsed short-wave diathermy

Some SWD machines allow the electromagnetic energy to be applied to the patient in short bursts of energy. When delivered in this way it is know as pulsed short-wave diathermy or PSWD. The physical characteristics of PSWD and SWD are identical, the only difference being that the field is interrupted or pulsed. Although continuous SWD is usually confined to a frequency of 27.12 MHz, pulsing results in the development of side bands; this can mean that the energy used ranges in frequency from 26.95 to 27.28 MHz with little, if any, of the energy being in the parent band. In terms of physiological effect on the tissues these side bands are of little clinical relevance, however.

When PSWD is used it means that there are periods when no SWD is delivered (Fig. 11.5) and the patient receives a lower dose of SWD; and consequently the tissues are subjected to a lower thermal load. Thus, the concept underpinning PSWD is to give the tissues an energy boost

in the form of an electromagnetic field without the tissues being required to tolerate a thermal load. Low (1995) theorises this as follows: 'energy simply "stirs" ions, molecules, membrane and metabolic activity of cells; thus increasing the overall rates of phagocytosis, transport across cell membranes, enzymatic activity and so forth'; evidence to support this is, however, lacking.

Depending on the features of the machine being used, it may be possible to vary the length of the SWD pulse or the length of the gap between SWD pulses. The three principal variables under the control of the therapist (Fig. 11.6, Table 11.1) are:

- pulse repetition rate (PRR)
- pulse duration (PD)
- peak pulse power (PPP).

The mean power is a product of these variables:

$$\text{Mean power} = \text{pulse duration} \times \text{pulse repetition rate} \times \text{peak pulse power.} \qquad [3]$$

Thermal changes: heating patterns produced with different application techniques

Debate exists as to which tissues are heated most during SWD and PSWD treatments. Tissues that have a high dielectric content and good conductivity should in theory absorb more energy from the SWD field. Muscle tissue and blood contain a high proportion of ions compared to adipose tissue. Thus, Kloth and Ziskin (1990) conclude that 'clinically, diathermy can be used to increase the temperature of skeletal muscle'. However, both Goats (1989) and Ward (1980) disagree and suggest that SWD may cause excessive heating of superficial adipose tissue. Their reasoning is that, although adipose tissue contains few ions for the efficient conversion of electromagnetic radiation energy into heat energy, living adipose tissue is permeated with many small blood vessels. The blood in these vessels provides appropriate conditions for the absorption of EM radiation and, further, the adipose tissue

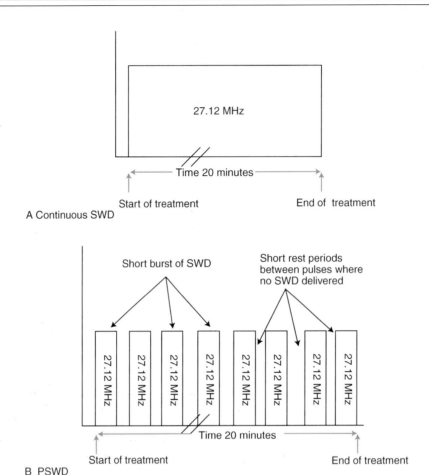

Figure 11.5 Diagrammatic illustration of the differences between A: continuous short-wave diathermy (SWD) and B: pulsed short-wave diathermy (PSWD).

surrounding the blood vessels acts as an insulator, preventing the dissipation of any heat produced.

Some authors also suggest that different application techniques will affect the depth at which the heating is produced. For example, Lehmann (1990) states that inductive SWD applications elevate the temperatures of deeper tissues selectively, with relatively smaller effects in surface tissues, and van der Esch and Hoogland (1991) consider the effect of the capacitive technique to occur mainly in superficial tissue (Table 11.2).

Verrier, Ashby and Crawford (1978) confirm that the capacitive (longitudinal contraplanar technique—see p. 159) and inductothermy (20 minutes at the maximum tolerable dose) lead to significant increases in cutaneous and intramuscular (IM) temperature, whereas a minimal dose of SWD inductothermy application produces significantly more heating than the capacitive technique. Thus the inductothermy method appears to be a more efficient means of energy tranfer.

Draper *et al.* (1999) also measured IM temperature in the medial head of gastrocnemius at a depth of 3 cm below the skin. The PSWD dose was: PRR 800 Hz, PD 400 μs, PPP 150 W, giving a mean power of 48 W for 20 minutes. The method of application was an induction drum. The average temperature increase was 3.9°C. This is a similar amount of heating as reported in studies of SWD (Table 11.3). This study used a

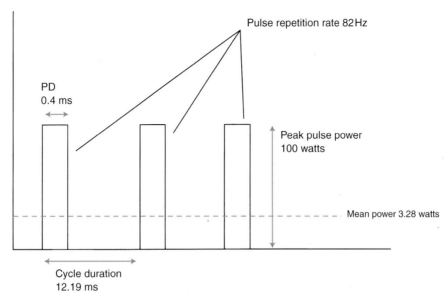

Figure 11.6 Illustration of the parameters required for calculating the mean power of PSWD treatments.

Table 11.1 Pulse SWD parameters

Parameters	Explanation	Range
Pulse reception rate (PRR)	The number of pulses delivered in 1 second	15–800 Hz
Pulse duration (PD)	The length of each pulse or 'on' period	25–400 μs
Peak pulse power (PPP)	The amplitude of the pulse (often referred to as intensity)	100–1000 W
Mean power (MP)	Gives a measure of the dose of PSWD that a patient receives, as illustrated in Figure 11.6	

Table 11.2 Figures estimating the ratio of superficial to deep heating for the capacitive and inductive methods

Application method	Superficial : deep	Reference
Capacitive	13 : 1	van der Esch and Hoogland, 1991
	10 : 1	van der Esch and Hoogland, 1991
	12–18 : 1	Hand, 1990
Inductive	1 : 1	van der Esch and Hoogland, 1991
	1 : 4	Hand, 1990

high dose (48 W), which explains the heating effect.

In a study by Murray and Kitchen (2000), a group of healthy students reported a definite thermal sensation when a mean power of 21.19 (±8.27) W was applied to the thigh using the inductive method. The mean skin temperature when a definite thermal sensation was reported was 31.14 (±1.04)°C, with a mean rise in temperature of 2.34°C. The PPP was maintained at 190 W and the pulse duration at 400 μs while the PRR was incrementally increased.

The part of the body heated will affect the perception of thermal sensation. Bricknell and Watson (1995) also found that subjects reported a definite thermal sensation during PSWD, but

Table 11.3   Summary of the studies that have reported the heating effect that can be produced by SWD

	Method	Skin	Subcutaneous	IM	Intraartic
Hollander and Hovarth (1950), $n = 5$ Dose: just perceptible	I	7.4°F	7.02°F	—	—
Abramson et al., $n = 14$ Dose: comfortably warm	C	1.3°C	1.5°C	1.9°C	—
Verrier et al. (1977), $n = 20$ Dose: maximum tolerable dose	I C	5.05°C 2.24°C	— —	4.40°C 3.28°C	— —
Verrier et al. (1978) Dose: comfortable	I	6.60°C	—	6.36°C	—
Oosterveld et al.(1992) Dose: just perceptible warmth	C	2.4°C	—	—	1.4°C

— indicates variables are not reported in paper. I = inductive. C = capacitive.

this time the mean power was only 10.88 W. The reason why a similar thermal sensation was reported at a lower dose to the Murray and Kitchen trial may be because this trial applied the PSWD continuously for 20 minutes, whereas Murray and Kitchen interrupted the PSWD every 2 minutes to take temperature readings, but also allowing some of the heat to dissipate. However, it may also highlight the view that no two PSWD and SWD treatments are exactly the same—depending on the part of the body treated, the equipment used and the dose selected, a different thermal load may be placed on the tissues.

What these studies do show is that PSWD is more than capable of producing a heating effect, contrary to popular notion that interrupted short-wave diathermy is designed to maximise mechanical and piezoelectric effects 'while minimising tissue heating' (Byl and Hoft, 1995).

Table 11.4 summarises the changes in tissue temperatures recorded in different body areas during PWSD treatments. To achieve a non-thermal treatment, therefore, the mean power output must be kept low.

In summary, both SWD or PSWD can be used to heat deep tissues, and both are more effective than conductive heating agents (heat packs or wax) at heating deeply situated IM tissues (Verrier, Ashby and Crawford, 1978).

Dose

The choice of dose when applying SWD and PSWD tends to be along the lines of a lower dose for more acute conditions and a higher dose for chronic conditions. Some authors have attempted to review completed trials to make decisions as to the most appropriate dose; however, Low (1995) was forced to admit, 'While this

Table 11.4   Summary of the changes in tissue temperature that have been recorded during PWSD treatments

	PRR (Hz)	PD (μs)	PPP (W)	MP (W)	Temperature increase (°C)
Erdman, 1960	400	65	—	16	0.5 (below treatment head) 2.0 (dorsum of foot)
Morrisey, 1966	600	50	—	40	2.2 (below treatment head)
	—	50	—	80	10.6 (below treatment head)
Silverman and Pendelton (1968)	—	—	—	15	3.1 (below treatment head) (no change on foot)
	—	—	—	65	5.3 (below treatment head) 1.9 (on foot)
				placebo	NS change

— indicates variables are not reported in paper.

may suggest that increasing amounts of energy are associated with better results it must be emphasised that it is based on some very tenuous assumptions since the trials are not comparable'. The need to establish the optimum dose for use in treatment is an example of the very basic information that needs to be established before clinical trials are undertaken, as an inappropriate dose may result in no treatment effects. For example, the large well-designed trial by Klaber-Moffett et al., 1996 has received some criticism (Low, 1997) because it was felt that the dose was too low to provide an effective intervention. Basic research to establish appropriate doses is fundamental to optimal use of this modality.

THERAPEUTIC EFFECTS OF SWD AND PSWD

Thermal effects

The main effect of both SWD and PSWD is tissue heating. The response of tissue to heat is similar no matter how the heat is applied. The only difference between diathermy and use of conductive heating agents is the depth at which the thermal effect occurs. The decision to use SWD may be appropriate if the desired treatment outcome is to produce heating within deep tissues, as it has been reported to:

- increase blood flow
- assist in the resolution of inflammation
- increase the extensibility of deep collagen tissue
- decrease joint stiffness
- relieve deep muscle pain and spasm (Kloth and Ziskin, 1990).

Further details of the effects of heating are to be found in Chapters 6, 9 and 10.

Non-thermal changes

As discussed earlier, depending on the dose, PSWD can produce a significant degree of heating (Bricknel and Watson, 1995; Murray and Kitchen, 2000). However, some authors have

suggested that PSWD may have an additional effect, which has been termed the *athermal effect* (Hayne, 1984). The term athermal effect is used to suggest that there is a physiological response to PSWD irradiation that is not due to the rise in tissue temperature. Issues around this topic were discussed in Chapter 7.

CLINICAL EFFECTS OF SWD AND PSWD

Although it is not precisely clear how SWD and PSWD work, these modalities are still used extensively in the clinical setting to treat a wide variety of conditions and pathologies (Kitchen and Partridge, 1992). The literature contains many anecdotal reports of conditions that will benefit from SWD and PSWD treatments—claims which are not currently supported by scientific evidence. The following section reviews some of the available evidence (for full details of the parameters the original articles should be consulted).

Soft tissue healing

Several trials using animal models have investigated the possible effects of SWD and PSWD on the rate of healing; however, there is conflicting evidence. Patino et al. (1996) showed a significant improvement in experimental wound healing in rats using pulsed magnetic energy (frequency of 50 Hz) for 35 minutes twice a day at an intensity of 20 mT. No other details were provided, however, making comparisons with PSWD and SWD modalities impossible. In studies using dogs, Bansal, Sobti and Roy (1990) concluded that SWD stimulated earlier maturation of the collagen fibres and more rapid regeneration of damaged muscle fibres, while Cameron (1961) credited PSWD with causing more rapid activity in collagen formation, white blood cell infiltration, phagocytosis, histocyte activity, fat activity and haematoma canalisation. In contrast, Constable, Scapicchio and Opitz (1971) conducted a series of three experiments, using PSWD, to examine wound repair in rabbits and guinea pigs; no benefit was reported. Finally, a study using a well-controlled double-blind experimental design (Krag *et al.*, 1979) reported that PSWD had no effect on the survival of experimental skin flaps in rats.

The directly conflicting findings reported in these studies may in part be attributed to poor methodologies or differences in doses used (none described dosage in sufficient detail to allow the trial to be repeated). This makes it impossible to draw firm conclusions about the most effective treatment dose to use.

Trials that have used humans as subjects tend to suggest that PSWD enhances the rate of skin healing. Cameron (1964) studied the effect of PSWD on the rate of healing of surgical wounds in a double-blind trial; once again little detail of the treatment parameters is provided and statistical analysis of the results was not undertaken.

Supporting this trend, PSWD was reported to increase the rate of healing of the donor site wound following medium-thickness skin grafts (Goldin *et al.*, 1981), while Itoh *et al.* (1991) and Salzberg and Cooper-Vastola (1995) in uncontrolled trials showed that PSWD enhanced the rate of resolution of chronic pressure ulcers. (The extremely powerful placebo response to PSWD has been demonstrated by Klaben-Moffett *et al.* (1996).) Some trials lack information about treatment dose, length of treatment or number of treatments, whereas others are uncontrolled. Some authors feel that too low a dose of PSWD will have no effect and too high a dose of PSWD may be detrimental (Klaber-Moffett *et al.*, 1996; Low, 1997). Applying a different protocol in the clinical setting may produce a completely different picture to the results reported here.

On the topic of wound healing, Badea *et al.* (1993) studied the effect of PSWD on bacterial growth in a tissue medium. They concluded that 'Diapulse action does not promote any increase of cell population, indicating the safety of this type of therapy for wound healing process'.

Resolution of haematomas

Two studies evaluated the effect of PSWD on the resolution of haematomas. A study by Fenn (1969) produced experimental haematomas in the ears of 60 rabbits. The treatment group received twice-daily PSWD. By the sixth day of the experiment the treated haematomas were significantly smaller and exhibited more advanced colour changes than the sham-treated haematomas. However, the clinical implications of this study are limited because the method used to produce haematomas did not involve any general trauma or tissue damage.

Another study by Brown and Baker (1987) produced experimental haematomas by injecting a myotoxic drug into the lateral head of the gastrocnemius muscle of 32 rabbits. Pulsed SWD was given to half of the animals with the rest acting as controls. Unfortunately, only a few details of the PSWD dose are provided, and one machine was used to treat two animals simultaneously. No differences in the rate of healing between the treated and control animals were found. However, the clinical relevance of this study must be questioned as treating two animals with one machine must have distorted the PSWD field shape, and thus the distribution of imparted energy.

The rate of healing, pain and swelling following oral surgery procedures were found to respond favourably to PSWD treatment, with earlier recovery in the 60 treated patients than in the control patients (Aronofsky, 1971). Furthermore, the effect of PSWD on swelling, disability and pain from recent hand injuries was studied, and PSWD was found to be a beneficial treatment (Barclay, Collier and Jones, 1983). However, both studies used a subjective assessment scale and the assessors were not blind to the treatment group, so this does not provide strong, reliable evidence.

In contrast, a well-controlled double-blind study by Grant *et al.* (1989) compared the effect of PSWD, ultrasound, placebo PSWD and placebo ultrasound on the recovery from perineal trauma in a trial of 414 postpartum women. Only a few details of the PSWD treatment parameters are given, but the treatment was applied for 10 minutes between 12 and 36 hours postdelivery. The mothers and the midwives were blind to the treatment groups and made assessments of the extent of bruising, oedema, use of analgesics and pain (on a visual analogue scale (VAS)). Analysis revealed that for all the parameters assessed there were no differences between the groups either immediately after the treatment, 10 days postpartum or at the 3 month follow-up. The active treatments were no better than the placebo treatments; however, placebo treatment may in itself offer considerable benefit over no treatment at all (Klaber-Moffett *et al.*, 1996).

A study by Livesley, Mugglestone and Whitton (1992), evaluated the effectiveness of PSWD in 48 patients with a minimally displaced fractured neck of the humerus. The trial was double blind and the patients were assigned randomly to either sham or active PSWD (0.4 ms, 35 Hz, 300 W, mean power = 4.2 W, 30 minutes daily for 10 consecutive working days). The results showed no significant difference between the pain levels in the two groups at 1, 2 and 6 months. However, it should be noted that 4.2 W is a low mean power.

A double-blind clinical trial by Gray *et al.* (1994) assessed the effects of four different physiotherapy treatments (SWD, mild thermal setting for 10 minutes; PSWD for 20 minutes; ultrasound; laser) and placebo on the symptoms of temporomandibular joint disorders ($n = 176$). No difference between the groups was found immediately after the treatments had finished, but at the 3 month post-treatment review the actively treated patients were significantly more improved than the placebo group. This warrants further work

In conclusion, there is only limited experimental evidence to make judgements on the anecdotal claims that SWD or PSWD has a positive effect on the rate of healing following soft tissue trauma. Those studies with poorer experimental design did tend to suggest a positive effect of SWD, which highlights the problems that may be encountered if suggestion and observer bias are not eliminated. In contrast, the results of the well-controlled studies (Grant *et al.*, 1989; Livesley, Mugglestone and Whitton, 1992) indicate that SWD has little beneficial effect on the resolution of soft tissue damage. However, each study used only one of the many possible treatment doses. It is quite possible that damaged cells or different tissues respond to a particular frequency or peak power (Kitchen and Partridge, 1992). It may be that too high a dose will cause a worsening of a condition or that too low a dose will have no effect.

Recent ankle injuries

The effect of SWD and PSWD has been investigated on recent ankle injury in six studies. Wilson (1972) found that active PSWD produced a significantly greater improvement in pain, swelling and disability than placebo treatment, while a second study (Wilson, 1974) confirmed that PSWD was a more effective treatment than SWD. Both studies used relatively high doses. The effectiveness of two different SWD machines were compared by Pasila, Visuri and Sundholm (1978) in a large study of 321 patients. No differences in strength, weight bearing, range of movement and volumetric measurements were found. However, after treatment, the ankle circumference of those treated with Curapulse was significantly less than in the placebo group, and the Diapulse group showed a significant improvement in gait compared with the placebo group.

In a randomised, double-blind study, Barker *et al.* (1985) investigated the effect of PSWD on the resolution of 73 recent, uncomplicated ankle injuries. Patients received 45 minutes treatment on three consecutive days. Assessments were made of the range of movement, gait, swelling and pain relief. No significant difference between the groups was identified after treatment.

McGill (1988) found no difference in the pain, swelling, or time to weight bearing in 31 patients receiving PSWD or placebo treatment; a double-blind protocol was used. Finally, Pennington *et al.* (1993) studied 50 grade 1 and 2 ankle injuries using a double-blind randomised design; PSWD was applied for 30 minutes to the medial and then the lateral side of the ankle followed by 10 minutes to the epigastrum. No details of the PSWD dose were provided. The active treatment group had significantly less swelling after treatment than the placebo group.

Of the six trials discussed, four reported using a double-blind protocol (Barker *et al.*, 1985; McGill, 1988; Pennington *et al.*, 1993; Wilson, 1972). However, the results of these four were inconclusive and even contradictory. An explanation for this may again lie in the doses used. In Wilson's 1972 study, a mean power of 40 watts was used and the treatment lasted for an hour. McGill (1988) on the other hand used a mean power of 19.6 watts for 15 minutes. Finally, the Barker *et al.* (1985) and Pennington *et al.* (1993) trials were flawed as they did not describe the dose fully. Thus, it could be that the far higher dose used by Wilson (1974) may have been sufficient to produce an effect whereas the lower dose used by McGill, was not.

Pain

In the clinical environment, SWD and PSWD may be used to relieve the pain associated with various conditions. In a review of physiotherapy modalities used in pain control, Chapman (1991) summarised that PSWD produces a significant relief of pain associated with acute injuries, but its value in the treatment of more chronic conditions remains to be proven.

Abramson, Chu and Tuck (1966) reported that SWD treatment, at a maximal tolerated dose, caused an increase in the conduction velocity of the median and ulnar motor nerves. Without further work the implications of this observation remain unclear, however.

Talaat, El-Dibany and El-Garf (1986) studied patients with myofacial pain dysfunction syndrome; SWD was found to reduce patients' pain and tenderness compared with a group of patients who received drug treatment. Reed *et al.* (1987) evaluated the effect of PSWD on post-operative wound pain in 43 patients undergoing inguinal hernia repair. Patients were allocated randomly to either a treatment or a sham-treatment group. The PSWD treatment consisted of 15 minutes of treatment twice daily (60 μs, 320 Hz, 1 W, mean power = 0.019 W). The PSWD was reported to have no beneficial effect. However, it must be noted that an extremely low power (0.019 W) of PSWD was used. Finally,

SWD was reported to ease the sensitivity of trigger points more so than hot packs (McCray and Patton, 1984). However, this trial did not use a double-blind protocol.

Back and neck pain

Low back pain (LBP) affects approximately 60–80% of adults and the disability associated with it is now reaching epidemic proportions (Waddell, 1998). In a survey by Foster *et al.* (1999), approximately 77% of therapists reported the use of electrotherapy, ultrasound, interferential therapy and PSWD being the most common; 11.2% of respondents used PSWD and 5.2% used SWD. However, there is little evidence to support this high level of use of electrotherapy.

Wagstaff, Wagstaff and Downey (1986) studied patients with back pain; they were allocated randomly to SWD, or PSWD (82 Hz, 700 W, mean power = 23.2 W), or a second PSWD group (200 Hz, 300 W, mean power = 23.4 W). Treatment was applied for 15 minutes twice a week for 3 weeks. The results indicated that all three groups showed a significant decrease in pain, using a 15 cm VAS, by the end of the trial. The PSWD groups showed a significantly greater reduction in pain than the SWD group. There was no difference in the improvement between the two PSWD groups. However, only limited interpretations can be made from these results because the study did not contain a placebo group.

The placebo effect of SWD on back pain has been demonstrated by Gibson *et al.* (1985) and Koes *et al.* (1992a, b). These authors concluded that their studies demonstrate the placebo response is induced by the renewed attention of healthcare professionals or the novelty of complex equipment. Whilst some may argue that it is acceptable to use the placebo response to gain a good treatment outcome, others argue that dependence on a passive treatment modality may encourage long-term problems and dependence (Waddell, 1998).

Finally Foley-Nolan *et al.* (1990), using low-dose PSWD (60 μs, 450 Hz, mean power = 1.5 mW/cm^2, 8 hours a day for 6 weeks), reported significantly improved symptoms in patients with persistent neck pain. A placebo group did not demonstrate the same improvement. The PSWD was delivered from small portable units that were placed inside surgical collars. This was a well-designed trial and this type of unit may warrant further investigation.

For managing LBP, the Clinical Standards Advisory Group (CSAG) guidelines indicate that, as LBP becomes chronic, passive treatments should be avoided and a more psychosocial approach allowing patients to develop active coping strategies to deal with their pain should be used (Waddell 1998). In view of the limited evidence to support the use of PSWD and SWD for treating LBP and neck pain (Gross et al., 1999) and the strong advice from the CSAG guidelines, electrotherapy modalities should not be used in the management of chronic back and neck conditions as passive modalities have the potential to cause long-term problems.

Nerve regeneration

Wilson and Jagadeesh (1976) reported regeneration of axons in the spinal cord of cats treated with PSWD. They also found that PSWD accelerated recovery of nerve conduction in rats. However, no statistical or histological analysis was undertaken in either study. Raji and Bowden (1983) demonstrated a significant acceleration in the recovery of injured peripheral nerves of rats. These studies provide interesting data. However, more work needs to be undertaken before the clinical importance of these findings can be established.

Osteoarthritis (OA)

SWD and PSWD often forms part of the physiotherapeutic management of patients with OA. However, its value has not yet been established. Some studies have shown an extremely positive response to SWD treatment, but poor methodology means that the results could also be explained by a placebo response similar to that for back pain (Lankhorst et al., 1982). Other studies have shown a negative response. For example,

the study by Klaber-Moffett et al. (1996) found that, although both active treatment and placebo treatment with PSWD were significantly better than no treatment (control), the placebo group reported more benefit from the treatment than did those in the active treatment group, at a marginally significant level. Low (1997) is critical of this study, suggesting that the treatment dose (mean wattage 23 W) was too low to produce a treatment effect. Klaber-Moffett (1997) acknowledges that different treatment doses may produce different outcomes, but conclude that the marginally significant improvement of the placebo group over the active group points to a placebo response. The results may also indicate a negative physiological response to active treatment that may be more marked with higher treatment doses. This is a matter for speculation that can be answered only by further rigorous clinical trials.

A comprehensive review by Marks et al. (1999) stated that 'although strong theoretical arguments can be made for the potential benefits of SWD on the underlying pathological process found in OA, the prevailing clinical studies … are essentially non-conclusive'. Many authors have in the past made a plea for further research; the review by Marks et al. (1999) usefully includes indications for possible lines of future research.

Conclusion

At present, the literature on SWD and PSWD is not sufficiently well developed to allow unequivocal conclusions to be drawn. The methodologies reported do not allow the exclusion of several variables as possible explanations of the results presented. Many trials even fail to describe the application parameters in sufficient detail to enable comparison between trials or replication of the study. The questions that still remain unanswered regarding PSWD and SWD include:

- How does PSWD and SWD work at a cellular level?

- What dose is effective in which circumstances?
- Which symptoms of what conditions are likely to respond to treatment?
- Are PSWD or SWD more effective than other treatments including placebo treatment?
- Do PSWD and SWD provide any long-term benefit?

APPLICATION OF SWD

During the application of SWD the patient is connected to the electrical circuit of the high-frequency generator by means of a capacitive applicator or an inductive coil.

The capacitive technique

There are two different types of electrodes for applying the capacitive method of SWD to the patient.

- **Flexible metal plates (malleable electrodes).** Flexible electrodes are flat metal sheets that are covered with a thick layer of rubber. They are often placed under or around the body part requiring treatment. A felt-like material is used to ensure that a sufficient spacing is retained between the electrode and the patient (Figure 11.7).
- **Rigid metal discs.** Disc electrodes are flat, round, metal electrodes that are encased with a clear plastic cover (Figure 11.8). They are used far more commonly than the flexible electrodes.

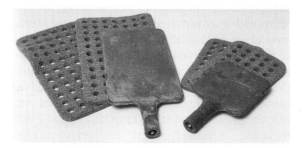

Figure 11.7 Flexible electrodes: three different sizes are available. Felt spacers are used to ensure sufficient electrode-to-skin distance.

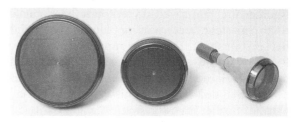

Figure 11.8 Disc electrodes: three different sizes are available. The electrode-to-skin distance can be altered by sliding the plate inside the plastic case.

The SWD machine has adjustable arms to position the electrodes close to the body part requiring treatment. The SWD field is generated between the two plates and the configuration of the electrodes influences the distribution of the SWD field within the tissues. It is therefore vitally important that the electrodes are positioned appropriately.

Guidelines for electrode selection and placement

- Electrodes should be of equal size. If electrodes of unequal size are used then stronger heating will occur close to the smaller electrode because the field will be concentrated over a smaller surface area. A very non-uniform electric field may be produced.
- Electrodes should be slightly larger than the body part because the electric field is less uniform at the edge of the plates. A weak or non-uniform field is not recommended for treatment purposes. Most SWD equipment has a choice of three different sizes of electrode that can be used: small, medium and large.
- Electrodes should be at right angles and so parallel to the skin surface. When the electrode is too close to the skin then intense superficial heating may occur. When the electrodes are placed further from the skin the distribution of the field will be more uniform. However, if the distance between the electrode and skin is too great the field strength will be severely reduced. Thus, a balance must be reached to prevent either excessive skin heating or insufficient energy absorption. A skin-to-electrode distance of

between 2 and 4 cm is optimal. It is the distance from the metal plate and not the plastic cover that is important. If the electrodes are not parallel to the skin then areas of intense heating will occur in the tissues closest to the electrodes and hot spots or burns could result.

Deviation from this ideal electrode configuration can lead to less-efficient field distribution or areas of intense heating.

Electrode arrangement

There are three principal electrode arrangements used with the capacitive techniques:

1. **Contraplanar application (transverse).** An electrode is placed on either side of the limb (Figure 11.9).
2. **Coplanar application.** Both electrodes are placed on the same side of the limb. The field follows the route of least resistance (e.g. through the blood vessels, which contain a high proportion of ions). If the electrodes are placed closer together than the distance between the electrodes and the skin, the field will pass directly between the electrodes and no tissue treatment will occur (Figure 11.10).
3. **Longitudinal application.** One electrode is placed at each end of the limb. The aim of this electrode placement is to allow the electric field to be oriented in the same direction as the tissues, thus providing good conditions for the current to flow through tissues of low resistance.

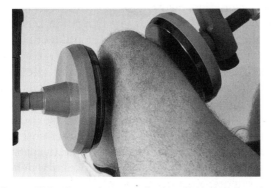

Figure 11.9 Contraplanar application. Note that the electrodes are of equal size, slightly larger than the body part to be treated, and equidistant from and parallel to the skin surface.

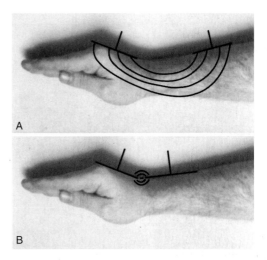

Figure 11.10 Coplanar application. A: Correct electrode arrangement. B: Electrodes placed too close together with the result that no tissue treatment will occur.

Inductive application

SWD can also be achieved using the inductive technique. Based on the law of electromagnetic induction, a magnetic field is generated whenever an electric current flows in a material. The lines of force of the magnetic field radiate at right angles to the direction of the current. This process has a converse, termed *magnetic induction*, in that the magnetic field induces secondary currents—*eddy currents*—in the material. The inductive SWD method uses magnetic induction to produce small eddy currents in the tissues. The eddy currents can result in an increase in tissue temperature, and conventional wisdom holds that the eddy currents produce the physiological effects. The role of the magnetic field is to act as a carrier medium into the tissues.

Inductive SWD can be administered using two different applicators. The most commonly used is an inductive (coil) applicator. Units available commercially include the Circuplode (Figure 11.11) and the Megaplode. The SWD cable is precoiled and encased in an insulated drum. The drum is placed close to the body part requiring treatment so that the coil is parallel with the skin surface. An electric current is generated inside the machine and passed through the coil. The magnetic field associated with

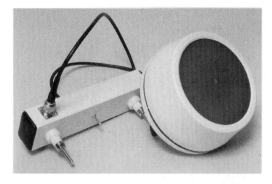

Figure 11.11 Circuplode. Inside the drum is a coiled electrode.

this current is set up at right angles to the direction of current flow, and it is therefore directed into the body part, where eddy currents are established.

The second method, now relatively rare, involves wrapping an insulated cable around the limb to be treated. The correct skin-to-coil distance is achieved by covering the limb with several layers of towelling.

Dosage

Thermal treatments

The parameters used to describe SWD should include:

- continuous wave therapy: frequency, power, time of irradiation, method of application and the type of field used
- pulsed therapy: as above, plus peak power, average power, pulse strength, and rest period or number of pulses per second.

The use of thermal sensation for assessing SWD dose

Knowledge of the theoretical patterns of heat production and information sought from the patient are used to inform the qualitative amount of heat that is being produced, but are more art than science (Ward, 1980). A standard method of determining dose is to ask the patient to report thermal sensation. Low and Reed (2000) suggest five SWD dose levels, ranging from imperceptible

heating at which the patient reports no sensation of heat, to a maximum tolerable heating dose. Delpizzo and Joyner (1987) divide doses for SWD into three categories—high, medium and low:

- high—clear increase in heat
- medium—thermal effects are weak but still apparent
- low—thermal effects are not noticeable, although physiological effects have been reported at these doses.

Monitoring dose by thermal sensation provides an extremely inaccurate measure of dose, however. The sensitivity to temperature change is vastly superior in the skin to that in deeper tissue. Patient statements of thermal sensation are, therefore, reports of temperature in the skin and not in deeper tissues. Odia and Aigbogun (1988) have also reported that certain areas of the body were more sensitive to changes in temperature than others; individuals were more accurate in reporting increases in temperature of the facial skin than in the skin of the lower limb.

Elder *et al.* (1989) report animal work that showed that temperature-induced cell injury occurred at a threshold level (42°C) that was below the threshold of thermally induced pain (45°C). Thus, Delpizzo and Joyner (1987) point out that when a patient is asked to report thermal sensation there is a possibility of high levels of heat and cell damage occurring in body areas with relatively low numbers of thermal receptors, including deeper tissue. Elder *et al.* (1989) extend this argument to state that cutaneous perception is not reliable in the prevention of potential damage from electromagnetic radiation.

Such arguments appear to limit the safe dose of SWD to those reported by a patient as *at most* 'a very mild sensation of warmth'. Even then, this dose level may be too high if the thermal sensory discrimination of the patient is less than optimum owing to pathology or to anatomical site. This is relevant particularly where the energy absorbed in superficial tissue may be lower than that absorbed in deep tissue. Certainly, the use of doses above this level of 'mild sensation' would appear to have potentially hazardous effects. Thus, at the present time, until more accurate methods of assessing dose are established, the therapist must be aware of the potential risk of causing tissue damage and ensure that the maximum dose that a patient receives causes only a mild sensation of warmth. (These exposure levels are based on work on recommendations for microwave irradiation, but may also be useful for short-wave frequencies until clearer guidelines are made available.)

PSWD dose

In theory, it is suggested that acute conditions should be treated with a low dose and more chronic conditions with a high dose (van der Esch and Hoogland, 1991). To give a patient a low dose of PSWD, the pulse repetition rate, the pulse duration and the peak pulse power should all be as low as possible. If the intention is to apply a high dose of PSWD, the above variables should be at their maximum (Table 11.5). However, the same mean power of PSWD can be delivered by using different combinations of the above variables (Table 11.6). Unfortunately, there is little information available to allow the importance of this to be determined. It is therefore essential that, when PSWD treatments are recorded, sufficient

information is given so that the treatment can be accurately repeated (Table 11.7).

Very few research trials investigating PSWD gave sufficient details of the treatment parameters, and comparison of studies is very difficult when such important details are absent. Also, it is impossible to evaluate whether there is a trend where a variable, such as mean power, influences the results.

Treatment procedures

The treatment procedure should ensure optimal safety for both patient and operator. The following procedure as outlined by the National Health and Medical Research Council of Australia in 1985 is suggested.

Prepare the patient

The operator should:

- examine the thermal and pain sensitivity of the patient
- exclude contraindications
- ensure that all metal objects (rings, jewellery, metal spectacles, etc.) are removed from the treatment area
- remove hearing aids
- remove all bandages and clothing
- ensure the skin is dry
- ask the patient to report immediately any sensation felt during treatment.

Prepare the machine

The operator should ensure that:

- cables are connected correctly
- cables or applicators are not rested on metal surfaces

Table 11.5 Examples of low dose and high dose PSWD

	Low dose	High dose
Pulse repetition rate	26 Hz	200 Hz
Pulse duration	0.065 ms	0.4 ms
Peak pulse power	100 W	1000 W
Mean power	1.7 W	80 W

Table 11.6 An example of how the same mean power (PSWD) can be delivered by using different pulse parameters

	Low dose	High dose
Pulse repetition rate	82 Hz	20 Hz
Pulse duration	0.4 ms	0.4 ms
Peak pulse power	200 W	800 W
Mean power	6.6 W	6.4 W

Table 11.7 Information required when recording PSWD treatments

Pulse repetition rate
Pulse duration
Peak pulse power
Length of treatment
Mode of delivery
Electrode type, spacing and size

- the applicator is aligned appropriately for maximum energy transfer
- the gonads are not subject to irradiation
- cables are not placed close to the patient's non-targeted tissue
- the patient support (e.g. chair or bed) is not metallic and that all metal objects are kept at least 3 m away from the applicator and cables.

During treatment

Once the unit has been activated the operator should:

- remain at least 1 m from the electrodes and 0.5 m from the cables (McDowell and Lunt, 1991)
- ensure that the patient maintains the correct position throughout the duration of the treatment
- ensure that the patient is not left alone during treatment unless supplied with a reliable cut-off switch
- ensure that the patient does not touch the machine
- ensure that no other person is in the vicinity of the machine.

SAFETY

Hazards

These include:

- burns
- exacerbation of symptoms, especially when thermal doses are used
- spread of existing pathologies, e.g. tumours, tuberculosis or infective pathogens
- cardiac failure due to electric shock or interference with cardiac pacemakers
- early pregnancy (first trimester).

Contraindications

The following factors contraindicate the use of SWD:

- implanted pacemakers (electromagnetic fields may interfere with these if screening is insufficient)

- metal in the tissues or external fixators (metal concentrates the magnetic field)
- impaired thermal sensation (burns and scalds may occur)
- uncooperative patients (e.g. uncooperative physically because of movement disorders or uncooperative mentally because of disability or age)
- pregnancy
- haemorrhaging areas (women who are menstruating should be warned that a temporary increase in bleeding may occur if the pelvis is irradiated)
- ischaemic tissue
- malignant tumours (Burr (1974) indicates that cancer cells proliferate in response to heating and the temperature in tumours tends to rise more than surrounding cells therefore not even a low dose of PSWD should be given)
- active tuberculosis
- recent venous thrombosis
- patient pyrexia
- areas of skin affected by courses of X-ray.

The following should be treated with caution:

- growing epiphysis: Doyle and Smart (1963) demonstrated that repeated exposure to SWD in the rat increased the rate of epiphyseal growth compared with the untreated legs. No histological abnormalities were identified.

Kitchen and Partridge (1999) and Kitchen (2000a, b) are establishing a system for reporting adverse effects of electrotherapy. Further contraindications may become apparent as this valuable work continues.

Safety of operator

Bearing in mind the presence of the electromagnetic field in the vicinity of the machine, the above-listed contraindications should apply to the machine operator as well as to the patient. Hamburger, Logue and Silverman (1983) investigated the association between non-ionising radiation and heart disease. Using a questionnaire to survey 3004 male physiotherapists they showed a link between heart disease (notably ischaemic heart disease) and high exposure to SWD. This incidence of heart disease was, however, smaller than in the general population—possibly because of higher socioeconomic status and better than average health in the physiotherapist population.

Kallen, Malmquist and Moritz (1982) carried out an epidemiological study of birth outcomes in physiotherapists in Sweden. They reported an above-normal incidence of death or malformations in babies born to those involved in operating SWD machines. In contrast Oullet Hellstrom and Stewart (1993) reported that the risk of miscarriage was not associated with reported use of SWD equipment.

A useful source of health and safety information regarding the safe use of PSWD and SWD can be found on the Chartered Society of Physiotherapists (CSP) members web site (CSP 1997).

REFERENCES

Abramson, DI, Bell, Y, Rejal, H et al. (1960) Changes in blood flow, oxygen uptake and tissue temperatures produced by therapeutic physical agents. II Effect of short-wave diathermy. American Journal of Physical Medicine 39: 87–95.

Abramson, DI, Chu, LSW, Tuck, S (1966) Effect of tissue temperatures and bloodflow on motor nerve conduction velocity. Journal of the American Medical Association 198(10): 1082–1088.

Aronofsky, DH (1971) Reduction of dental postsurgical symptoms using non-thermal pulsed high-peak-power electromagnetic energy. Oral Surgery 32(5): 688–696.

Badea, MA, Roxana, VD, Sandru, D, Paslaru, L, Jieanu, V, Comorosan, S (1993) The effect of pulsed electromagnetic field (Diapulse) on cellular systems. Romanian Journal of Physiology 30(1–2): 65–71.

Bansal, PS, Sobti, VK, Roy, KS (1990) Histomorphochemical effects of shortwave diathermy on healing of experimental muscular injury in dogs. Indian Journal of Experimental Biology 28: 766–770.

Barclay, V, Collier, RJ, Jones, A (1983) Treatment of various hand injuries by pulsed electromagnetic energy (diapulse). Physiotherapy 69(6): 186–188.

Barker, AT, Barlow, PS, Porter, J et al. (1985) A double blind clinical trial of low power pulsed shortwave therapy in the treatment of a soft tissue injury. Physiotherapy 71(12): 500–504.

Bricknell, R, Watson, T (1995) The thermal effects of pulsed shortwave diathermy. British Journal of Therapy and Rehabilitation 2: 430–443.

Brown, M, Baker, RD (1987) Effect of pulsed short-wave diathermy on skeletal muscle injury in rabbits. Physical Therapy 67(2): 208–214.

Burr, B (1974) Heat as a therapeutic modality against cancer. Report no. 16. US National Cancer Institute, Bethesda, MD.

Byl, N, Hoft, H (1995) The use of oxygen in wound healing. In: McCulloch, JM, Kloth, LC, Feeder, JA (eds) Wound Healing Alternatives in Management. FA Davis, Philadelphia, pp 365–404

Cameron, B (1961) Experimental acceleration of wound healing. American Journal of Othopaedics 3: 336–343.

Cameron, BM (1964) A three-phase evaluation of pulsed, high frequency, radio short waves (Diapulse) on 646 patients. American Journal of Orthopaedics 6: 72–78.

Chapman, EC (1991) Can the use of physical modalities for pain control be rationalized by the research evidence? Canadian Journal of Physiology and Pharmacology 69: 704–712.

Clinical Standards Advisory Group (1994) Back Pain Report. HMSO, London.

Constable, JD, Scapicchio, AP, Opitz, B (1971) Studies of the effects of diapulse treatment on various aspects of wound healing in experimental animals. Journal of Surgical Research 11: 254–257.

CSP (1997) Electrotherapy health and safety briefing pack no. www.csp.org.uk (member centre, electronic library, health and safety, safe practice with electrotherapy (shortwave therapies)).

Delpizzo, V, Joyner, KH (1987) On the safe use of microwave and shortwave diathermy units. Australian Journal of Physiotherapy 33(3): 152–162.

Doyle, JR, Smart, BW (1963) Stimulation of bone growth by shortwave diathermy. Journal of Bone and Joint Surgery 45(A1): 15–23.

Draper, DO, Knight, K, Fujiwara, T, Castel, C (1999) Temperature change in human muscle during and after pulsed short-wave diathermy. Journal of Orthopaedic and Sports Physical Therapy 29(1): 13–22.

Elder, JA, Czerski, PA, Stuchly, MA et al. (1989) Radiofrequency radiation. In: Suess, MJ, Benwell-Morison, DA (eds) Nonionizing Radiation Protection, 2nd edn. WHO Regional Publications, European Series, no. 25, Ottawa, pp. 117–174.

Erdman, WJ (1960) Peripheral blood flow measures during application of pulsed high frequency currents. American Journal of Orthopaedics 2: 196–197.

van der Esch, M, Hoogland, R (1991) Pulsed shortwave diathermy with the Curapulse 419. Delft Instruments Physical Medicine BV, Delft.

Fenn, JE (1969) Effect of electromagnetic energy (Diapulse) on experimental haematomas. Canadian Medical Association Journal 100: 251–253.

Foley-Nolan, D, Barry, C, Coughlan, RJ et al. (1990) Pulsed high frequency (27 MHz) electromagnetic therapy for persistent neck pain. A double blind, placebo-controlled study of 20 patients. Orthopedics 13(4): 445–451.

Foster, NE, Thompson, KA, Baxter, GD, Allen, JM (1999) Management of nonspecific low back pain by physiotherapists in Britain and Ireland: A descriptive questionnaire of current clinical practice. Spine 24(13): 1332–1342.

Gibson, T, Harkness, J, Blagrave, P et al. (1985) Controlled comparison of short wave diathermy treatment with osteopathic treatment in nonspecific low back pain. *The Lancet* **i**(8440): 1258–1261.

Goats, CG (1989) Pulsed electromagnetic (short-wave) energy therapy. *British Journal of Sports Medicine* **23**(4): 213–216.

Goldin, JH, Broadbent, NRG, Nancarrow, JD et al. (1981) The effects of Diapulse on the healing of wounds: a double blind randomised control trial in man. *Brtitish Journal of Plastic Surgery* **34**: 267–270.

Grant, A, Sleep, J, McIntosh, J et al. (1989) Ultrasound and electromagnetic energy treatment for the perineal trauma. A randomised placebo control trial. *British Journal of Obstetrics and Gynaecology* **96**: 434–439.

Gray, RJ, Quayle, AA, Hall, CA, Schofield, MA (1994) Physiotherapy in the treatment of temporal mandibular joint disorders: a comparative study of four treatment methods. *British Dental Journal (ASW)* 9 April, 176 (**7**: 257–261).

Gross, AR, Aker, PD, Goldsmith, CH, Peloso, P (1999) Physical medicine modalities for mechanical neck disorders. *Cochrane Library—Issue 4*.

Guy, AW, Chou, CK, Neuhaus, B (1984) Average SAR and distribution in man exposed to 450 Mhz radiofrequency radiation. *IEEE transactions on microwave theory and techniques*. **MTT-32**: 752–762.

Hamburger, S, Logue, JN, Silverman, PM (1983) Occupational exposure to non-ionising radiation and an association with heart disease. An exploratory study. *Journal of Chronic Diseases* **36**: 791–802.

Hand, JW (1990) Biophysics and technology of electromagnetic hypothermia. In: Gauthier, M (ed) *Methods of External Hyperthermic Heating*. Springer-Verlag, Berlin.

Hayne, CR (1984) Pulsed high frequency energy—its place in physiotherapy. *Physiotherapy* **70**(12): 459–466.

Hollander, JL, Hovarth, SM (1949) The influence of physical therapy procedures on the intra-articular temperature of normal and arthritic subjects. *American Journal of Medical Science* **218**: 543–548.

Itoh, M, Montemayor, JS, Matsumoto, E et al. (1991) Accelerated wound healing of pressure ulcers by pulsed high peak power electromagnetic energy (Diapulse). *Decubitus* **4**(1): 24–34.

Kallen, B, Malmquist, G, Moritz, U (1982) Delivery outcome among physiotherapists in Sweden: is non-ionising radiation a fetal hazard? *Archives of Environmental Health* **37**: 81–85.

Kitchen, S (2000a) Audit of the unexpected effects of electrophysical agents. Interim report: responses to December 1999. *Physiotherapy* **86**: 152–155.

Kitchen, S (2000b) Audit of the unexpected effects of electrophysical agents. Interim report: responses January to June 2000. *Physiotherapy* **86**: 509–511.

Kitchen, S, Partridge, C (1992) Review of shortwave diathermy. Continuous and pulsed patterns. *Physiotherapy* **78**: 4, 243–252.

Kitchen, S, Partridge, C (1999) Adverse effect of electrotherapy used by physiotherapists. *Physiotherapy* **85**(6): 298–303.

Klaber Moffett, JA, Richardson, PH, Frost, H, Osborn, A (1996) A placebo controlled double blind trial to evaluate the effectiveness of pulsed short wave therapy for osteoarthritic hip and knee pain. *Pain* **67**: 121–127.

Klaber-Moffett, J (1997) Response to Low. *Pain* **71**(2): 207.

Kloth, LC, Ziskin, MC (1990) Diathermy and pulsed electromagnetic fields. In: Michlovitz, SL *Thermal Agents in Rehabilitation*, 2nd edn. FA Davis, Philadelphia, pp 175–193.

Koes, BW, Bouter, LM, van Maneren, H et al. (1992a) The effectiveness of manual therapy physiotherapy and treatment by the general practitioner for nonspecific back and neck complaints. *Spine* **17**(1): 28–35.

Koes, BW, Bouter, LM, van Mameren, H et al. (1992b) Randomised clinical trial of manipulative therapy and physiotherapy for persistent back and neck complaints: results of one year follow up. *British Medical Journal* **304**: 601–605.

Krag, C, Taudorf, U, Siim, E, Bolund, S (1979) The effect of pulsed electromagnetic energy (Diapulse) on the survival of experimental skin flaps. A study on rats. *Scandinavian Journal of Plastic and Reconstructive Surgery* **13**: 377–380.

Lankhorst, GJ, van de Stadt, RJ, van der Korst, JK et al. (1982) Relationship of isometric knee extension torque and functional variables in osteo-arthrosis of the knee. *Scandinavian Journal of Rehabilitation Medicine* **14**: 7–10.

Lehmann, JF (1990) *Therapeutic Heat and Cold*, 4th edn. Williams and Wilkins, Baltimore, MD.

Livesley, PJ, Mugglestone, A, Whitton, J (1992) Electrotherapy and the management of minimally displaced fracture of the neck of the humerus. *Injury* **23**(5): 323–327.

Low, J (1995) Dosage of some pulsed shortwave clinical trials. *Physiotherapy* **81**(10): 611–616.

Low, J (1997) Response to Moffett, Richardson, Frost, Osborn. *Pain* **71**(2): 207.

Low, J, Reed, A (2000) *Electrotherapy Explained, Principles and Practice*, 3rd edn. Butterworth-Heinemann, London.

McCray, RE, Patton, NJ (1984) Pain relief at trigger points; a comparison of moist heat and shortwave diathermy. *Journal of Orthopaedic and Sports Physical Therapy* **5**(4): 175–178.

McDowell, AD, Lunt, MJ (1991) Electromagnetic field strength measurements on Megapulse units. *Physiotherapy* **77**(12): 805–809.

McGill, SN (1988) The effects of pulsed shortwave therapy on lateral ligament ankle sprains. *New Zealand Journal of Physiotherapy* **16**: 21–24.

Marks, R, Ghassemi, M, Duarte, R, van Ngyuyen, JP (1999) A review of the literature on shortwave diathermy as applied to osteo-arthritis of the knee. *Physiotherapy* **85**(6): 304–316.

Morrissey, LJ (1966) Effect of pulsed short-wave diathermy upon volume blood flow through the calf of the leg. *Journal of the American Physical Therapy Association* **46**(9): 946–952.

Murray, CC, Kitchen, S (2000) Effect of pulse repetition rate on the perception of thermal sensation with pulsed shortwave diathermy. *Physiotherapy Research International* **5**(2): 73–84.

Odia, GI, Aibogun, OS (1988) Thermal sensation and the skin sensation test: regional differences and their effects on the issue of reliability of temperature ranges. *Australian Journal of Physiotherapy* **34**(2): 89–93.

Oosterveld, FGJ, Rasker, JJ, Jacobs, JWG et al. (1992) The effects of local heat and cold therapy on the inraarticular and skin surface temperature of the knee. *Arthritis and Rheumatism* **35**(2): 146–151.

Oullet Hellstrom, R, Stewart, WF (1993) Miscarriages among female physical therapists who report using radio- and microwave-frequency eletromagnetic radiation. *American Journal of Epidemiology* **138**(10): 774–786.

Pasila, M, Visuri, T, Sundholm, A (1978) Pulsating shortwave diathermy; value in treatment of recent ankle and foot sprains. *Archives of Physical Medicine and Rehabilitation* **59**: 383–386.

Patino, O, Grana, D, Bolgiani, A *et al.* (1996) Pulsed electromagnetic fields in experimental cutaneous wound healing in rats. *Journal of Burn Care and Rehabilitation* **17**(6): 528–531.

Pennington, GM, Danley, DL, Sumko, MH *et al.* (1993) Pulsed, non-thermal, high frequency electromagnetic energy (Diapulse) in the treatment of grade I and grade II ankle sprains. *Military Medicine* **158**: 101–4.

Pope, G (1999) The trouble with electrotherapy… *Physiotherapy* **85**(6): 290, 293.

Pope, GD, Mocket, SP, Wright, JP (1995) A survey of electrotherapeutic modalities: ownership and use in the NHS in England. *Physiotherapy* **81**(2): 82–91.

Raji, ARM, Bowden, REM (1983) Effects of high-peak pulsed electromagnetic field on the degeneration and regeneration of the common peroneal nerve in rats. *Journal of Bone and Joint Surgery* **65B**(4): 478–492.

Reed, MWR, Bickerstaff, DR, Hayne, CR *et al.* (1987) Pain relief after inguinal herniorrhaphy. Ineffectiveness of pulsed electromagnetic energy. *British Journal of Clinical Practice* **41**(6): 782–784.

Salzberg, CA, Cooper-Vastola, SA (1995) The effects of non-thermal pulsed electromagnetic energy on wound healing of pressure ulcers in spinal cord-injured patients: A randomised double-blind study. *Ostomy/wound Management* **41**(3): 42–51.

Silverman, DR, Pendleton, L (1968) A comparison of the effects of continuous and pulsed shortwave diathermy on circulation. *Archives of Physical Medicine and Rehabilitation* **49**: 429–436.

Talaat, AM, El-Dibany, MM, El-Garf, A (1986) Physical therapy in the management of myofacial pain dysfunction syndrome. *Annals of Otology, Rhinology and Laryngology* **95**: 225–228.

Verrier, M, Falconer, K, Crawford, JS (1977) A comparison of tissue temperature following two shortwave diathermy techniques. *Physiotherapy Canada* **29**: 21–25.

Verrier, M, Ashby, P, Crawford, JS (1978) Effects of thermotherapy on the electrical and mechanical properties of human skeletal muscle. *Physiotherapy Canada* **30**(3): 117–120.

Waddell, G (1998) *Back Pain Revolution*. Churchill Livingstone, New York.

Wagstaff, P, Wagstaff, S, Downey, M (1986) A pilot study to compare the efficacy of continuous and pulsed magnetic energy (shortwave diathermy) on the relief of low back pain. *Physiotherapy* **72**(11): 563–566.

Ward, AR (1980) *Electricity, Fields and Waves in Therapy*. Science Press, Marrickville.

Wilson, DH (1972) Treatment of soft-tissue injuries by pulsed electrical energy. *British Medical Journal* **2**: 269–270.

Wilson, DH (1974) Comparison of shortwave diathermy and pulsed electromagnetic energy in treatment of soft tissue injuries. *Physiotherapy* **60**(10): 309–310.

Wilson, DH, Jagadeesh, P (1976) Experimental regeneration in peripheral nerves and the spinal cord in laboratory animals exposed to a pulsed electromagnetic field. *Paraplegia* **14**: 12–20.

BIBLIOGRAPHY

Allberry, J, Manning, FRC, Smith, EE (1974) Short-wave diathermy for herpes zoster. *Physiotherapy* **60**(12): 386.

Astrand, PO, Rodhal, K (1986) *Textbook of Work Physiology*, 3rd edn. McGraw-Hill, New York.

Balogun, JA, Okonofau, FE (1988) Management of chronic pelvic inflammatory disease with shortwave diathermy. *Physical Therapy* **68**(10): 1541–1545.

Barker, P, Allcut, D, McCollum, CN (1984) Pulsed electromagnetic energy fails to prevent postoperative ileus. *Journal of the Royal College of Surgeons of Edinburgh* **29**(3): 147–150.

Comorosan, S, Pana, L, Pop, L *et al.* (1991) The influence of pulsed high peak power electromagnetic energy (Diapulse) treatment on posttraumatic algoneurodystrophies. *Review of Rheumatology Physiology* **28**(3–4): 77–81.

Forster, A, Palastanga, N (1985) *Clayton's Electrotherapy*. Baillière-Tindall, London.

Ginsberg, AJ (1961) Pulsed short wave in the treatment of bursitis with calsification. *International Record of Medicine* **174**(2): 2936, 71–75.

Goats, CG (1989) Continuous short-wave (radio frequency) diathermy. *British Journal of Sports Medicine* **23**(2): 123–127.

Hovind, H, Nielson, SL (1974) The effects of short-wave and microwave on blood flow in subcutaneous and muscle tissue in man. *Proceedings of the 7th WCPT*, Montreal, Canada 147–151.

Michlovitz, SL (1990) *Thermal Agents in Rehabilitation*, 2nd edn. FA Davis, Philadelphia.

O'Dowd, WJ (1989) Pulse mythology. *Physiotherapy* **75**(3): 97–98.

Oliver, DE (1984) Pulsed electro-magnetic energy—what is it? *Physiotherapy* **70**(12): 458–459.

Raji, AM (1984) An experimental study of the effects of pulsed electromagnetic field (Diapulse) on nerve repair. *Journal of Hand Surgery* **9B**(2): 105–112.

Santiesteban, AJ, Grant, C (1985) Post-surgical effect of pulsed shortwave therapy. *Journal of the American Pediatric Association* **75**(6): 306–309.

Selsby, A (1985) Physiotherapy in the management of temporomandibular joint disorders. *Australian Dental Journal* **30**(4): 273–280.

Wells, PE, Frampton, V, Bowsher, D (1988) *Pain Management and Control in Physiotherapy*, 2nd edn. Heinemann, London.

Wright, GG (1973) Treatment of soft tissue and ligamentous injuries in professional footballers. *Physiotherapy* **59**(12): 385–387.

PART 2
MICROWAVE DIATHERMY

INTRODUCTION

Microwave diathermy, although deeper than superficial (surface) heating, is not as deep as capacitive shortwave or ultrasonic heating. In addition, microwaves produce some non-thermal effects.

In order to address concerns regarding hazardous exposure to electromagnetic radiation, exposure standards have been developed by international and national authorities including the Canadian Department of Health and Welfare (1983), Australian National Health and Medical Research Council (1985) (reproduced in Delpizzo and Joiner, 1987), National Radiation Protection Board (1989), De Domenico *et al.* (1990), and Australian Standards Association (1992).

Nature of microwaves

The group of *electromagnetic radiations* known as microwaves occupy that part of the electromagnetic spectrum extending from wavelength 1 m (frequency 300 MHz) to 1 mm (300 GHz) (see Fig. 1.20, Ch. 1, p. 19). The operating specification for apparatus in Australia, the United Kingdom and Europe is 122.5 mm (2450 MHz), whilst physiotherapeutic microwaves in North America also operate at 327 mm (915 MHz) and 690 mm (433.9 MHz).

Microwave apparatus

The core of the microwave apparatus, a multi-cavity magnetron valve, transmits microwave energy to one of a variety of different-sized circular or rectangular directors (antennae) via a shielded coaxial cable. In turn, the director radiates microwaves to the surface of the region to be treated in the same manner as a simple bar radiator.

Physical behaviour

On reaching the surface of the body (or other material) the initially radiated microwaves may be *absorbed, transmitted, refracted* or *reflected* according to the optical laws of radiations (see Ch. 1). These behaviours determine the distribution of the energy within the body.

The propagation characteristics of microwaves are first determined by the wavelength and frequency of the energy. Whilst the penetration of microwaves is inversely proportional to their wavelength, this is not a simple (linear) relationship because other factors such as tissue composition contribute to the final pattern of absorption (Fig. 11.12).

Tissue composition and microwave absorption

Microwave energy is predisposed to penetrate tissues with low electrical conductivity and be absorbed in tissues with high conductivity. In essence, high electrical conductivity equates with high fluid content—typically blood vessels, muscle, moist skin, internal organs and eyes. Microwaves of 122.5 mm (2450 MHz) heat the skin at least to the same extent as the deeper tissues.

Heating occurs by means of dipole rotation and molecular distortion (see SWD, p. 148).

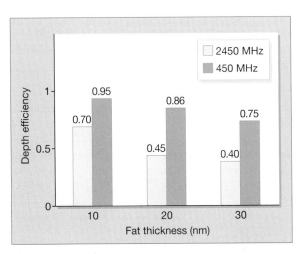

Figure 11.12 The relationship of efficiency of penetration (where maximum = 1) for microwaves at 2450 and 450 MHz at three different thicknesses of superficial fat.

Muscle contains more dipole molecules than fatty tissue, leading to a greater rise in muscle temperature when microwave diathermy is used (McMeeken and Bell, 1990). The effect of microwaves on tissues with low fluid content such as fat is to produce *molecular distortion*, leading to some heating in these relatively avascular tissues, but not as much as in tissues where dipole rotation occurs.

The proportion of reflected energy at the meeting point of different surfaces is determined by the magnitude of the difference between the dielectric properties of the two surfaces, and by the angle of the incident microwave radiations (Fig. 11.13). Relatively large differences in dielectric properties enhances energy absorption at these sites, which include skin–air, muscle–fat, and bone–soft tissue interfaces.

The skin–air interface is the most significant interface limiting the deep heating capacity of microwaves (Schwan and Piersol, 1954, 1955). Reflection can also augment the heating of fat immediately overlying muscle. For example, a subcutaneous fat layer thicker than 20 mm may be heated even more than the underlying muscle (Lehmann *et al.*, 1962).

Although, in theory, microwaves are capable of passing through bone, in practice the energy is largely prevented from entering bone owing to significant reflection at its surface.

Relationship between wavelength and microwave absorption

The degree of penetration of microwaves is proportional to their wavelength and, hence, inversely proportional to their frequency. As the wavelength increases, penetration increases and absorption occurs in deeper tissues. Two wavelengths are available for physiotherapeutic use: 122.5 mm (2450 MHz) and 327 mm (915 MHz). The former produces more superficial heating because of its lesser degree of penetration.

The ratio of heat developed in muscle to the total heating of fat and muscle, the *penetration depth*, is a convenient means of measuring the

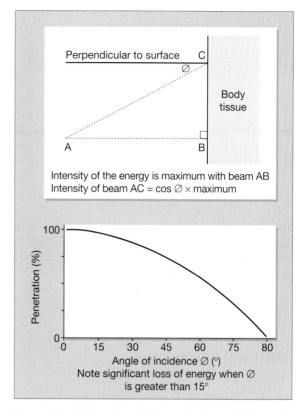

Intensity of the energy is maximum with beam AB
Intensity of beam AC = cos ∅ × maximum

Note significant loss of energy when ∅ is greater than 15°

Figure 11.13 The effect of the cosine law on the intensity of microwave energy at the body surface.

efficacy of deep heating. A depth efficiency of 1.0 represents perfect deep heating (Ward, 1986). Representative examples of depth efficacy are given in Figure 11.12, which also shows that there is a relationship with the thickness of the fat layer.

Laws of microwave radiations

Only radiations which are absorbed can be considered to have any potential for therapeutic effect. Transmission, refraction and reflection change only the site at which the energy is eventually absorbed. In practice, the director is always placed at a short fixed distance (2–6 cm) from the part, hence the influence on the reflection, penetration or absorption by tilting the director is relatively small.

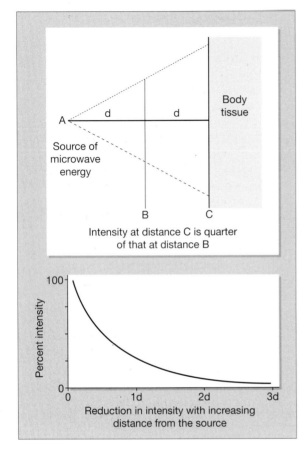

Figure 11.14 The effect of the inverse square law on the intensity of microwave energy at the body surface.

Microwaves obey the inverse square law of distance (Fig. 11.14):

The intensity of radiation falling on unit surface area of the body is inversely proportional to the square of the distance of the source of energy from the surface.

Since the director is placed close to the part, and the intensity is varied by adjusting the variable power control, the operation of the inverse square law results in small changes in the distance between the director and the body part causing large changes in the power. Accordingly, care should be taken with skin–director distances. Furthermore, when using apparatus with a potentially large power output, where a small increase in the variable power

control causes a large increase in power, this should be offset by increasing the distance between the director and the body part.

BIOLOGICAL EFFECTS OF MICROWAVES

Thermal effects

The effects of heating on tissue have been detailed in Chapter 6, including some experimental evidence of effects due to microwave heating.

Non-thermal effects

Non-thermal biological reactions may be isolated using the pulsed mode of microwave at levels where the patient does not feel warmth. Whether or not heat is perceived in pulsed mode depends on the amount of energy absorbed. Energy absorption is dependent on the factors previously mentioned, the frequency and duration of pulses and the total power. Useful athermal effects remain ill defined. Moreover, it has not been established whether a low continuous dose has the same effects as the same average dose derived from pulsed microwave. Although there is some evidence of non-thermal microwave effects, including the *pearl chain effect* (alignment of molecules in the tissues), and neural excitability changes unrelated to the heating effect, there is no evidence at present that these have any physiotherapeutic relevance (Lehmann and de Lateur, 1990, 1999). (See Ch. 7 for a further discussion.)

Evidence of clinical efficacy

The few published clinical trials involving microwave irradiation did not describe the effects from readily available clinical apparatus. Weinberger *et al.* (1989), using 237 mm (915 MHz) microwave, achieved increased intra-articular tissue temperature to 41.3°C, reduced joint pain and increased walking time in patients with rheumatoid arthritis. They suggested that the heat may have potentiated the effects of the concurrent anti-inflammatory agents. Increased extensibility of collagenous tissue (Lehmann *et al.*, 1970) and reduced joint stiffness (Wright and Johns, 1961) have been reported following heating of a magnitude that might reasonably be expected from microwave apparatus. Using direct-contact 915 MHz microwave in conjunction with stretching activities, de Lateur, Stonebridge and Lehmann (1978) demonstrated lengthening of shortened quadriceps muscle.

PRINCIPLES OF APPLICATION IN CLINICAL PRACTICE

The principles of treatment are similar to those for short-wave diathermy.

Treatment preparation

Metal objects can function as aerials when acted on by microwave radiations. Therefore, metal furniture should not be used during microwave treatments. Microwaves may also interfere with other electronic equipment in the vicinity such as computers. Metal furniture and electronic equipment should be at least 3 m away.

Dosage

Safe microwave treatment first requires that the patient has normal skin pain and temperature sensation. As the patient's thermal sensation is the most important indicator of dosage, this must be tested in the area to be treated before commencing the first treatment. The chosen dosage, which should be based on the severity, type and progress of the disorder, is determined in the same way as for shortwave diathermy.

Hazards of microwaves

Microwave apparatus should be tested regularly for output and safety. (See Appendix.) The potential hazards of microwave treatments in physiotherapy are:

1. burns from:
   a. poor technique
   b. inability of tissues to dissipate heat
   c. inability of patient to detect heat (decreased thermal sensation)
   d. treatment over areas with surface or implanted metal
   e. treatment of moist open wounds, or over wet dressings—water concentrates microwaves
   f. treatment near the eyes, including the sinuses and temporomandibular joint (both 1e and 1f constitute a hazard owing to the high fluid volume; the high dielectric constant and conductivity of fluids increases the temperature locally)

2. exacerbation of symptoms following treatment of:
   a. inflammatory conditions
   b. infective disorders
   c. areas of increased fluid tension such as bursitis, oedema, synovial effusion
   d. haemorrhagic conditions—menstruation is unlikely to be affected by microwaves due to their limited penetration
   e. severe cardiac disease

3. cardiac failure due to electric shock or interference with cardiac pacemakers
4. spread of existing pathologies including tumours, active tuberculosis and acute infections
5. early pregnancy (first 3 months)—heat may be teratogenic.

Contraindications

Contraindications are identical to those for short-wave diathermy. The treating physiotherapist should not remain in the direct line of the beam or within 2 m of the director. Operators should also be conscious that reflection may be from 50 to 75% from the patient and nearly 100% from the metal of the apparatus.

REFERENCES

Australian National Health and Medical Research Council (1985) *Code of Practice for the Safe Use of Microwave Diathermy Units.* ANHMRC, Canberra.

Australian Standards Association (1992) *Australian Standard AS 3200.2.6 Particular Requirements for Safety—Microwave Therapy Equipment.* ASA, Sydney.

Canadian Department of Health and Welfare (1983) Shortwave diathermy guidelines for limited radio-frequency exposure, safety code 25. 83-EHD 98. DHW, Ottawa.

de Lateur, BJ, Stonebridge, JB, Lehmann, JF (1978) Fibrous muscular contractures: treatment with a new direct contact microwave applicator operating at 915MHz. *Archives of Physical Medicine and Rehabilitation* **59**: 488–490.

De Domenico, GD, Foord, I, Hadley, J, McMeeken, JM, Richardson, C (1990) Clinical standards for the use of electrophysical agents. *Australian Journal of Physiotherapy* **36**: 39–52.

Delpizzo, V, Joiner, KH (1987) On the safe use of microwave and shortwave diathermy units. *Australian Journal of Physiotherapy* **33**: 152–161.

Lehmann, JF, de Lateur, BJ (1990) Therapeutic heat. In: Lehmann, JF (ed) *Therapeutic Heat and Cold,* 4th edn. Williams & Wilkins, Baltimore, MD, pp 417–581.

Lehmann, JF, de Lateur, BJ (1999) Ultrasound, shortwave, microwave, laser, superficial heat and cold in the treatment of pain. In: Wall, PD, Melzack, R (eds) *Textbook of Pain,* 4th edn. Churchill Livingstone, New York, pp 1383–1397.

Lehmann, JF, McMillan, JA, Brunner, GD *et al.* (1962) Heating patterns produced in specimens by microwaves of the frequency of 2456 megacycles when applied with the 'A', 'B' and 'C' directors. *Archives of Physical Medicine and Rehabilitation* **43**: 538–546.

Lehmann, JF, Masock, A, Warren, CG *et al.* (1970) Effect of therapeutic temperatures on tendon extensibility. *Archives of Physical Medicine and Rehabilitation* **51**: 481–487.

McMeeken, JM, Bell, C (1990) Effects of microwave irradiation on blood flow in the dog hindlimb. *Experimental Physiology* **75**: 367–374.

National Radiation Protection Board (1989) Guidance as to restrictions on exposure to time varying electromagnetic fields and the 1988 recommendations of the International Non-ionising Radiation Committee. *NRPB Report GS 11.* HMSO, London.

Schwan, HP, Piersol, GM (1954) The absorption of electromagnetic energy in body tissues. Part 1: Biological aspects. *American Journal of Physical Medicine* **33**: 371–404.

Schwan, HP, Piersol, GM (1955) The absorption of electromagnetic energy in body tissues. Part 2: Physiological and clinical aspects. *American Journal of Physical Medicine* **34**: 425–448.

Ward, AR (1986) *Electricity Fields and Waves in Therapy.* Marrickville, Science Press, pp 232–234.

Weinberger, A, Fadilah, R, Lev, A *et al.* (1989) Treatment of articular effusions with local deep hyperthermia. *Clinical Rheumatology* **8**: 461–466.

Wright, W, Johns, RJ (1961) Quantitative and qualitative analysis of joint stiffness in normal subjects and in patients with connective tissue diseases. *Annals of Rheumatic Diseases* **20**: 30–46.

12

Low-intensity laser therapy

David Baxter

BRIEF HISTORY

The term 'laser' is an acronym for Light Amplification by Stimulated Emission of Radiation. Although Albert Einstein originally outlined the principles underlying the generation of such light in the early part of this century, it was not until 1960 that Theodore Maiman produced the first burst of ruby laser light at Hughes Laboratories in the USA. In the intervening decades, various laser devices based upon Maiman's original prototype have found applications ranging from laser pointers and bar code readers to military range finders and target acquisition systems.

Since their inception, lasers have found application in medicine and particularly in surgery: ophthalmic surgeons were the first specialty to use the pulsed ruby laser successfully for the treatment of detached retina in humans. In general, most medical applications to date have relied upon the photothermal and photoablative interactions of laser with tissue; thus lasers are routinely used to cut, weld and even destroy tissue. The use of lasers as alternatives to metal scalpels, as well as for tumour ablation and tattoo removal, are all based upon such tissue reactions. In contrast, interest has also focused on the potential clinical applications of the non-thermal interactions of laser light with tissue, principally based upon initial work carried out by Professor Endre Mester's group in Budapest during the late 1960s and early 1970s. Results of this work indicated the potential of relatively low-intensity laser irradiation applied directly to tissue to modulate certain biological processes—in particular to photobiostimulate wound-healing processes (Mester, Mester and Mester, 1985). Based upon Mester's work in animals and in patients, the ensuing decade saw the promotion of He–Ne laser radiation as the treatment of choice for a variety of conditions throughout the countries of the former Soviet Union, and in the Far East, particularly China. Within the last 10–15 years, the introduction of small, compact laser-emitting photodiodes has produced an increase in the use of this therapy, known as low-level or low-intensity laser therapy (LILT) in the West. Although the Food and Drug Administration (FDA) in the USA has still to approve laser therapy, the modality has found increasing application by physiotherapists (for human and animal use), dentists, acupuncturists, podiatrists, and some physicians, for a range of conditions including the treatment of open wounds, soft tissue injuries, arthritic conditions and pain associated with various aetiologies (see Baxter *et al.*, 1991).

DEFINITIONS AND NOMENCLATURE

Low-intensity laser therapy (Baxter, 1994) or low-(reactive)level laser therapy (Ohshiro and Calderhead, 1988), is a generic term that defines the therapeutic application of relatively low-output ($< 500\,$mW) lasers and monochromatic superluminous diodes for the treatment of disease and injury at dosages (usually $< 35\,$J/cm^2) generally considered to be too low to effect any detectable heating of the irradiated tissues. Low-intensity laser therapy is thus an athermal treatment modality. For this reason, this modality has also sometimes (inappropriately) been termed 'soft' or 'cold' laser therapy to distinguish the devices (and the resulting applications) from high-power sources of the type used in surgery and in other medical and dental applications; however, such terms are misleading and inappropriate, and are therefore best avoided.

This modality is also frequently referred to as laser (photo)biostimulation, particularly in the USA, where the term is sometimes abbreviated to 'biostim'. The use of such terminology is essentially based upon the early observations of Mester's group and others, which suggested the potential of such devices to accelerate selectively various wound healing processes and cellular functions. However, the term is inappropriate to define the modality for two reasons. In the first instance, the applications of the modality exceed merely the treatment of wounds. Furthermore, and more importantly, lasers also have the potential, even at therapeutic intensities, to inhibit cellular processes (i.e. laser *photobioinhibition*; see section on Arndt–Schultz law below); thus a more accurate generic term for the biological effects of low intensity laser irradiation is laser photobiomodulation.

PHYSICAL PRINCIPLES

Light emission and absorption, and the production of laser radiation

The basis of production of stimulated emission is summarised in Figure 12.1.

- In non-laser sources, light is typically produced by *spontaneous emission of radiation* (Fig. 12.1A). In such circumstances, the atoms and molecules comprising the central emitter in such devices (e.g. the element/filament in a typical household light bulb) are stimulated with (electrical) energy so that the electrons shift to higher energy orbits. Once in such orbits, the electrons are inherently unstable and fall spontaneously within a short period of time to lower energy levels and in so doing release their extra energy as photons of light. The properties of the emitted photons are determined by the difference in energy levels (or valence bands) through which an excited electron 'dropped', as the difference in energy will be exactly the same as the quantal energy of the photon produced. As, for a given photon of light, the quantal energy (specified in electron-volts) is inversely related to the wavelength (in nm), the wavelength is effectively determined by the difference in valence bands; and in turn, molecules produce typical

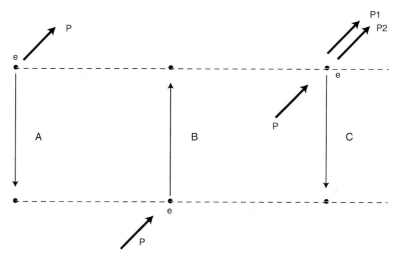

Figure 12.1 Spontaneous emission, absorption and stimulated emission of light. A: Spontaneous emission: excited electron (e) drops to lower (resting) level, emitting a single photon (P). B: Absorption: incident photon is absorbed by resting electron, which moves to higher level. C: Stimulated emission: incident photon interacts with already excited electron to produce two identical photons (P1, P2).

ranges of wavelengths or emission spectra when appropriately stimulated.

- *Absorption of radiation* occurs when a photon of light interacts with an atom or molecule in which the difference in energy of the valence bands exactly equals the energy carried by the photon (Fig. 12.1B). This has two consequences: for a photon of a given quantal energy (and thus wavelength) only certain molecules will be capable of absorbing the light radiation; conversely, for a given molecule, only certain quantal energies (and thus wavelengths) can be absorbed (this is termed the *absorption spectrum* for the molecule). Thus absorption is said to be *wavelength specific*. This is an important concept in LILT applications, as this wavelength specificity of absorption effectively determines which types of tissue will preferentially absorb incident radiation, and (in turn) the depth of penetration of a particular treatment unit.

- *Stimulated emission of radiation* is a unique event which occurs when an incident photon interacts with an atom which is already excited (i.e. where the electron(s) are already in a higher energy orbit); additionally, the quantal energy of the incident photon must exactly equal the difference in energy levels between the electron's excited and resting states (see Figure 12.1C). Under these exceptional circumstances the electron, in returning to its original orbit, gives off its excess energy as a photon of light with exactly the same properties as the incident photon, and completely in phase. In laser devices, the unique circumstances which give rise to stimulated emission of radiation are produced through the selection of an appropriate material or substance which, when electrically stimulated, will produce large numbers of identical photons through the rapid excitation of the medium. In order to produce such stimulated emission of radiation, laser treatment devices rely upon three essential components:

1. *A lasing medium* is capable of being 'pumped' with energy to ultimately produce stimulated emission; for therapeutic systems, the energy source is invariably electrical, and the energy is delivered to the medium typically from the mains or (less commonly) from a battery (see below). The two media most commonly used in LILT applications are the gaseous mixture of helium and neon (He–Ne) operating at a wavelength of 632.8 nm (i.e. red light), or gallium arsenide (Ga–As) or gallium–aluminium–arsenide

(GaAIAs) semiconductors typically producing radiation at 630–950 nm (i.e. visible red to the near infrared). Although He–Ne systems were the first to be used for LILT applications, and a significant percentage of the papers published within this area are based upon such devices, their use has diminished considerably over the last decade; thus, very few He–Ne lasers, which can be regarded as the 'first generation' of laser therapy systems, currently find application in routine physiotherapeutic practice, at least in Britain or Ireland. This is due to the relative expense of such units, and the comparatively low power output associated with He–Ne systems. In addition, the relatively greater collimation (see below) of these units when applied without fibre-optic applicators poses a significant hazard to the unprotected eye compared with the average semiconductor-diode-based treatment unit.

2. *A resonating cavity* or chamber consisting of a structure to contain the lasing medium and incorporating a pair of parallel reflecting surfaces or mirrors. Within this chamber, photons of light produced by the medium are reflected back and forth between the 'mirrors' to ultimately produce an intense photon resonance. As one of the reflecting surfaces (also termed the output coupler) is not a 'pure' mirror and so does not reflect 100% of the light striking its surface, some of the radiation is allowed to pass through as the output of the device. While the resonating cavity for an He–Ne unit can be relatively large and cumbersome, those for diode-based units are tiny, being the lasing medium itself (i.e. the semiconductor diode), the ends of which are carefully polished to form reflecting surfaces. This has important implications for the routine use of these units in clinical practice, as the treatment 'head' or 'probe' is usually not much larger than the size of a pen and represents another reason why diode-based units, which may be regarded as the 'second generation' of laser therapy system development, are so popular with clinicians. Furthermore, several manufacturers incorporate a number of diodes (up to 180 diodes) into multisource 'cluster' arrays in order to allow simultaneous treatment of larger lesions

and (in some cases) to allow several wavelengths of radiation to be used in parallel (Fig. 12.2). Such multisource cluster units may be usefully regarded as the 'third generation' of development for therapeutic lasers. More recently, several manufacturers have introduced 'fourth-generation' flexible multisource arrays to allow more efficient delivery of light to tissue surfaces with 'hands-free' application.

It should be noted that, for He–Ne based systems, because the resonating cavity is usually more cumbersome to apply, the laser radiation from the output coupler is normally delivered to the tissue to be treated by means of a fibre-optic applicator. This allows the operator to direct the radiation to the target tissue more easily.

3. A *power source* to 'pump' the lasing media to produce stimulated emission. In most cases, therapeutic devices have tended to be mains supplied and incorporate a base unit to contain the transformer and control unit (Fig. 12.2). More recently, however, a number of manufacturers have produced rechargeable and battery-powered units to enhance the portability of their laser devices (e.g. for sports injuries applications).

Characteristics of laser radiation

The radiation generated by therapeutic laser devices differs from that produced by other

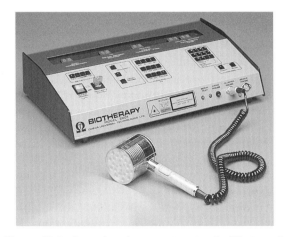

Figure 12.2 A modern laser treatment unit. (Photograph courtesy of Central Medical Equipment, Nottingham.)

similar sources (e.g. infrared lamps) in the following three respects.

Monochromaticity

The light produced by a laser is 'single coloured', the majority of the radiation emitted by the treatment device being clustered around a single wavelength with a very narrow band width. In contrast, light generated by other sources comprises a wide variety of wavelengths, sometimes ranging from the ultraviolet to the infrared, which result in the sensation of the colour white when the light strikes the retina of a human observer. Wavelength is a critical factor in determining the therapeutic effects produced by laser treatments, as this parameter determines which specific biomolecules will absorb the incident radiation, and thus the basic photobiological interaction underlying any given treatment effect.

Collimation

In laser light, the rays of light or photons produced by the laser device are for all practical purposes parallel, with almost no divergence of the emitted radiation over distance. This property keeps the optical power of the device 'bundled' on to a relatively small area over considerable distances, and, to a degree, even when passing through tissue.

Coherence

The light emitted by laser devices is also in phase, so in conjunction with the two unique properties already outlined above, the troughs and peaks of the emitted light waves match perfectly in time (temporal coherence) and in space (spatial coherence). The biological and clinical relevance of this property is still debated (e.g. see Karu, 1998; Tuner and Hode, 1999), not least because of the availability of so-called 'superluminous diodes' which possess all the qualities of a 'true' laser diode, less the coherence, but which are a fraction of the cost of the latter. Multisource third- and fourth-generation cluster

treatment units incorporating some 30 or 40 diodes would be prohibitively expensive for routine clinical use if they comprised nothing other than true laser diodes; thus these units typically incorporate no more than several laser diodes, the remainder being superluminous diodes.

Laser–tissue interaction

As already indicated above, laser–tissue interaction is typically associated with the potentially destructive effects of irradiation at relatively high power and energy levels; in these circumstances, high densities of laser light from highly collimated or focused sources with output in the watt range can easily produce photothermal reactions in tissues, including ablative or explosive effects. However, in low-intensity laser therapy, the emphasis is by definition upon the non-thermal (or athermal) reactions of light with tissue. Light from a laser or monochromatic light therapy treatment device can interact with irradiated tissue in two ways:

1. **Scattering of incident light.** This is essentially a change in the direction of propagation of the light as it passes through the tissues, and is due to the variability in the refractive indices of tissue components relative to water. Such scattering will cause a 'widening' of the beam as it passes through irradiated tissue, and result in the rapid loss of coherence.

2. **Absorption of incident light by a chromophore.** A chromophore is a biomolecule which is capable, through its electronic or atomic configuration, of being excited by the incident photon(s). Light at the wavelengths typically employed in LILT are readily absorbed by a variety of biomolecules including melanin and haemoglobin; as a consequence, the penetration depth associated with treatment devices is limited to no more than several millimetres. It should be noted that, as the absorption is dependent upon the wavelength of incident light, the depth of penetration is similarly wavelength dependent.

Of these two modes of interaction, absorption may be regarded as the most important in terms of the photobiological basis of laser therapy, as without absorption no photobiological, and thus clinical, effects would be possible.

Conceptual basis of laser photobiomodulation: the Arndt–Schultz law

The photobiological effects of laser or mono-chromatic light upon tissue are many and complex, and to a large degree still poorly understood, particularly in terms of the variable stimulative/inhibitory reactions which may be effected by such irradiation. In providing a theoretical basis for the observed biological and clinical effects of this modality, the Arndt–Schultz law has been proposed as a suitable model; the main tenets of this law are illustrated in Figure 12.3. It should be stressed, however, that although this model can account for such phenomena as the 'inverse' dosage dependency reported in some papers (e.g. Lowe *et al.*, 1994) it essentially applies to radiant exposure (or energy density—see below); the putative relevance of manipulation of other irradiation parameters such as pulse repetition rate or power output remains, at least for the time being, a matter of debate.

BIOLOGICAL AND PHYSIOLOGICAL EFFECTS

Investigations of the biological and physiological effects of low-intensity laser radiation can usefully be considered under three main areas: cellular studies involving the use of well-established cell lines and explanted cells, studies in various species of animals (in vivo and in vitro), and finally research in healthy human volunteers.

Whilst the following provides an overview of the findings to date in these areas, a full and comprehensive review of the literature on the biological and physiological effects of low-intensity laser radiation is beyond the scope of this book; for further detail the reader is directed to the reviews of Basford (1989, 1995), Baxter (1994), Karu (1998), King (1990), Kitchen and Partridge (1991), Shields and O'Kane (1994), and Tuner and Hode (1999).

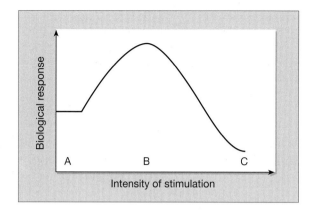

Figure 12.3 The Arndt–Schultz law. A: Prethreshold: no biological activation (resting). B: Biostimulation: activation of biological processes. C: Bioinhibition: inhibition of biological processes.

Cellular research

A range of studies have examined the effects of low-intensity laser irradiation in a variety of cell lines and explanted cells to establish the photobiological basis for the clinical use of this modality, especially for the promotion of wound healing. In these studies a number of possible indicators have been used to assess the photobiomodulatory effects of laser irradiation, including cell proliferation (Bolton, Young and Dyson, 1995; Boulton and Marshall, 1986; Hallman *et al.*, 1988; Loevschall and Arenholt-Bindslev, 1994), collagen production (Castro *et al.*, 1983; Lam *et al.*, 1986) and ultrastructural changes (Bosatra *et al.*, 1984; Manteifel and Karu, 1992). Because of their importance in wound repair, the cells most commonly used to date have been fibroblasts and macrophages (e.g. O'Kane *et al.*, 1994; Pogrel, Chen and Zang, 1997). However, it should be stressed that although findings from such studies are generally positive, the findings are not exclusively favourable nor straightforward; results in some cell types have tended to be more variable—for instance, research on lymphocytes has shown variable effects as a result of laser irradiation (Hallman *et al.*, 1988; Manteifel & Karu, 1992; Ohta *et al.*, 1987; Yamaguchi, Trukamoto and Matono, 1994).

Cellular studies such as those outlined above are important in two respects. In the first instance they provide a scientific basis for the clinical application of low-intensity lasers for the management of wounds, through demonstration of the photobiological mechanisms underlying such treatments (Karu, 1998). Secondly, by using such well-controlled laboratory research techniques, systematic investigations by some groups have demonstrated the importance of laser irradiation parameters such as wavelength, dosage, and pulse repetition rate to the observed effects (e.g. Agaiby *et al.*, 1996; O'Kane *et al.*, 1994; Rajaratnam, Bolton and Dyson, 1994; van Breugel, Engels and Bar, 1993).

This notwithstanding, the extrapolation of findings from this type of study to the clinical setting is difficult, as the precise relevance of the reported observations to clinical treatments is not always entirely clear. For example, where photobiostimulatory effects are reported at a radiant exposure of $1.5 J/cm^2$ in a laboratory study involving the direct irradiation of artificially maintained murine macrophage-like cell lines, what direct relevance has this for dosage selection in the laser treatment of a venous ulcer in a 67-year-old patient? Given such problems, particularly the vast difference between the cell lines and the highly complicated microenvironment of the clinical wound, a number of groups have employed animal studies and experimental studies on healthy human volunteers to further assess the biological and physiological effects of this modality in the laboratory.

Animal studies

To date, animal studies have concentrated on two main areas of research: the photobiostimulative effects of laser irradiation upon wound healing and tissue repair in experimentally induced lesions, and the neurophysiological and in particular the antinociceptive effects of such irradiation. For the former studies, small loose-skinned animals such as rats and mice have been most commonly used (e.g. Lyons *et al.*, 1987; Mester, Mester and Mester, 1985); in these species, a range of experimental wounds have been employed including muscle injuries (Mester *et al.*, 1975), burns (Rochkind *et al.*, 1989), tendon

injuries (Enwemeka *et al.*, 1990) and open skin wounds of various types (Abergel, Lyons and Castel, 1987; Haina *et al.*, 1982; Mester, Mester and Mester, 1985; Walker *et al.*, 2000). Although these studies have typically reported positive effects of laser irradiation (in terms of increased rates of healing, wound closure, enhanced granulation tissue formation, etc.), the experimental lesions in these animals are considered to represent a poor model for wounds in humans because of the species differences in tegument compared with humans (Basford, 1989; King, 1990). As a consequence, some investigators have preferred to use porcine wound healing as a more appropriate experimental assay to study the potential benefits of laser irradiation for management of wounds in humans, with more variable findings (Abergel, Lyons and Castel, 1987; Hunter *et al.*, 1984). Thus, although findings from animal research has generally demonstrated biostimulative effects upon wound healing, particularly in rodents, the findings are not exclusively positive. The effects of laser irradiation upon tissue repair in experimental muscle lesions has also been investigated, with positive results (Morrone *et al.*, 1998); this represents an important finding, particularly given the widespread use of laser therapy in sports rehabilitation.

Perhaps the most interesting aspect of this type of animal work has been reports, principally by Rochkind's group, of the potential of laser irradiation to accelerate regeneration of nerves, together with associated electrophysiological and functional recovery, after various types of experimental lesions (e.g. Khullar *et al.*, 1994; Rochkind *et al.*, 1989). If such effects are also possible in humans, the implications for future applications of this modality would be enormous; interestingly, Rochkind's group has conducted some limited clinical work in humans using relatively high dosages ($>100 J/cm^2$) with encouraging preliminary results in both peripheral and central nerve lesions (Rochkind *et al.*, 1994a, b).

Neurophysiological and antinociceptive effects of laser irradiation have also been investigated in a variety of species. In particular, withdrawal and avoidance behaviours such as the tail-flick and hot-plate tests have been used to assess hypoalgesic effects of laser irradiation, its mechanism of action and dependence upon the pulse repetition rate used (e.g. Ponnudurai et al., 1988; Ponnudurai, Zbuzek and Wu, 1987; Wu, 1983). These studies consistently demonstrated a significant hypoalgesic effect of laser irradiation, in terms of increased latency to tail flick or paw lick, which was found to be most pronounced at the lower pulse repetition rates (4 Hz; Ponnudurai, Zbuzek and Wu, 1987). Furthermore, the hypoalgesia was found not to be reversible when the opiate antagonist naloxone was administered, which suggests that the observed pain relief was not mediated by endogenous opiates (Ponnudurai et al., 1988). However, the hypoalgesic effects of laser irradiation, at least in animals, are not straightforward, as one group has also reported laser-mediated *hyperalgesic* effects in experimental mice using a hot-plate paradigm to assess pain relief (Zarkovic et al., 1989).

It can thus be seen that animal studies have provided some evidence of beneficial effects of laser irradiation upon experimental wounds and pain. Although studies in animals such as those outlined above do go some way towards bridging the gap between cellular work and clinical practice, some of the problems in extrapolating and applying the findings to humans remain. As a consequence, several groups have used controlled studies in healthy human volunteers as a useful means of investigation without recourse to patients and the considerable problems inherent in undertaking controlled clinical research.

Controlled studies in humans

Studies in this area have focused principally on the physiological and hypoalgesic effects of laser radiation. This approach has been particularly useful in investigating the effects of laser upon peripheral nerves; while early studies provided contradictory findings (e.g. Greathouse et al., 1985; Snyder-Mackler and Bork, 1988; Walker and Akhanjee, 1985; Wu et al., 1987), more recent studies have demonstrated significant

effects upon peripheral nerve conduction in the median and superficial radial nerves which would appear to be critically dependent upon the dosage and pulse repetition rate of the laser source (Basford et al., 1993; Baxter et al., 1994; Lowe et al., 1994; Walsh, 1993). Although these papers typically report changes in nerve conduction latencies or velocities in response to laser irradiation applied to the skin overlying the course of the nerve, the precise relevance of such observations to the clinical applications of this modality are debatable. Of more direct relevance to clinical practice, a number of studies have assessed the effects of laser upon various types of experimentally induced pain in humans. These studies have essentially relied upon two main types of pain induction: thermal pain threshold and the submaximal effort tourniquet technique. Noxious heat stimulation has been used by several groups to assess the efficacy of single-diode laser application, applied directly to the site of noxious stimulation or to appropriate acupuncture points, with variable findings (e.g. Brockhaus and Elger, 1990; Seibert and Gould, 1984); in particular the latter study found the hypoalgesic effects of needle acupuncture to be significantly superior to laser acupuncture. Variable findings have also been obtained with experimentally induced ischaemic pain; significant hypoalgesic effects upon this model of pain have been reported with combined phototherapy/low-intensity laser therapy using a multiwavelength, multisource 'cluster' array at radiant exposures of over $30 \, \text{J/cm}^2$ (e.g. Mokhtar et al., 1992), but not with low-intensity laser applied using a single (830 nm) diode (Lowe et al., 1997).

CLINICAL STUDIES

Although a large number of clinical studies have been completed and published in this area, in the main with positive results, reviewers have consistently noted the following problems with the literature:

- most studies have been published in foreign language journals, often without English abstracts, making the work inaccessible to anglophone researchers and clinicians

- the studies reported in the literature (regardless of language) are often poorly controlled with only very limited blinding; indeed a significant proportion of the studies is merely anecdotal in nature
- the irradiation parameters and treatment protocols used are frequently inadequately specified, thus limiting comparison of results and rendering replication and application in the clinical setting impossible. Even where irradiation parameters are specified, the bewildering number of possible permutations and combinations of wavelength, irradiance, pulse repetition rate, etc. will often mean that precise replication is problematic.

This notwithstanding, it is important to stress that the published database of clinical studies on low-intensity laser therapy represents a significant body of anecdotal evidence in favour of the modality; while the constraints of the current text precludes an exhaustive review of this literature, the following at least provides an overview of some of the most relevant papers to date.

Wound healing

The popularity of laser therapy among physiotherapists for the treatment of various types of wounds is witnessed by the results of the only large scale survey of current clinical practice in this field (Baxter et al., 1991). Treatment of various types of chronic ulceration was the first application for low-intensity laser to be trialled in humans during the late 1960s and early 1970s (see Mester and Mester, 1989), using He–Ne sources and dosages of up to 4 J/cm^2; it was based upon the reported success of these early studies, in terms of enhanced rates of wound healing and pain reduction, that the modality quickly achieved popularity in this application. In the ensuing decades, laser therapy has been assessed in the treatment of a variety of wounds and ulcerated lesions with positive results, especially when applied in more chronic, intractable cases (e.g. Karu, 1985; Lagan, Baxter

and Ashford, 1998; Robinson and Walters, 1991; Sugrue et al., 1990). However, given that many of the reports to date are poorly controlled and based upon relatively small numbers, and furthermore that results are not exclusively positive (e.g. Santioanni et al., 1984), additional studies are warranted to establish definitively the benefit of this modality for the promotion of wound healing, and particularly the relevance of irradiation parameters to such effects.

Arthritic conditions

The potential benefit of laser therapy in the management of such conditions as rheumatoid arthritis, osteoarthritis and arthrogenic pain has been assessed by a number of groups with varying degrees of success reported. Although several papers have reported decreased joint pain and inflammation coupled with increased functional status in rheumatoid joints after treatment with a low output Nd–YAG laser (Goldman et al., 1980; Vidovich and Olson, 1987), it is important to stress that such units, which are typically used at higher output levels for surgical applications, are not suitable for routine use in physiotherapeutic laser therapy. Using the more commonly available He–Ne and diode-based units, a number of groups have reported significant decreases in pain with concomitant improvements in function as a result of laser treatment of these patients (Lonauer, 1986; Palmgren et al., 1989; Trelles et al., 1991; Walker et al., 1987). Equally, however, several groups have failed to find any significant benefit of laser treatment in well-controlled and reported trials (Basford et al., 1987; Bliddal et al., 1987; Jensen, Harreby and Kjer, 1987). While the precise reasons for such discrepancies are not entirely clear, it may be due in part to the differences in laser parameters employed in these studies and in particular the relatively low-power output units used in some of the latter studies (<1 mW). Thus, despite some promising findings, this is another area in which further research would appear to be indicated before more definitive pronouncements on efficacy are possible (Brosseau *et al.*, 2000; Marks and de Palma, 1999).

Musculoskeletal disorders

Given the evidence of the potential biostimulative effects of laser irradiation at the cellular and clinical level, it is not surprising that a number of groups have assessed the efficacy of these devices in the management of a range of musculoskeletal disorders. Laser therapy for tendinopathies has been investigated by several groups with both positive (England *et al.*, 1989) and negative (Siebert *et al.*, 1987) findings being reported. However, the disparate findings between these two studies may in part be explained by the irradiation techniques used, in that the investigators in the latter study inappropriately employed a non-contact technique (see below), using the laser source at a distance of some 10 cm from the target tissue; this would have significantly reduced the intensity of radiation on the tissue (i.e. irradiance) and thus the effectiveness of the applied laser treatment in this trial. Similarly, the use of inappropriately low dosage levels may in part explain the non-significant results reported by some groups in the laser treatment of other musculoskeletal conditions such as myofascial pain (Waylonis *et al.*, 1988) and lateral epicondylitis (Lundeberg, Haker and Thomas, 1987), compared with the typically positive findings at other centres (Choi, Srikantha and Wu, 1986; Glykofridis and Diamantopoulos, 1987; Li, 1990). However, it should be stressed that, although the former studies may be criticised on the basis of their use of inappropriate irradiation parameters, these studies were in the main better designed and controlled than many of the case-series type of paper typically published in this area.

Pain

Early observations of concomitant reductions in reported pain in wound patients treated with laser led to attempts at exploitation and investigation of the analgesic effects of this modality. Apart from decreases in pain associated with the laser-mediated treatment effects documented in those studies already indicated above, a number of groups have also reported analgesic effects of laser irradiation in various types of chronic pain as well as in neuropathic and neurogenic pain syndromes (Amoils and Kues, 1991; Lukashevich, 1985; Moore *et al.*, 1988; Shiroto, Ono and Onshiro, 1989; Walker, 1983). However, and despite such positive reports, the treatment of pain remains one of the most contentious areas of laser application, particularly in terms of the management of chronic pain syndromes; while the reasons for scepticism are essentially those already identified, the lack of an obvious mechanism of action further confounds acceptance of the pain-relieving effects of this modality (see Devor, 1990). This notwithstanding, the modality has become a popular treatment method with physiotherapists for the relief of pain, and one which is highly rated against alternative electrotherapeutic modalities (Baxter *et al.*, 1991). Furthermore, a recent report from Basford's centre indicates potential benefits in the management of low back pain, at least with the use of defocused high-power sources at therapeutic intensities (Basford, Sheffield and Harmsen, 1999).

PRINCIPLES OF CLINICAL APPLICATION

Indications

Laser therapy finds a variety of applications in clinical practice; these can be usefully summarised under the following headings:

1. stimulation of wound healing in various types of open wounds
2. treatment of various arthritic conditions
3. treatment of soft tissue injuries
4. relief of pain.

These are considered in outline below, after an overview of the principles underlying effective laser treatment. As a basis for subsequent sections and to aid the reader in more critical review of the work published in this area, the method of calculating dosage and the importance of other irradiation parameters are presented below.

Dosage and irradiation parameters

Apart from wavelength, which is determined by the lasing medium used in the device, the other irradiation parameters that appear to be important in laser treatments are as follows.

Power output

The power output of a unit is usually expressed in milliwatts (mW), or thousandths of a watt. This is usually fixed and invariable. However, some machines allow operator selection of the percentage of the total power output (e.g. 10%, 25%, etc.); in addition, where pulsing of the output is provided as an option by the manufacturer, this can have profound effects upon the power output of the unit in some instances. Over the last decade, the trend in commercially available units has been towards higher-output devices (30–200 mW), rather than the once-popular 1–10 mW devices, not least because higher-output units can deliver a specified treatment in a much shorter period of time.

Irradiance (power density)

The power per unit area (mW/cm^2) is an important irradiation parameter, which is usually kept as high as possible for a given unit by the so-called 'in-contact' treatment technique, and applying a firm pressure through the treatment head during treatment. It should be noted that, even with the small degrees of divergence associated with laser treatment devices, treatment out of contact with the target tissue will significantly reduce the effectiveness of treatment as the irradiance falls owing to the inverse square law (see Fig. 11.14, p. 168) and because of increased reflection from the skin or tissue interface. For in-contact treatments, the irradiance is simply calculated by dividing the power output (or average power output for a pulsed unit) by the spot size of the treatment head; typical values for the latter are 0.1–0.125 cm^2.

Energy

This is given in joules (J) and is usually specified per point irradiated, or sometimes for the 'total' treatment where a number of points are treated. It is calculated by multiplying the power output in watts by the time of irradiation or application in seconds. Thus a 30 mW (i.e. 0.03 W) device applied for 1 minute (i.e. 60 s) will deliver 1.8 J of energy. Dosage is recorded in joules per point, as well as total joules for the treatment.

Radiant exposure (energy density)

This is generally considered to be the best means of specifying dosage, at least for research papers, and is given in joules per unit area (i.e. J/cm^2); typical values for routine treatments may range from less than one to over 30 J/cm^2; however 1–12 J/cm^2 would be most commonly used (see below). Energy density is usually calculated by dividing the energy delivered (in joules) by the spot size of the treatment unit (in cm).

Pulse repetition rate

Although a large percentage of the laser units routinely used in clinical practice are continuous wave (CW) output (i.e. the output power is essentially invariable over time), most units currently available in the UK allow some form of pulsing of their output. For pulsed units, the pulse repetition rate is expressed in hertz (Hz, pulses per second). Typical values for pulse repetition rate can vary from 2 to tens of thousands of Hz. Although the potential biological and clinical relevance of pulse repetition rate is still far from being universally accepted, cellular research would suggest that this parameter is critical to at least some of the biological effects of this modality (e.g. Rajaratnam, Bolton and Dyson, 1994).

Importance of the use of contact technique

Although the method of application may vary depending on the presenting condition, wherever possible the treatment head or probe should be applied with a firm pressure to the area of tissue to be treated (Fig. 12.4). In the first instance, this makes the laser treatment inherently safer by reducing the potential for accidental intrabeam viewing, as indicated elsewhere. However, the primary reason for using so-called contact technique is to maximise the irradiance or power density on the tissue surface, and thus the light flux within the target tissue, which are important in ensuring the effectiveness of laser treatment. Where the treatment head is used out of contact, the light flux within the tissue is reduced owing to several factors; most importantly, the inverse square law applies to such non-contact applications, leading to reduced incident irradiance on surface of the irradiated tissue. Furthermore, more reflection of incident photons will occur where the probe is not maintained directly in contact with the tissue (Fig. 12.4).

Apart from producing the highest levels of light flux within the tissue, application of contact technique will also allow the operator to press the treatment probe into the tissues to treat deeper-seated lesions more effectively. As well as compensating for the relatively limited penetration of therapeutic laser devices by approximating the treatment probe with the target tissue, the deep pressure will drive red blood cells from the area of tissue directly under the probe head and thus reduce the attenuation of light due to absorption by such cells.

Application of the laser treatment probe also affords the opportunity of applying pressure treatments to key points (e.g. trigger or acupoints) and thus effectively combines laser with acupressure-type treatments; indeed, 'laser acupuncture' has long been proposed as a viable alternative (and non-invasive) means of stimulating acupuncture points (Wong and Fung, 1991). Despite the above, there are situations where laser treatment cannot be applied using contact technique; principally these are where such application would be too painful or aseptic technique is required (e.g. in cases of open wounds). Less commonly, the contours of the tissue to be treated may not allow use of a so-called 'cluster' head in full contact, thus non-contact technique must be used. Where this is the case, the treatment head should not be held more than 0.5–1 cm from the surface of the target tissue.

Treatment of open wounds and ulcers

The treatment of open wounds and ulcers represents the cardinal application for low-intensity laser devices, and combined phototherapy/low-intensity laser therapy units (Fig. 12.5). For comprehensive treatment of such conditions,

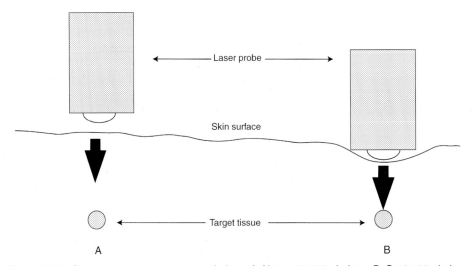

Figure 12.4 Contact versus non-contact technique. A: Non-contact technique. B: Contact technique.

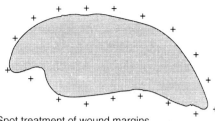

Spot treatment of wound margins

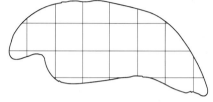

Gridding technique for wound bed

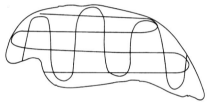

Treatment of wound margins and bed with 'cluster' array

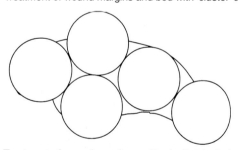

Treatment of wound margins and bed with 'cluster' array

Figure 12.5 Laser treatment of wounds. Wound margin is treated with single probe using contact technique (1 cm from wound; 2 cm intervals); wound bed is treated using non-contact technique, using either gridding or scanning technique (single-diode probe) or multidiode 'cluster' unit.

irradiation is applied in two stages: the first using standard contact technique around the edges of the wound, the second during which the wound bed is treated using non-contact technique.

Treatment of wound margins

For this a single-diode probe is the ideal unit to apply treatment around the circumference of

wound at approximately 1–2 cm from its edges. Points of application should be no more than 2–3 cm apart, and the treatment unit should be applied with a firm pressure to the intact skin within the patient's tolerances.

For such treatments of the wound margins, dosages should be of no more than 1 J per point, or approximately 10 J/cm^2.

Treatment of the wound bed

As already indicated above, treatment of the wound bed will invariably be completed using non-contact technique. As the wound lacks the usual protective layer of dermis, the dosages applied during treatment will be much lower than during application over intact skin, and typically cited radiant exposures are somewhere in the range of 1–10 J/cm^2, with 4 J/cm^2 being most commonly recommended as the so-called 'Mester protocol' based upon the pioneering work of Professor Endre Mester's group.

However, the problem of applying such a dosage in a standardised fashion across the surface of an open wound is obvious and has led to several means of application being recommended in these conditions. At the simplest level, where only a single probe or fibre-optic applicator is available, the wound may be 'mapped' with a hypothetical grid of equal-sized squares (typically 1–2 cm square), each of which may be regarded as an individual area of target tissue and treatment applied accordingly at the recommended dosage. In order to standardise the 'grid', some therapists have employed acetate sheets marked with a grid, upon which the outline of the wound can also be traced at regular intervals as a method of recording the progress of the patient's lesion to treatment. Alternatively, a clear plastic sheet with holes drilled in a regular grid has also been successfully used in some units as a means of standardising wound treatments; in such cases, the size of the holes corresponds to the circumference of the tip of the laser treatment probe, which is applied in sequence to each of the holes overlying the wound, for the time required to deliver the prescribed dosage.

Apart from such gridding, some therapists have also employed some variant of scanning technique to treat the wound bed where single-diode or fibre-optic applicators are used. In these cases, the probe is moved slowly over the area of the lesion using a non-contact technique while taking care to deliver a standardised radiant exposure to all areas, and to maintain the head at a distance of no more than 1 cm from the wound bed. Perhaps not surprisingly, most therapists find this technique difficult to perform, and thus it is increasingly rare to find units where manual scanning treatments are performed.

Special devices for treatment of wounds

Given the problems inherent in performing effective standardised laser irradiation of wound beds, a number of special devices have been produced and marketed in an attempt to simplify and improve the efficacy of such treatments. In the first instance, several manufacturers have produced scanning devices that may be used in conjunction with their treatment units; these scanners mechanically direct the output of the device over an area defined by the operator by means of controls on the scanning unit. While such devices have been popular in some circles in offering a 'hands off' approach to providing a well-standardised treatment across the whole wound area, particularly in cases of more extensive wounds (e.g. burns), the relatively high cost and potentially greater hazards associated with these units have prevented them becoming as popular as they perhaps might otherwise be.

As an alternative to scanners, a number of manufacturers now provide the option of so called 'cluster' units, typically incorporating an array of diodes in a single hand-held unit. The number of diodes provided in these clusters varies between 3 and almost 200, but it is generally true that the larger units incorporate a mixture of superluminous (monochromatic) diodes as well as (true) laser sources in their arrays, due to the prohibitive cost of the latter. Such cluster units allow simultaneous treatment of an area of tissue, the extent of which is decided by the number and configuration of the diodes included in the array. Furthermore, several manufacturers have incorporated diodes operating at a variety of wavelengths (i.e. multisource/multiwavelength arrays) in their cluster units, claiming enhanced clinical effects through parallel (and possibly synergistic) wavelength-specific effects. In routine clinical practice, the relative difficulty in treating extensive ulceration with single-diode units has led to cluster units being frequently cited as the most popular units by therapists (see Baxter *et al.*, 1991). In treating wound beds, cluster units can be used in isolation or in conjunction with single probes to access deeper or recessed areas, and in either case present a more time efficient means of treatment than single probes units used in isolation.

Treatment of other conditions

As already indicated, when treatment is applied to intact skin, contact technique is the application of choice. For such treatment of general musculoskeletal conditions, laser therapy can usefully be applied in a number of ways.

Direct treatment of the lesion

In such cases, the laser probe is applied directly to the lesion (area of bruising, site of pain, etc.) using a firm pressure within the patient's tolerance. Where extensive bruising/haematoma is present, an 'in contact' version of wound treatment (as already summarised above) is applied; for these cases, dosages applied are correspondingly higher than those used for the treatment of open wounds, given the presence of the skin as a barrier to laser irradiation.

Treatment of acupuncture and trigger points

In China and Japan, the main method of laser application is as an alternative to needles for acupuncture. Although the comparative efficacy of such application with respect to needles or other non-invasive alternatives (e.g. TENS, acupressure, etc.) is still to be determined definitively and is a matter for intense debate, there are many reports in the literature of successful application of laser in this area (see Baxter, 1989; Ellis, 1994; Wong and Fung, 1991). Taut muscles with associated, well-localised areas of pain upon palpation (i.e. trigger points; Baldry, 1993) may also be treated with laser irradiation; although no definitive recommendations can be made on dosage for such trigger-point therapy, in the author's experience the best results are achieved when a relatively high-power unit (i.e. 50–200 mW) is employed to deliver initial dosages of around 2–5 J per point.

Irradiation over nerve roots, trunks, etc.

In the laser treatment of pain syndromes, or in cases where pain represents a major feature of the clinical presentation of the condition to be treated, irradiation may usefully be applied to the skin overlying the appropriate nerve root, plexus or trunk. For example, in treating upper limb pain, laser therapy might be applied over the relevant cervical nerve roots, the brachial plexus by irradiation over Erb's point, as well as to points where the nerves in the arm are relatively superficial such as the radial, median or ulnar nerves at the elbow or wrist.

Key points on laser treatment of some selected conditions

Soft tissue injuries

In such conditions, treatment should be initiated as early as is practically possible within the acute stage, using relatively low dosages in the region of 4–8 J/cm^2 applied directly to the site of injury and any areas of palpable pain. Within the first 72–96 hours after injury, such treatment may be applied up to three times daily with no risk of overtreatment, provided that dosages are kept low. It is important to reiterate that low-intensity laser treatment is by definition athermal and thus eminently suitable for treatment in these situations. As the condition resolves, the frequency of laser treatment may be reduced and dosage correspondingly increased, up to a

maximum of 30 J/cm^2. Where pulsed systems are available, early treatments should be initiated with relatively low pulse repetition rates (<100 Hz) and increased into the kilohertz range as treatment progresses. Where haematoma or bruising is present, it should be treated using the general principles already outlined for the treatment of open wounds, although in this case a firm contact technique should be used within the patient's tolerance, particularly where the lesion is relatively deep.

Recommended initial dosages should be in the region of 4–8 J/cm^2 around the margins of the lesion, and using a grid technique or a multi-source array applied over the centre of the bruise. In the treatment of muscle tears and injuries, laser therapy can be highly effective in accelerating the repair process and thus the return to normal function. This, coupled with its ability to be applied early in the acute stage—in some cases immediately after injury—makes it a popular modality in the treatment of sports injuries.

Neuropathic and neurogenic pain

Where the patient presents with chronic neurogenic pain, laser irradiation is typically applied in a systematic fashion to all relevant nerve roots, plexus and trunks, using a middle-range dosage (10–12 J/cm^2) to initiate treatment. Where trigger or tender points are identified, these are also treated, using an initial dosage of at least 10–20 J/cm^2, which is increased to achieve desensitisation of the point upon repalpation. Irradiation is also applied directly to any areas of referred pain, and to the affected dermatome, etc.

Arthrogenic pain

Arthralgia of various aetiologies may be effectively managed with laser treatment when applied in a comprehensive manner to the affected joints; for this, care should be taken (especially with regard to patient positioning) to ensure that all aspects of the joint are systematically treated.

HAZARDS

Classification of lasers and ocular hazard

Under an internationally agreed classification system which grades laser devices on a scale from 1 to 4 according to the associated dangers to the unprotected skin and eye, the units typically used in LILT are classed as class 3B lasers, although much lower output class 1 and 2 devices have also been used in the past. This essentially means, for the majority of systems used in physiotherapy applications (i.e. class 3B units), that although the laser's output may be considered harmless when directed on to the unprotected skin, it poses a *potential* hazard to the eye if viewed along the axis of the beam (i.e. intrabeam viewing) owing to the high degree of collimation of the laser light. For this reason the use of protective goggles, which must be appropriate for the wavelength(s) used, is recommended for operator and patient. Care is also recommended in ensuring that the beam is never directed towards the unprotected eye; the patient should be specifically warned about the ocular hazard associated with the device and asked not to stare directly at the treatment site during application. Furthermore, the laser treatment unit should ideally be used only in an area specifically designated for this purpose; outside this area, the appropriate laser warning symbols should be clearly displayed. Having outlined these fundamental safety rules, it is important to stress that the ocular hazard associated with therapeutic units is (for all practical purposes) negligible, especially where the treatment head or probe is used with the recommended 'in-contact' technique (see 'Principles of application'). In addition to the above, the output of the treatment unit should be regularly tested to ensure the optimal operation (and thus effectiveness) of the device; this is particularly important as recent research would indicate that a large proportion of laser units in routine use may not be providing adequate power output to be effective (Nussbaum, Van Zuylen and Baxter, 1999).

Contraindications

(See Chartered Society of Physiotheraphy (1996) *Safety of electrotherapy guidance*, for additional information.)

Apart from direct treatment of the eye (for whatever reason), the use of low-intensity laser therapy is also contraindicated in the following cases.

• **In patients with active or suspected carcinoma.** (With the exception of treatment in hospice care.) Studies at the cellular level testify to the potential photobiostimulatory effects of laser radiation; given this, it is possible that therapeutic laser application could accelerate carcinogenesis in patients where carcinoma is present. Despite this potential danger, it should be stressed that laboratory studies in normal cells have consistently failed to demonstrate any carcinogenic effects of laser radiation; indeed, recent results would suggest that laser irradiation might affect DNA repair mechanisms (Logan, Craig and Barnett, 1994).

• **Direct irradiation over the pregnant uterus.** In the absence of hard evidence to show no associated hazard to fetus or mother, avoiding treatment directly over the pregnant uterus represents a prudent and standard precaution that applies to all forms of electrotherapy.

• **Areas of haemorrhage.** This represents an absolute contraindication to laser treatment due to the possibility of laser-induced vasodilatation, which would exacerbate the condition.

• **Cognitive difficulties or unreliable patient.** The patient should be able to understand the explanation and mandatory warnings, and to comply with instructions.

Other safety considerations

Whilst the above are usually regarded as the cardinal contraindications to treatment with low-intensity laser therapy, the Chartered Society of Physiotherapy's Safety of Electrotherapy Equipment Working Group have also recommended the exercise of caution in a number of other situations. Principally these include the following.

- **Treatment of infected tissue (e.g. infected open wounds).** As laser light has the potential to stimulate the bacteria *Escherichia coli* in culture (Karu, 1998; Shields and O'Kane, 1994), it would seem only prudent to recommend caution in the application of laser therapy to infected tissue, and especially infected open wounds. However, the situation is far from clear, as there is evidence to suggest that clinicians have successfully treated such conditions with laser therapy, and in some cases regard the presence of infection as an *indication* for such treatment (Baxter *et al.*, 1991).
- **Treatment over the sympathetic ganglia, vagus nerves and cardiac region in patients with heart disease.** The possibility of laser-mediated alterations in neural activity resulting in adverse effects upon cardiac function can represent an unacceptable risk for these patients.
- **Treatment over photosensitive areas.** Patients with a history of photosensitivity (e.g. adverse reactions to sunlight) should be treated with care, and in such cases the use of a test dose is recommended. In addition, the current use of photosensitising drugs should also be excluded.
- **Treatment of patient with epilepsy.** Care should be exercised when treating patients with a history of epilepsy.
- **Treatment of areas of altered skin sensation.** Although laser treatment is athermic, and is recommended in the treatment of peripheral nerve lesions, care should be exercised in such cases.

REFERENCES

Abergel, RP, Lyons, RF, Castel, JC (1987) Biostimulation of wound healing by lasers; experimental approaches in animal models and fibroblast cultures. *Journal of Dermatological Surgery Oncology* **13**: 127–133.

Agaiby, A, Ghali, L, Dyson, M (1996) Laser modulation of angiogenic factors production by T-lymphocytes. *Lasers in Surgery and Medicine* **Suppl 8**: 46.

Amoils, S, Kues, J (1991) The effect of low level laser therapy on acute headache syndromes. *Laser Therapy* **3**: 155–157.

Baldry, P (1993) *Acupuncture, Trigger Points and Musculoskeletal Pain*, 2nd edn. Churchill Livingstone, New York.

Basford, JR (1989) Low-energy laser therapy: controversies and new research findings. *Lasers in Surgery and Medicine* **9**: 1–5.

Basford, JR (1995) Low intensity laser therapy: still not an established clinical tool. *Lasers in Surgery and Medicine* **16**: 331–342.

Basford, JR, Sheffield, CG, Mair, SD *et al.* (1987) Low energy helium neon laser treatment of thumb osteoarthritis. *Archives of Physical Medicine and Rehabilitation* **68**: 794–797.

Basford, JR, Hallman, JO, Matsumoto, JY *et al.* (1993) Effects of 830 nm laser diode irradiation on median nerve function in normal subjects. *Lasers in Surgery and Medicine* **13**: 597–604.

Basford, JR, Sheffield, CG, Harmsen, WS (1999). Laser therapy: a randomised, controlled trial of the effects of low-intensity Nd:YAG laser irradiation on musculoskeletal back pain. *Archives of Physical Medicine and Rehabilitation* **80**: 647–652.

Baxter, GD (1989) Laser acupuncture analgesia: an overview. *Acupuncture in Medicine* **6**: 57–60.

Baxter, GD (1994) *Therapeutic Lasers: Theory and Practice.* Churchill Livingstone, New York.

Baxter, GD, Bell, AJ, Ravey, J *et al.* (1991) Low level laser therapy: current clinical practice in Northern Ireland. *Physiotherapy* **77**: 171–178.

Baxter, GD, Walsh, DM, Lowe, AS *et al.* (1994) Effects of low intensity infrared laser irradiation upon conduction in the human median nerve in vivo. *Experimental Physiology* **79**: 227–234.

Bliddal, H, Hellesen, C, Ditlevsen, P *et al.* (1987) Soft laser therapy of rheumatoid arthritis. *Scandinavian Journal of Rheumatology* **16**: 225–228.

Bolton, P, Young, S, Dyson, M (1995) The direct effect of 860 nm light on cell proliferation and on succinic dehydrogenase activity of human fibroblasts in vitro. *Laser Therapy* **7**: 55–60.

Bosatra, M, Jucci, A, Olliano, P *et al.* (1984) In vitro fibroblast and dermis fibroblast activation by laser irradiation at low energy. *Dermatologica* **168**: 157–162.

Boulton, M, Marshall, J (1986) He–Ne laser stimulation of human fibroblast proliferation and attachment in vitro. *Lasers in Life Sciences* **1**: 125–134.

Brockhaus, A, Elger, CE (1990) Hypoalgesic efficacy of acupuncture on experimental pain in man. Comparison of laser acupuncture and needle acupuncture. *Pain* **43**: 181–186.

Brosseau, L, Welch, V, Wells, G *et al.* (2000) Low level laser therapy (classes I, II, III) in the treatment of rheumatoid arthritis. *Cochrane Database Systemic Review* 2, CD002049.

Castro, DJ, Abergel, P, Meeker, C *et al.* (1983) Effects of Nd-Yag laser on DNA synthesis and collagen production in human skin fibroblast cultures. *Annals of Plastic Surgery* **11**: 214–222.

Chartered Society of Physiotherapy (1991) Guidelines for the safe use of lasers in physiotherapy. *Physiotherapy* **77**: 169–170.

Choi, JJ, Srikantha, K, Wu, W-H (1986) A comparison of electroacupuncture, transcutaneous electrical nerve stimulation and laser photobiostimulation on pain relief and glucocorticoid excretion. *International Journal of Acupuncture Electrotherapeutics Research* **11**: 45–51.

Devor, M (1990) What's in a beam for pain therapy? *Pain* **43**: 139.

Ellis, N (1994) *Acupuncture in Clinical Practice: a Guide for Health Professionals*. Chapman and Hall, London.

England, S, Farrell, AJ, Coppock, JS et al. (1989) Low power laser therapy of shoulder tendonitis. *Scandinavian Journal of Rheumatology* **18**: 427–431.

Enwemeka, CS, Rodriquez, O, Gall, NG et al. (1990) Correlative ultrastructural and biomechanical changes induced in regenerating tendons exposed to laser photostimulation. *Lasers in Surgery and Medicine* **Suppl 2**: 12.

Glykofridis, S, Diamantopoulos, C (1987) Comparison between laser acupuncture and physiotherapy. *Acupuncture in Medicine* **4**: 6–9.

Goldman, JA, Chiapella, J, Casey, H et al. (1980) Laser therapy of rheumatoid arthritis. *Lasers in Surgery and Medicine* **1**: 93–101.

Greathouse, DG, Currier, DP, Gilmore, RL (1985) Effects of clinical infrared laser on superficial radial nerve conduction. *Physical Therapy* **65**: 1184–1187.

Haina, D, Brunner, R, Landthaler, M et al. (1982) Animal experiments in light induced wound healing. *Laser Basic Biomedical Research* **22**: 1.

Hallman, HO, Basford, JR, O'Brien, JF et al. (1988) Does low energy He–Ne laser irradiation alter in vitro replication of human fibroblasts? *Lasers in Surgery and Medicine* **8**: 125–129.

Hunter, JG, Leonard, LG, Snider, GR et al. (1984) Effects of low energy laser on wound healing in a porcine model. *Lasers in Surgery and Medicine* **3**: 328.

Jensen, H, Harreby, M, Kjer, J (1987) Is infrared laser effective in painful arthrosis of the knee? *Ugeskr Laeger* **149**: 3104–3106.

Karu, TI (1985) Biological action of low intensity visible monochromatic light and some of its medical applications. In: *International Congress on Lasers in Medicine and Surgery, June 26–28, Bologna*. Monduzzi Editore, Bologna, pp 25–29.

Karu, T (1998) *The Science of Low Power Laser Therapy*. Gordon & Breach, Amsterdam.

Khullar, SM, Brodin, P, Hanaes, HR (1994) The effects of low level laser therapy (LLLT) on function and neurophysiological activity in the injured rat sciatic nerve. *Laser Therapy* **6**: 19.

King, PR (1990) Low level laser therapy: a review. *Physiotherapy Theory and Practice* **6**: 127–138.

Kitchen, SS, Partridge, CJ (1991) A review of low level laser therapy. *Physiotherapy* **77**: 161–167.

Lagan, KM, Baxter, GD, Ashford, RL (1998). Combined phototherapy/low intensity laser therapy in the management of diabetic ischaemic and neuropathic ulceration: a single case series investigation. *Laser Therapy* **10**: 103–110.

Lam, T, Abergel, P, Meeker, C et al. (1986) Low energy lasers selectively enhance collagen synthesis. *Lasers in Life Sciences* **1**: 61–77.

Li, XH (1990) Laser in the department of traumatology. With a report of 60 cases of soft tissue injury. *Laser Therapy* **2**: 119–122.

Loevschall, H, Arenholt-Bindslev, D (1994) Effects of low level diode laser (GaAlAs) irradiation of fibroblasts of the human oral mucosa *in vitro*. *Laser in Surgery and Medicine* **14**: 347–354.

Logan, ID, Craig, HE, Barnett, Y (1994) Low intensity laser irradiation induces DNA repair in X-ray damaged friend erythroleukaemia and HL-60 cells. *Laser Therapy* **6**: 30.

Lonauer, G (1986) Controlled double blind study on the efficacy of He–Ne laser beams versus He–Ne plus infrared laser beams in the therapy of activated osteoarthritis of finger joints. *Lasers in Surgery and Medicine* **6**: 172.

Lowe, AS, Baxter, GD, Walsh, DM et al. (1994) The effect of low intensity laser (830 nm) irradiation upon skin temperature and antidromic conduction latencies in the human median nerve: relevance of radiant exposure. *Lasers in Surgery and Medicine* **14**: 40–46.

Lowe, AS, McDowell, BC, Walsh, DM et al. (1997) Failure to demonstrate any hypoalgesic effect of low intensity laser irradiation of Erb's Point upon experimental ischaemic pain in humans. *Lasers in Surgery and Medicine* **14**: 40–46.

Lukashevich, IG (1985) Use of a helium-neon laser in facial pains. *Stomatologia* **64**: 29–31.

Lundeberg, T, Haker, E, Thomas, M (1987) Effects of laser versus placebo in tennis elbow. *Scandinavian Journal of Rehabilitation Medicine* **19**: 135–138.

Lyons, RF, Abergel, RP, White, RA et al. (1987) Biostimulation of wound healing in vivo by a helium neon laser. *Annals of Plastic Surgery* **18**: 47–50.

Manteifel, VM, Karu, TI (1992) Ultrastructural changes in human lymphocytes under He-Ne laser radiation. *Lasers in Life Sciences* **4**: 235–248.

Marks, R, de Palma, F (1999). Clinical efficacy of low power laser therapy in osteoarthritis. *Physiotheraphy Research International* **4**: 141–157.

Mester, AF, Mester, A (1989) Wound healing. *Laser Therapy* **1**: 7–15.

Mester, E, Korenyi-Both, A, Spiry, T et al. (1975) The effect of laser irradiation on the regeneration of muscle fibers. *Zeitschrift Experimentelle Chirurgie* **8**: 258–262.

Mester, E, Mester, AF, Mester, A (1985) The biomedical effects of laser application. *Lasers in Surgery and Medicine* **5**: 31–39.

Mokhtar, B, Walker, D, Baxter, GD et al. (1992) A double blind placebo controlled investigation of the hypoalgesic effects of low intensity laser irradiation of the cervical nerve roots using experimental ischaemic pain. In: *Proceedings, Second Meeting, International Laser Therapy Association* **61**.

Moore, KC, Hira, N, Kumar, PS et al. (1988) A double blind crossover trial of low level laser therapy in the treatment of post herpetic neuralgia. *Laser Therapy*, Pilot Issue, 7–9.

Morrone, G, Guzzardella, GA, Orienti, L et al. (1998) Muscular trauma treated with a GaAlAs diode laser: *in vivo* experimental study. *Lasers in Medical Science* **13**: 293–298.

Nussbaum, E, Van Zuylen, V, Baxter, GD (1999) Specification of treatment dosage in laser therapy: unreliable equipment and radiant power determination as confounding factors. *Physiotherapy Canada* **51**: 159–167.

Ohshiro, T, Calderhead, RG (1988) *Low Level Laser Therapy: A Practical Introduction*. Wiley, Chichester.

Ohta, A, Abergel, RP, Vltto, J et al. (1987) Laser modulation of human immune system: Inhibition of lymphocyte proliferation by Gallium-Arsenide laser at low energy. *Lasers in Surgery and Medicine* **7**: 199–201.

O'Kane, S, Shields, TD, Gilmore, WS et al. (1994) Low intensity laser irradiation inhibits tritiated thymidine incorporation in the haemopoietic cell lines HL-60 and U-937. *Lasers in Surgery and Medicine* **14**: 34–39.

Palmgren, N, Jensen, GF, Kaae, K et al. (1989) Low power laser in rheumatoid arthritis. *Lasers in Medical Science* **4**: 193–196.

Pogrel, MA, Chen, JW, Zang, K (1997) Effects of low-energy gallium-aluminium-arsenide laser irradiation on cultured fibroblasts and keratinocytes. *Lasers in Surgery and Medicine* **20**: 426–432.

Ponnudurai, RN, Zbuzek, VK, Wu, W (1987) Hypoalgesic effect of laser photobiostimulation shown by rat tail flick test. *International Journal of Acupuncture Electrotherapeutics Research* **12**: 93–100.

Ponnudurai, RN, Zbuzek, VK, Niu, H-L et al. (1988) Laser photobiostimulation-induced hypoalgesia in rats is not naloxone reversible. *International Journal of Acupuncture Electrotherapeutics Research* **13**: 109–117.

Rajaratnam, S, Bolton, P, Dyson, M (1994) Macrophage responsiveness to laser therapy with varying pulsing frequencies. *Laser Therapy* **6**: 107–112.

Robinson, B, Walters, J (1991) The use of low level laser therapy in diabetic and other ulcerations. *Journal of British Podiatric Medicine* **46**: 10.

Rochkind, S, Rousso, M, Nissan, M et al. (1989) Systemic effects of low power laser irradiation on the peripheral and central nervous system, cutaneous wounds and burns. *Lasers in Surgery and Medicine* **9**: 174–182.

Rochkind, S, Alon, M, Dekel, S et al. (1994a) Peripheral nerve and brachial plexus injuries: results of surgery and/or low level laser therapy. *Laser Therapy* **6**: 53.

Rochkind, S, Alon, M, Sosnov, Y et al. (1994b) Severe spinal cord or cauda equina injuries: results of low level laser therapy. *Laser Therapy* **6**: 55.

Santionnai, P, Monfrecola, G, Martellotta, D et al. (1984) Inadequate effect of Helium–Neon laser on venous leg ulcers. *Photodermatology* **1**: 245–249.

Seibert, DD, Gould, WR (1984) The effect of laser stimulation on burning pain threshold. *Physical Therapy* **64**: 746.

Shields, D, O'Kane, S (1994) Laser photobiomodulation of wound healing. In: Baxter, GD (ed) *Therapeutic Lasers: Theory and Practice*. Churchill Livingstone, Edinburgh, 89–138.

Shiroto, C, Ono, K, Ohshiro, T (1989) Retrospective study of diode laser therapy for pain attenuation in 3635 patients: detailed analysis by questionnaire. *Laser Therapy* **1**: 41–48.

Siebert, W, Siechert, N, Siebert, B et al. (1987) What is the efficacy of 'soft' and 'mid' lasers in therapy of tendinopathies? *Archives of Orthopaedic and Traumatic Surgery* **106**: 358–363.

Snyder-Mackler, L, Bork, CE (1988) Effect of Helium–Neon laser irradiation on peripheral sensory nerve latency. *Physical Therapy* **68**: 223–225.

Sugrue, ME, Carolan, J, Leen, EJ et al. (1990) The use of infra-red laser therapy in the treatment of venous ulcerations. *Annals of Vascular Surgery* **4**: 179–181.

Trelles, MA, Rigau, J, Sala, P et al. (1991) Infrared diode laser in low reactive-level laser therapy (LLLT) for knee osteoarthrosis. *Laser Therapy* **3**: 149–153.

Tuner, J, Hode, L (1999) *Low Level Laser Therapy. Clinical Practice and Scientific Background*. Prima Books, Spjutvagen, Sweden.

van Breugel, HHF, Engels, C, Bar PR (1993) Mechanisms of action in laser-induced photo-biomodulation depend on the wavelength of the laser. *Lasers in Surgery and Medicine* **Suppl. 5**: 9.

Vidovich, D, Olson, DR (1987) Neodymium YAG laser stimulation as a treatment modality in acute and chronic pain syndromes and in rheumatoid arthritis. *Lasers in Surgery and Medicine* **7**: 79.

Walker, J (1983) Relief from chronic pain by low power laser irradiation. *Neuroscience Letters* **43**: 339–344.

Walker, J, Akhanjee, LK (1985) Laser-induced somatosensory evoked potential: evidence of photosensitivity in peripheral nerves. *Brain Research* **344**: 281–285.

Walker, J, Akhanjee, LK, Cooney, MM et al. (1987) Laser therapy for pain of rheumatoid arthritis. *Clinical Journal of Pain* **3**: 54–59.

Walker, MD, Rumpf, S, Baxter, GD et al. (2000). Effect of low-intensity laser irradiation (660 nm) on a radiation-impaired wound-healing model in murine skin. *Lasers in Surgery and Medicine* **26**: 41–47.

Walsh, DM (1993) *Investigations of the Neurophysiological and Hypoalgesic Effects of Low Intensity Laser Therapy and Transcutaneous Electrical Nerve Stimulation*. DPhil Thesis, University of Ulster.

Waylonis, GW, Wilkie, S, O'Toole, D et al. (1988) Chronic myofascial pain: management by low output helium-neon laser therapy. *Archives Physical Medicine and Rehabilitation* **69**: 1017–1020.

Wong, TW, Fung KP (1991) Acupuncture: from needle to laser. *Family Practitioner* **8**: 168–170.

Wu, W (1983) Recent advances in laserpuncture. In: Atsumi, K (ed) *New Frontiers in Laser Medicine and Surgery*. Elsevier, Amsterdam.

Wu, W-H, Ponnudurai, R, Katz, J et al. (1987) Failure to confirm report of light-evoked response of peripheral nerve to low power Helium-Neon laser light stimulus. *Brain Research* **401**: 407–408.

Yamaguchi, N, Trukamoto, Y, Matono, S (1994) The effects of semiconductor laser irradiation on the immune activities of human lymphocytes in vitro. *Lasers in Life Sciences* **6**: 143–149.

Zarkovic, N, Manev, H, Pericic, D et al. (1989) Effect of semiconductor GaAs laser irradiation on pain perception in mice. *Lasers in Surgery and Medicine* **9**: 63–66.

13

Ultraviolet therapy

Brian Diffey
Peter Farr

INTRODUCTION

The foundation of modern-day ultraviolet (UV) phototherapy began with the work of the Danish physician Niels Finsen, who was awarded the Nobel Prize for Medicine in 1903 for his successful treatment of cutaneous tuberculosis. Following his pioneering work there was a rapid expansion of heliotherapy (using the sun as the source of radiation) and actinotherapy (using lamps as the source), for the treatment of many skin diseases. Most of the irradiation protocols for the countless number of diseases described in *Actinotherapy Technique*, first published by Sollux in 1933, are now of historical interest only. The advent of effective antibiotics and the realisation that the successes claimed in many of these diseases were little more than anecdotal have resulted today in a much reduced role of UV radiation in clinical medicine.

One of the major contributions to dermatological practice in the past 30 years has been the introduction of a treatment for several skin diseases, including psoriasis, known as photochemotherapy; the combination of ultraviolet radiation (UVR) and photoactive drugs producing a beneficial effect in the skin.

The first sources of artificial ultraviolet radiation were carbon arc lamps of the type developed by Finsen at around the turn of the century. These lamps were unpopular in clinical practice because of their noise, odour and sparks, and were superseded by the development of mercury arc lamps. Fluorescent lamps were developed in the late 1940s and, since then, a variety of phosphor and envelope materials have been used to produce lamps with different emissions in the ultraviolet spectrum.

THE NATURE OF ULTRAVIOLET RADIATION

Ultraviolet radiation covers a small part of the electromagnetic spectrum (See Fig. 1.20). Other regions of this spectrum include radiowaves, microwaves, infrared radiation (heat), visible light, X-rays and gamma radiation. The feature that characterises the properties of any particular region of the spectrum is the wavelength of the radiation.

Ultraviolet radiation spans the wavelength region from 400 to 100 nm. Even in the ultraviolet portion of the spectrum the biological effects of the radiation vary enormously with wavelength and, for this reason, the ultraviolet spectrum is further subdivided into three regions:

1. UVA: 400–320 nm
2. UVB: 320–290 nm
3. UVC: 290–200 nm.

The divisions between the different wavebands are not rigidly fixed, and 315 nm is sometimes taken as the boundary between UVA and UVB, and 280 nm as that between UVB and UVC.

PRODUCTION OF ULTRAVIOLET RADIATION

Ultraviolet radiation is produced artificially by the passage of an electric current through a gas, usually vaporised mercury. For lamps containing mercury vapour at about atmospheric pressure (medium-pressure mercury arc lamps), radiation is emitted with several different wavelengths in the UVC, UVB and UVA. The mercury atoms become excited by collisions with the electrons flowing between the lamp's electrodes. These excited electrons return to particular electronic states in the mercury atom and in doing so release some of the energy they have absorbed in the form of radiation, that is, ultraviolet, visible and infrared radiation.

The spectrum of the radiation emitted consists of a limited number of discrete wavelengths (so-called 'spectral lines') corresponding to electron transitions which are characteristic of the mercury atom; the relative intensity of the different wavelengths in the spectrum depends upon the pressure of the mercury vapour. Another common way of producing ultraviolet radiation is by fluorescent lamps, or tubes. A fluorescent lamp is a low-pressure mercury vapour lamp which has a phosphor coating applied to the inside of the glass tube (sometimes referred to as the *envelope*). At low pressures in mercury vapour there is a predominant spectral line at a wavelength of 253.7 nm, and radiation of this wavelength is efficiently absorbed by the phosphor. The results in the re-emission of radiation of longer wavelengths by the phenomenon of fluorescence. The wavelength range of the fluorescent radiation will be a property of the chemical nature of the phosphor material. Phosphors are available which produce their fluorescence radiation mainly in the visible region (for artificial lighting purposes), the UVA, or the UVB regions.

Spectral power distribution

It is common practice to talk loosely of 'UVA lamps' or 'UVB lamps'. However, such a label does not characterise ultraviolet lamps adequately since nearly all phototherapy lamps will emit UVA and UVB, and even UVC, visible light, and infrared radiation. The only correct way to specify the nature of the emitted radiation is by reference to the spectral power distribution. Figure 13.1 indicates the radiated power as a function of wavelength and shows the spectral power distribution of ultraviolet radiation emitted by a medium-pressure mercury arc lamp. Fluorescent lamps reach their full output within 1 minute of switching on, and yield maximum radiation output when the lamp is running in free air at an ambient temperature of about 25°C. As the temperature increases, the output decreases, and this can be a problem in irradiation units which incorporate large numbers of fluorescent lamps packed closely

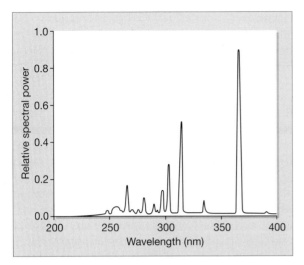

Figure 13.1 The spectral power distribution of ultraviolet radiation from a medium-pressure mercury arc lamp of the type used in an Alpine Sunlamp. The graph shows the intensity of the radiation emitted at each wavelength. The specific wavelengths are characteristic of mercury and are the same irrespective of the manufacturer of the mercury lamp, although the intensity at the different wavelengths may differ. The prominent wavelengths (*spectral lines*) in the ultraviolet region from a mercury lamp are at 254, 265, 280, 297, 302, 313, 334 and 365 nm. There are also spectral lines in the visible spectrum (not shown on the graph) which occur at 405 (violet), 436 (blue), 546 (green), and 578 (yellow) nm, which combine to give these lamps a bright white light.

together (unless adequate, forced-air cooling is incorporated into the unit).

The output from ultraviolet lamps deteriorates with time. There is a 'running-in' time with all lamps during which period the rate of fall in radiation output is considerably greater than for later times. For fluorescent lamps, the running-in period is about 100 hours, but is only about 20 hours for medium- and high-pressure lamps. The useful lifetime of most ultraviolet lamps is between 500 and 1000 hours. After this period, the output will have fallen to around 80% of the value at the end of the running-in period.

The UV output of medium- and high-pressure lamps deteriorates more rapidly than the visible light output. With fluorescent lamps, however, the relative decrease in radiation output with usage is more or less independent of wavelength—in other words, the spectrum of the radiation remains approximately constant even though the absolute radiation output decreases.

BIOLOGICAL EFFECTS OF ULTRAVIOLET RADIATION

Effects on skin

Erythema

Erythema, or redness of the skin due to dilatation of superficial dermal blood vessels, is one of the commonest and most obvious effects of ultraviolet exposure ('sunburn'). The potential for development of erythema is the major factor that limits the exposure that may be given during phototherapy. Erythema is usually encountered only when UVB treatment is used, as without psoralen sensitisation (see the section Psoralen photochemotherapy below), the skin is between 100 and 1000 times less sensitive to UVA than to UVB.

The mechanism of erythema production following ultraviolet exposure is understood poorly. It is known that erythema from UVB is mediated, at least in part, by the release from the epidermis of pharmacologically active compounds, such as prostaglandins, which diffuse to act on dermal blood vessels. The erythemal response may also be related to the DNA-damaging effects of UVR, as patients with the rare condition of xeroderma pigmentosum, in which there are defective mechanisms to repair UVR-induced DNA damage, also have abnormal erythemal responses to UVR. Further details of this and other light-related disorders can be found in Hawk (1999).

Following UVR exposure, there is usually a latent period of 2–4 hours before erythema develops, although after sufficient exposure to UVA some immediate erythema may occur. Ultraviolet-induced erythema reaches maximum intensity between 8 and 24 hours after exposure, but may take several days to resolve completely. If a high-enough exposure has occurred, the skin will also become painful and oedematous, and blistering may result.

The smallest dose of UVR to result in erythema that is just detectable by eye at between 8 and 24 hours after exposure is termed the *minimal erythema dose* (MED). A test dose to determine the MED is measured normally by exposing small areas of normal skin, usually on the back, to different doses of UVR. Ideally, a series of doses increasing geometrically is used (e.g. successive doses increasing by 40%). This is a widely used indicator of an individual's sensitivity to UVR, and is a useful clinical measure of exposure as the goal of many phototherapy regimens is to achieve a mild degree of erythema. The MED shows a wide variation between individuals: even within Caucasians, a four- to six-fold difference in MED will occur between those who burn easily in sunlight and those who rarely burn. At doses higher than the MED, the intensity of erythema increases rapidly, for example, an exposure of twice the MED (2 MED) would result in erythema of moderate intensity, but 3 MED might cause a severe and painful response. The characteristics of erythema induced in psoralen-sensitised skin during PUVA therapy are different in a number of important respects (see the section Psoralen photochemotherapy).

Tanning

Another consequence of exposure to UVR is the delayed pigmentation of the skin known as *tanning*, or melanin pigmentation. Melanin pigmentation of skin is of two types: constitutive (the colour of the skin seen in different races and determined by genetic factors only), and facultative (the reversible increase in tanning in response to UVR and other external stimuli).

Individuals may be classified according to their self-reported erythemal and pigmentary response to natural sunlight exposure. This skin-type system is used widely to choose a starting dose of UVR at the beginning of a course of phototherapy. However, wide variation in MED values occurs both within each skin-type category and between categories, limiting its clinical usefulness. The categories of this skin type system are as follows:

- group I—always burns, never tans;
- group II—always burns, sometimes tans;
- group III—sometimes burns, always tans;
- group IV—never burns, always tans;

- group V—moderate racial pigmentation (e.g. Asian skin)
- group VI—marked racial pigmentation (black skin).

Hyperplasia

In addition to tanning, the skin is capable of another response, which limits damage from further ultraviolet exposure—epidermal thickening or hyperplasia. This begins to occur around 72 hours after exposure, is a result of an increased rate of division of basal epidermal cells, and results eventually in thickening of both the epidermis and stratum corneum which persists for several weeks (for further details see Johnson, 1984). This adaptive process, unlike tanning, occurs with all skin types, and is the major factor that protects those who tan poorly in sunlight (skin types I and II). That epidermal hyperplasia occurs mainly following UVB exposure, rather than UVA, is shown by the poor sunburn protection achieved with a UVA-only-induced tan (e.g. from a sunbed) compared with an equivalent tan achieved from natural sunlight exposure (UVA and UVB).

The adaptive processes of tanning and epidermal hyperplasia that occur during a course of phototherapy treatment mean that, in order to maintain an effective dose of UVR at the key target site in the skin (considered for most disorders to be around the basal layer of the epidermis), the exposure dose to the skin surface needs to be gradually increased (see the sections on treatment regimens in Phototherapy and Psoralen photochemotherapy below).

Production of vitamin D

The skin absorbs UVB radiation in sunlight and converts sterol precursors in the skin, such as 7-dehydrocholesterol, to vitamin D_3. Vitamin D_3 is further transformed by the liver and kidneys to biologically active metabolites such as 25-hydroxyvitamin D; these metabolites then act on the intestinal mucosa to facilitate calcium absorption, and on bone to facilitate calcium exchange.

Ageing of the skin

Chronic exposure to sunlight can result in an appearance of the skin often referred to as premature ageing or actinic damage. The clinical changes associated with skin ageing include a dry, coarse, leathery appearance, laxity with wrinkling, and various pigmentary changes. These changes are believed to be due mainly to exposure to the ultraviolet component of sunlight.

Skin cancer

The three common forms of skin cancer, listed in order of seriousness, are: basal cell carcinoma, squamous cell carcinoma and malignant melanoma. Exposure to UVR is considered to be a major aetiological factor for all three forms of cancer. For basal cell carcinoma and malignant melanoma, neither the wavelengths involved nor the exposure pattern that results in risk have been established with certainty, whereas for squamous cell carcinoma both UVB and UVA are implicated, and the major risk factors seem to be cumulative lifetime exposure to UVR and a poor tanning response (e.g. skin types I and II). The development of squamous cell carcinoma is a significant risk for patients treated for long periods with psoralen photochemotherapy (see the section Psoralen photochemotherapy below).

Effects on eyes

Photokeratitis and conjunctivitis

The acute effects of exposure to UVC and UVB radiation are primarily those of conjunctivitis and photokeratitis.

Conjunctivitis is an inflammation of the membrane that lines the insides of the eyelids and covers the cornea; it may often be accompanied by an erythema of the skin around the eyelids. There is the sensation of 'gritty eyes' and also varying degrees of photophobia (aversion to light), lacrimation (tears), and blepharospasm (spasm of the eyelid muscles) may be present.

Photokeratitis is an inflammation of the cornea that can result in severe pain. Ordinary clinical photokeratitis is characterised by a period of latency that tends to vary inversely with the severity of UV exposure. The latent period may be as short as 30 minutes or as long as 24 hours, but it is typically 6–12 hours. The acute symptoms of visual incapacitation usually last from 6–24 hours. Almost all discomfort usually disappears within 2 days and rarely does exposure result in permanent damage. Unlike the skin, the ocular system does not develop tolerance to repeated exposure to UVR. Many cases of photokeratitis have been reported following exposure to UVR produced by welding arcs and by the reflection of solar radiation from snow and sand. For this reason, the condition is sometimes referred to as 'welder's flash', or 'arc eye', or 'snow blindness'.

Cataract

In PUVA therapy (see the section Psoralen photochemotherapy below) patients are administered photosensitising drugs called psoralens which are deposited in the lens. Evidence from animal studies shows that subsequent UVA irradiation can lead to cataract formation and, for this reason, adequate eye protection should always be worn for 12 hours or so following the ingestion of psoralens.

PHOTOTHERAPY/ PHOTOCHEMOTHERAPY

Treatment of skin disease by exposure to UVR is termed *phototherapy*, and is often used in combination with agents applied topically (e.g. dithranol plus UVB phototherapy for psoriasis). When treatment with UVR is combined with a photosensitising agent (e.g. psoralen plus UVA exposure), the term *photochemotherapy* is used.

Diseases that are treated by ultraviolet phototherapy

Diseases that are treated with ultraviolet phototherapy are:

- psoriasis
- eczema

- acne
- vitiligo
- pityriasis lichenoides chronica;
- polymorphic light eruption (and other photosensitive disorders);
- pruritus (particularly related to renal disease).

The vast majority of patients treated with ultraviolet phototherapy will have psoriasis or eczema (particularly atopic eczema). UVB phototherapy is also used to treat a number of photosensitive skin disorders, only one of which (polymorphic light eruption) is at all common. Increased tolerance to sun exposure is achieved by tanning and skin thickening and, probably of equal importance, by immunological and pharmacological actions (see, for example, Farr and Diffey, 1988).

Spectrum of therapeutic response

The erythemal or 'sunburn' sensitivity of the skin varies greatly with the wavelength of ultraviolet radiation; UVB being 100–1000 times more potent at inducing erythema than UVA. The variation in erythemal sensitivity may be depicted graphically as an action spectrum (Fig. 13.2); other effects of ultraviolet exposure can be described in a similar way, for example the relative effectiveness of different wavelengths at healing skin disease. Unfortunately, at present, only the action spectrum for the clearance of psoriasis with ultraviolet phototherapy is established with any degree of certainty (Parrish and Jaenicke, 1981). Figure 13.2 shows that for wavelengths shorter than 290 nm, even when doses are used that are considerably in excess of the MED, no healing of psoriasis occurs. With wavelengths longer than 290 nm, the action spectrum for clearance of psoriasis is very similar to that for the development of erythema. This has important implications for the selection of ultraviolet lamps to treat psoriasis: lamps with a large component of UVC will produce erythema easily but will not clear psoriasis. Based on this therapeutic action spectrum, lamps have been designed specifically to treat psoriasis (such as the Philips TL01), and have been shown to be more effective

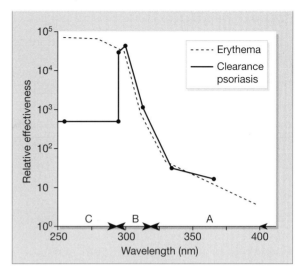

Figure 13.2 A plot of effectiveness of radiation against wavelength (action spectrum) for erythema (dashed line) and for the clearance of psoriasis with daily phototherapy (solid line). The two curves diverge at wavelengths shorter than 290 nm where even doses greater than ten times the MED fail to result in clearance of psoriasis. A logarithmic scale has been used for the vertical axis in order to allow the large change in response of the skin with wavelength to be visible, together with relatively small but biologically important differences between the two curves.

than conventional UVB lamps. It is to be hoped that more efficient treatment will become available for the other diseases in which ultraviolet phototherapy is used once further disease-specific action spectra have been determined.

Ultraviolet lamps for phototherapy

A survey of the practice of phototherapy in the UK carried out in 1993 (Dootson et al., 1994) showed that 70% of treatment machines for whole-body irradiation incorporate fluorescent lamps, rather than arc lamps. In this survey, the machine used most frequently was the Theraktin ultraviolet bath or tunnel. This unit has several drawbacks, which include low irradiance and uneven skin exposure, often with relative sparing of the lower legs and sides of trunk. It has no place in a modern phototherapy service. More efficient units are either:

- semicylindrical or cylindrical cubicles incorporating up to 48 fluorescent lamps,

extending for 2 m in length, and mounted vertically around the inner circumference
- a bed and canopy incorporating up to 28 fluorescent lamps for simultaneous anterior and posterior irradiation with patients lying supine (Fig. 13.3).

Some cylindrical cubicles incorporate a mixture of UVB and UVA fluorescent lamps (Fig. 13.4). The advantage of such a cubicle is that the one machine can be used for phototherapy (when the UVB lamps are switched on) or PUVA therapy (when the UVA lamps are switched on). The disadvantage is that both UVB and UVA irradiances are lower than can be obtained from a unit incorporating just one type of lamp. Consequently, longer treatment times are necessary, but this may not be a problem in a department with a low throughput of patients.

There are several types of UVB fluorescent lamps with varying spectral emissions, as indicated in Table 13.1.

Irradiation with lamps such as the Sylvania UV21 and Philips TL12 requires shorter exposure times than with lamps such as the Sylvania UV6, Wolff Helarium or Philips TL01 in which the spectrum is shifted to longer wavelengths and considerably less UVC is present. However, for a given degree of erythema the latter three lamps will be more effective because they emit much less erythemally effective, but therapeutically ineffective, radiation at wavelengths shorter than 290 nm. An appraisal of the different lamps used for phototherapy has been given by Diffey and Farr (1987).

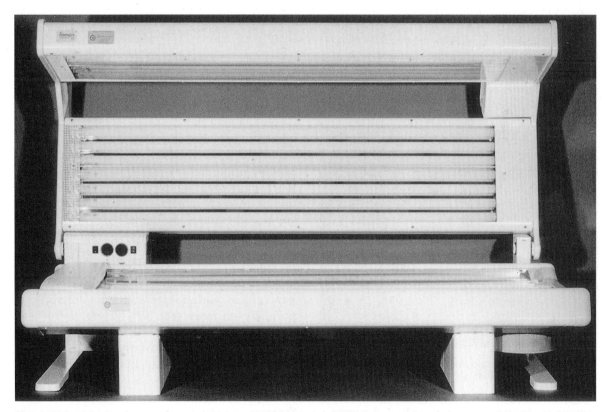

Figure 13.3 A bed and canopy incorporating a total of 28 Helarium (UVB) fluorescent lamps (courtesy of Sun Health Services Ltd, Crowborough, England).

Table 13.1 Spectral properties of different UVB fluorescent lamps used in phototherapy

Type of UVB fluorescent lamp	Wavelength range and spectral peak (% of total ultraviolet)				
	Range (nm)	Peak (nm)	UVA	UVB	UVC
Philips TL12	276–380	313	34	60	6
Sylvania UV21	276–380	313	34	60	6
Sylvania UV6	286–370	313	40	59	<1
Wolf Helarium	295–400	340	92	8	0
Philips TL01	300–320	311	10	90	0

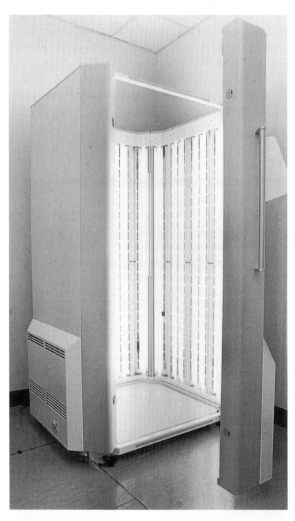

Figure 13.4 A whole-body cubicle incorporating 27 UVA lamps (shown illuminated) and 13 UVB fluorescent lamps (not illuminated) which can be used for either UVB or PUVA therapy (model 7001K, Waldmann GmbH, Schwenningen, Germany).

Treatment times

Treatment times depend not only upon the spectrum of the radiation, but also upon factors such as electrical power, number of lamps, lamp-to-skin distance and differences in patient susceptibility to UVR. Initial treatment times with most phototherapy lamps are about 0.5–3 minutes. Treatment times need to be increased throughout a course of phototherapy in order to maintain an erythema on increasingly acclimatised skin (see section on treatment regimens in Phototherapy).

Uniformity of irradiation

Most modern phototherapy units incorporate several lamps and are designed for partial- or whole-body irradiation. Studies have shown that the vertical distribution of ultraviolet radiation in phototherapy cabinets is non-uniform when fluorescent lamps are used, with a reduction in intensity of between 20 and 50% near the ends of the tubes compared with the middle, resulting in significantly lower radiation doses at the extremities. In contrast, when columns incorporating five or six high-pressure metal halide lamps are used, as shown in Figure 13.5, the vertical variation of radiation intensity is normally no more than 10% (Chue, Borok and Lowe, 1988).

Phototherapy lamps of the type shown in Figure 13.5 have the advantage that not all of the lamps need to be switched on, so that partial-body irradiation is possible. This is not the case with fluorescent lamp systems, although fluorescent lamps are available in a variety of

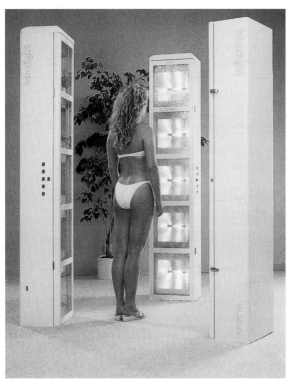

Figure 13.5 Three columns, each incorporating five high-pressure metal halide lamps (courtesy of Uvalight Technology Ltd, Birmingham, England).

lengths ranging from 30 cm to 2 m so that units designed for treating small areas, such as the hands or feet, are available.

In addition to geometrical problems associated with the lamps, variation in irradiance over a patient's skin will depend also on the topology and self-shielding of the patient's body. Measurements of the ultraviolet dose received at different body sites have shown that a large fraction of the body surface area receives more than 70% of the maximum dose which occurs on the trunk, while areas such as the groin and axillae receive a smaller fraction, as expected (Diffey, Harrington and Challoner, 1978).

Treatment regimens

Psoriasis

For psoriasis, UVB phototherapy may be given on a daily basis, although less-frequent exposures, for example three times weekly, may be equally effective (Dawe *et al.*, 1998). Ideally, the initial exposure dose will be based on the outcome of a test dose establishing the minimal erythema dose established for each patient (e.g. 70% of the MED). If this is not possible or practical, the first exposure time should be selected according to the skin type of the patient and the degree of any pre-existing melanin pigmentation. Once erythema has developed, exposure times should be increased cautiously (for example, by 10–20%) to maintain an effective treatment dose as the skin adapts. If severe or symptomatic erythema is present, further exposure should be avoided until the skin returns to normal.

Treatment is continued until the desired clinical response is obtained, or until no further improvement is occurring. Complete clearance of psoriasis may take several weeks of phototherapy.

Other disorders

Protocols for the treatment of other skin disorders should be agreed in line with evidence available in the literature and through discussion with experts in the area. Erythema and skin irritation from phototherapy may be a significant problem for patients with atopic eczema and photosensitivity disorders, such as polymorphic light eruption.

Adjunctive agents

Both tar and emollients are used topically in an attempt to improve the effectiveness of phototherapy for psoriasis. Several ointment preparations (e.g. emulsifying ointment, white soft paraffin and yellow soft paraffin) and products containing the keratolytic agent salicylic acid, have a sunscreening action and may reduce the effectiveness of phototherapy (Hudson-Peacock, Diffey and Farr, 1994).

Ultraviolet phototherapy is often used in addition to dithranol treatment and, when given optimally, can reduce by around one-third the number of days of treatment required for clearance (Farr, Diffey and Marks, 1987).

Side-effects

The main side-effect of UVB phototherapy is the development of erythema or, in more severe cases, blistering and subsequent peeling of the skin. Severe erythema can usually be avoided, providing further exposure is not given if the patient has any residual erythema from the previous day's treatment. Once symptomatic erythema has developed, treatment with emollients may provide some relief and topical corticosteroids are often prescribed.

Although sun exposure is the major risk factor for the development of skin carcinoma, particularly squamous carcinoma, no additional risk from UVB phototherapy has been reported and, on theoretical grounds, any risk is likely to be minimal (Studniberg and Weller, 1993).

PSORALEN PHOTOCHEMOTHERAPY (PUVA)

Psoralen photochemotherapy is the combined treatment of skin disorders with a photosensitising drug (**p**soralen) and **u**ltraviolet **A** radiation. Psoralens are naturally occurring plant compounds and their therapeutic potential for the treatment of vitiligo has been recognised for many thousands of years. Photochemotherapy of psoriasis, using synthetic psoralen compounds such as 8-methoxypsoralen (8-MOP) or 5-methoxypsoralen (5-MOP), was introduced in the 1970s and is now widely used as a second-line form of treatment, being available in approximately 100 dermatology units in the UK (Farr and Diffey, 1991).

Diseases that respond to PUVA

Although used principally to treat psoriasis, many disorders show partial or complete response to PUVA:

- psoriasis
- vitiligo
- eczema
- lichen planus
- graft-versus-host disease
- pityriasis lichenoides chronica

- cutaneous T-cell lymphoma (mycosis fungoides)
- urticaria pigmentosa
- photosensitive disorders (polymorphic light eruption, actinic prurigo, chronic actinic dermatitis).

Further details on the role of PUVA in the treatment of these diseases can be found in the guidelines prepared by the British Photodermatology Group (Norris *et al.*, 1994).

Pharmacology and mechanism of action

Psoralen is usually given orally using a dose system based on body weight or surface area ($0.6\,mg/kg$ or $25\,mg/m^2$ for the crystalline form of 8-MOP; $1.2\,mg/kg$ or $50\,mg/m^2$ for 5-MOP). Absorption and resulting plasma concentrations show considerable variation between subjects, but UVA exposure is given usually 2 hours after ingestion at the average time of peak plasma concentration (Stevenson *et al.*, 1981). PUVA may also be given using topical psoralen, either painted on to the skin surface or, more frequently, using a bath delivery system in which the patient soaks for 15 minutes in a weak psoralen solution (e.g. $3.75\,mg/L$ of 8-MOP), followed immediately by UVA exposure. Significant concentrations of psoralen in plasma are not achieved with topical psoralen. Detailed information concerning methods for using bath or topical psoralen may be found in the guidelines produced by the British Photodermatology Group (Halpern *et al.*, 2000).

Psoralen molecules, when activated by UVA radiation, form cross-links between adjacent strands of DNA, thus interfering with DNA and cellular replication. Although it has been assumed that this is the mechanism of action of PUVA in disorders associated with increased cell division (such as psoriasis), PUVA also has other important actions on the skin, including induction of pigmentation and epidermal hyperplasia, suppression of certain components of the immune system and release of reactive oxygen and free radicals which damage cell membranes and cytoplasmic structures.

Unlike ultraviolet phototherapy, the therapeutic wavelength response (or action spectrum for clearance of psoriasis) for PUVA has not yet been fully established. However, there is some evidence that lamps which emit shorter wavelengths (around 320–330 nm) may be more effective than conventional lamps (Farr *et al.*, 1991).

Psoralen erythema

Following oral administration of 8-MOP, the cutaneous photosensitivity to UVA parallels the plasma psoralen concentration—maximally sensitive after around 2 hours and gradually returning to normal by 8–12 hours. The photosensitivity from topical psoralen lasts for a much shorter period (< 4 hours). Unlike UVB erythema (or UVA erythema without psoralen), PUVA erythema has a delayed onset, being first noticeable 24–48 hours after irradiation, and does not reach maximum intensity until 72–96 hours (Ibbotson and Farr, 1999). The smallest dose of UVA required to achieve erythema in psoralen-sensitised skin is referred to usually as the *minimal phototoxic dose* (MPD), the term phototoxic indicating that an external agent has been used to increase the sensitivity of the skin. Unlike UVB erythema, where doses above the MED cause severe burning easily, two or three times the MPD results only in mild or moderate erythema when psoralen has been given orally. Burning may happen more easily with topical psoralen however.

Treatment apparatus

Photoirradiation systems designed for PUVA therapy of psoriasis and other skin diseases normally incorporate UVA fluorescent lamps (e.g. Philips Performance, Sylvania FR90T12/PUVA) emitting a continuous distribution from about 315–400 nm and peaking at around 352 nm. The spectrum from this lamp is shown in the upper half of Figure 13.6. Although it would seem that the true peak is at 365 nm (one of the characteristic spectral lines of mercury vapour), there is actually very little energy present in this spectral line. A variety of treatment

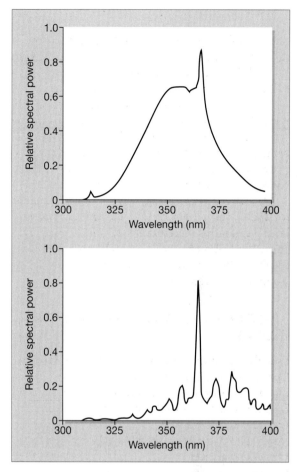

Figure 13.6 The spectral power distribution of the ultraviolet radiation emitted by two different types of lamp used for PUVA therapy. Upper curve—UVA fluorescent lamps; note that the spectrum lies almost entirely between 320 and 400 nm (the UVA waveband) and peaks at 350 nm. Lower curve—optically filtered high-pressure metal-halide lamps; note that most of the radiation is emitted at wavelengths longer than 360 nm.

units are available, ranging from small area (Fig. 13.7) to whole-body cabinets (Fig. 13.4).

Some centres use high-pressure metal halide lamps behind glass filters to remove the UVB and UVC components of the radiation and allow UVA to be transmitted, similar to the unit shown in Figure 13.5. The UVA irradiance from this arrangement at typical treatment distances can be two to three times higher than can be achieved in conventional UVA fluorescent lamp units and might be thought to be a positive

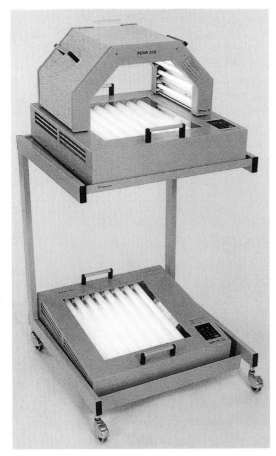

Figure 13.7   Small area PUVA units used for treating hands and feet (courtesy of Athrodax Surgical Ltd, Ross-on-Wye, England).

feature in favour of this type of unit. However, high-pressure metal halide lamps behind glass filters emit a spectrum as shown in the lower half of Figure 13.6. Whereas the spectrum from UVA fluorescent lamps peaks at around 350 nm, the optically filtered metal halide lamps used in the high-power units emit much of their ultraviolet radiation in the band between 360 and 380 nm. The action spectrum for the clearance of psoriasis by psoralen photochemotherapy is such that shorter UVA wavelengths are more effective than radiation at the long-wavelength end of the UVA spectrum (see section on Pharmacology and mechanism of action above). The apparent advantage of higher UVA irradiances from high-pressure lamp systems may be

more than offset by the relative lack of radiation in the shorter wavelength interval (320–340 nm) of the UVA spectrum compared with the commonly used UVA fluorescent lamps.

Treatment regimens

For psoriasis, PUVA treatment regimens are now well established. Protocols for treatment of other disorders, however, remain to be developed.

Treatment for psoriasis in the UK has been given usually three times per week. However, as PUVA erythema does not reach a maximum until at least 72 hours after exposure, treatment on a Monday, Wednesday and Friday, leaving only 48 hours between some exposures, considerably increases the risk of burning. Consequently, many dermatology units in the UK are changing to twice-weekly treatment. This has been shown to be effective for psoriasis (Sakuntabhai, Sharpe and Farr, 1993), is considerably more convenient for patients than treatment three times a week, and allows greater efficiency of operation of a PUVA unit.

Starting doses of UVA are often based on the skin type of the patient, such as:

- skin type I: 0.5J/cm^2
- skin type II: 1.0J/cm^2
- skin type III: 1.5J/cm^2
- skin type IV: 2.0J/cm^2.

However, the additional factor of variable skin photosensitivity due to differences between patients in psoralen pharmacokinetics means that skin typing is even less useful as a method of prediction of erythemal sensitivity for PUVA than with UVB phototherapy. Measurement of each patient's minimal phototoxic dose (MPD) at the start of a course of treatment allows high-dose treatment regimens to be used without increased risk of burning, and results in faster clearance of psoriasis. The MPD may be measured by exposing small areas of normal skin (e.g. 1 cm diameter sites) on the forearm or back to increasing doses of UVA (e.g. 1, 2, 4 and 8J/cm^2 for oral 8-MOP treatment), and then observing which, if any, of the sites become erythematous at 72 hours (Diffey *et al.*, 1993).

Whole-body treatment is given using between 40 and 70% of the MPD. Doses are increased usually weekly by between 10 and 40% to maintain the response to treatment as the skin adapts by pigmentation and epidermal thickening. Using a twice-weekly protocol with MPD measurement to choose the starting dose, it is typically possible to clear psoriasis with 12 exposures and a cumulative UVA dose of around $50 J/cm^2$. The response to treatment is quite variable, however, and some patients will clear faster than this, whilst others show a slower response. For topical (bath) PUVA, smaller UVA doses are used, as the skin is more photosensitive than with oral PUVA. Typical starting doses are $0.2–0.5 J/cm^2$.

Once clearance of psoriasis has been achieved, it was common practice to continue with PUVA for a variable period to maintain remission. With the long-term side-effects of PUVA now well defined, however, many dermatologists prefer to avoid maintenance treatment wherever possible.

Adjunctive agents

Vitamin A derivatives (retinoids), given orally, are sometimes used in conjunction with PUVA therapy for psoriasis. They may reduce the cumulative UVA dose required for clearance, particularly in patients who are poor or slow responders to PUVA.

Side-effects

The main short-term side-effects of PUVA are erythema and nausea. PUVA erythema has a delayed onset compared with UVB erythema, can persist for a week or more, and may be associated with severe itching, blistering and local skin pain. The risk of burning is minimised if care is taken not to treat patients who have any residual erythema from the previous treatment. Once symptomatic erythema has developed, emollients and topical corticosteroids may aid resolution. Severe erythema may be followed by the development of new lesions of psoriasis arising within areas of damaged skin.

Nausea is quite common with oral 8-methoxypsoralen, lasting 1–4 hours after ingestion. In some patients, this problem can be overcome if the drug is taken with a light meal. For the 5% of patients in whom nausea prevents the use of 8-methoxypsoralen, 5-methoxypsoralen may be substituted, although this drug may be less effective at clearing psoriasis.

Many patients who have received PUVA in high doses over long periods will have some signs of skin damage. Multiple, small hyperpigmented lesions, termed PUVA freckles (or PUVA lentigines), are seen in up to 70% of high-dose patients. They have not been shown to have malignant potential, but may be perceived by some patients as a cosmetic problem. More worrying is the development of warty, keratotic lesions (PUVA keratoses), usually up to 1 cm in diameter, which may show premalignant features on histological examination. It is now clearly established that long-term PUVA treatment results in an increased risk of cutaneous squamous cell carcinoma (Stern and Laird, 1994). This risk has been shown to be dose dependent: a cumulative UVA dose received through PUVA of $< 500 J/cm^2$ is unlikely to result in significant risk; above $1000 J/cm^2$ is associated with definite risk, and around 50% of patients who have received $> 2000 J/cm^2$ will have PUVA keratoses or squamous carcinoma (Lever and Farr, 1994). In some centres, malignant tumours have occurred on the male genitalia and it is now recommended that this area should be protected by clothing whenever possible during a course of treatment. There has also been one report suggesting that PUVA treatment may be associated with an increased risk of malignant melanoma (Stern, Nichols and Vakeva, 1997). The very real risk of serious skin damage through PUVA emphasises the importance of accurate dosimetry and careful selection of patients for PUVA treatment.

ULTRAVIOLET DOSIMETRY

Accurate UV dosimetry in photo(chemo)therapy is important for two reasons:

- to ensure that patients receive the correct prescribed dose of UVB or UVA, thus allowing treatment regimens to be optimally effective.

- to maintain accurate records of patients' lifetime UV exposure received during treatment, which is especially important when the risk of PUVA-related malignancy is considered.

There are several makes of UV dosemeter that are used in photo(chemo)therapy. A dosemeter consists of two parts:

- a *sensor* incorporating a detector which is primarily sensitive to either UVB or UVA
- a *meter* which displays the irradiance in units of milliwatts per square centimetre (mW/cm^2).

A simple calculation allows exposure time to be determined for a prescribed dose in joules per square centimetre (J/cm^2) and a dosemeter reading in mW/cm^2:

$$\text{Treatment time} = (1000 \times \text{prescribed dose} \\ \text{(minutes)} \quad (J/cm^2))/(60 \times \text{measured} \\ \text{irradiance } (mW/cm^2))$$

The UV irradiance in whole-body photo(chemo)-therapy cubicles normally ranges from 3 to $20\,mW/cm^2$ depending upon the number and type of installed lamps and their age.

Many UV machines have a built-in sensor that controls patient exposure. Yet there can be dangers with this approach:

1. The sensor inside the UV cabin may only 'see' a small fraction of the lamps and the output from these may not be representative
2. The patient may shield the sensor either inadvertently or deliberately
3. The sensor may accumulate dust and skin with the consequence that it gives a falsely low measurement of irradiance, which results in patients receiving an overdose of radiation
4. Exposure to radiation inside the UV cabin will cause the sensitivity of the sensor to change with time.

Ideally, therefore, one or more hand-held UV dosemeters (depending on whether a centre has just UVB or UVA, or both) should be available so that regular checks can be made on the integrity of built-in sensors. It is a sound policy to have the dosemeter recalibrated annually.

Measuring irradiance inside PUVA machines

The purpose of monitoring inside the unit is to determine a representative irradiance to which patients are exposed, although it should be remembered that irradiance will vary over the body surface due to topology and spatial uniformity. Lamps should be switched on at least 5 minutes before measurement to allow stability of output. One of two methods may be used.

Direct method

The operator should measure the irradiance while standing in the unit at waist level. The irradiance values should be determined with the operator facing the door and repeated after facing each panel in turn. The mean irradiance of the four to six readings is taken as the working value. Care must be taken to ensure that the field of view of the sensor is not restricted by any part of the body or clothing, and that the operator is protected against UV exposure, especially in UVB cabins.

Indirect method

The irradiance should be measured in the UV cabin while it is unoccupied. The sensor should be clamped at 20 cm from the lamps at mid-height, directed at each bank of lamps. The mean value of these measurements is multiplied by a correction factor to obtain a representative irradiance. The correction factor should be determined by operators for their own cabin; values between 0.80 to 0.85 are typical. It is important to use a correction factor in an unoccupied cabin, as the irradiance will be increased by approximately 20% because the shielding effect of the body is not present.

Most centres prefer to use the direct method of monitoring irradiance. The frequency with which this is done varies considerably: from daily to annually, and sometimes never. We recommend weekly monitoring by the direct method as a compromise between limiting operator exposure in the UV cabin and keeping check of the changes in output as the lamps age.

SAFETY

Considerations of safety relate to both patients and staff (Diffey, 1990).

Patient safety

There must be adequate protection against electrical hazards. Patients (and physiotherapists) should not be able to touch any live electrical parts, and all metal components, such as handrails and safety grids, must satisfy national electrical safety standards and codes of practice.

Patients should not be able to come in contact with bare lamps. In high-pressure units this is achieved by interposing a glass filter(s) between the patient and lamps. However, in whole-body phototherapy units incorporating large numbers of fluorescent lamps, it is normally possible for patients to touch the lamps. The main risk is that from flying glass if a fluorescent lamp implodes. Although the occurrence is rare, it does happen.

Other features that relate to patients' safety include hand rails to support patients during treatment, a cord within the cabinet that can be pulled by the patient to summon help, doors that can be opened easily by the patient from inside the irradiation cabinet, non-skid flooring in the cabinet, and adequate air flow to maintain patient comfort during the irradiation period.

Finally, there is one potential hazard associated with high-pressure lamp phototherapy units that incorporate optical filters to allow either UVA or UVA plus UVB irradiation. If only UVA irradiation is intended but the operator fails to ensure that the correct filter is in place, the patient may be exposed to high doses of UVB (depending on the treatment times), which can lead to severe, painful erythema. A similar hazard exists with combination units incorporating both UVA and UVB fluorescent lamps.

Because psoralens are deposited in the lens of the eye there is the possibility of cataract induction if the eyes are exposed to UVA irradiation in the 12 hours or so following the ingestion of the drug. Consequently, patients should avoid unnecessary exposure to sunlight for the remainder of the day after taking the psoralens, and should be instructed to wear UVA-opaque spectacles or sunglasses for the following 12 hours. (Some dermatology units recommend wearing eye protection for 24 hours.) The effectiveness of spectacles in blocking UVA should ideally be measured in a spectrophotometer (a laboratory instrument for measuring light transmission on a wavelength-by-wavelength basis). Staff can check spectacles by using the radiation from a PUVA unit and a hand-held UVA dosemeter. Spectacles are acceptable only if there is a zero or near-zero reading on the dosemeter.

Staff safety

Exposure to ultraviolet radiation can produce harmful effects in the eyes and the skin, and measurements have shown that an ultraviolet exposure hazard exists in the vicinity of many lamps used for phototherapy; the maximum permissible exposure for 8 hour working periods recommended by national regulatory authorities can be exceeded in less than 2 minutes. For this reason, operators should always keep away from the primary beam as much as is practicable when working with unenclosed lamps. Measures which can be taken to minimise the unnecessary exposure of staff to ultraviolet radiation include: proper engineering design of ultraviolet apparatus; wearing of appropriate goggles or face shields, accompanied, if necessary, by suitable UVR-opaque clothing; limiting access to the area to persons directly concerned with the work; and ensuring that staff are aware of the potential hazards associated with exposure to ultraviolet radiation sources.

Patients undergoing UV irradiation are often given green-tinted, occlusive goggles (e.g. Portia Actinotherapy Goggles, Solport Ltd), whereas staff may prefer to wear clear spectacles with side shields which have negligible transmission of UVR (e.g. Blak-Ray Contrast Control Spectacles Model No UVC-303, Ultraviolet Products Ltd, Cambridge).

It is not acceptable for staff to experience either skin erythema or photokeratitis. If this does occur, working practices should be examined and steps taken to ensure that over-exposure is unlikely in the future (Diffey, 1989).

Hazards from ozone

Ozone is a colourless, toxic, irritant gas formed by a photochemical reaction between short-wavelength UVR and the oxygen present in the air. It is possible to find ozone near ultraviolet lamps, especially those where radiation of wavelengths shorter than about 250 nm is transmitted through the envelope of the lamp. Most modern phototherapy lamps are so-called 'ozone-free'; that is, the lamp envelope is opaque to wavelengths below about 260 nm, thus preventing shorter-wavelength UVR from forming ozone in the air. If ozone is suspected, either by measurement or smell, the gas should be removed by adequate ventilation.

PURCHASING AND INSTALLATION REQUIREMENTS

Phototherapy equipment is purchased relatively infrequently and the pace of technological improvements means that when new equipment is needed it will almost certainly be a different model from existing equipment. A number of factors should be considered in selecting equipment including cost, fitness for intended application, safety, reliability and service support. Further guidance on these and other factors can be found in *Medical Device and Equipment Management for Hospital and Community-based Organisations* published by the Medical Devices Agency (1998).

Single lamps require no special electrical supply or room modification. With whole-body systems, however, it will normally be necessary to install a high-current mains electrical supply. Consideration should also be given to maintaining a satisfactory environmental temperature by installing air-conditioning units.

In the United Kingdom, phototherapy equipment should be installed in accordance with the MDA publication *Checks and Tests for Newly Delivered Medical Devices* (Medical Devices Agency, 1999). It will normally be the responsibility of the hospital engineering department to ensure that appropriate requirements are followed and the equipment is thoroughly checked for electrical safety before handing over the equipment to the Physiotherapy Department.

MAINTENANCE AND REPAIR

Keeping phototherapy equipment both safe and effective needs both routine maintenance procedures and planned preventative maintenance (PPM) carried out by competent staff.

There is very little required in the way of routine maintenance of phototherapy units. Lamp surfaces should be cleaned regularly to remove dust and skin, both of which will attenuate the radiation. Lamps should be replaced when the irradiance has dropped sufficiently low that treatment times become unacceptably long. When this point occurs is very much dependent on local circumstances and workload. For example, if using a TL01 phototherapy unit at a maximum dose of around 4J/cm^2 for no longer than 20 minutes, a change of lamps will be required when the irradiance has fallen to:

$$(4 \times 1000)/(20 \times 60) \text{ mW/cm}^2,$$

which is

$$3.3 \text{ mW/cm}^2.$$

It is the responsibility of the Physiotherapy Manager to ensure that a PPM programme, which includes electrical safety checks on equipment, is in place.

REFERENCES

Chue, B, Borok, M, Lowe, NJ (1988) Phototherapy units: comparison of fluorescent ultraviolet B and ultraviolet A units with a high-pressure mercury system. *Journal of the American Academy of Dermatology* **18**: 641–645.

Dawe, RS, Wainwright, NJ, Cameron, H, Ferguson J (1998) Narrow-band (TL-01) ultraviolet B phototherapy for chronic plaque psoriasis: three times or five times weekly treatment? *British Journal of Dermatology* **138**: 833-839.

Diffey, BL (1989) Ultraviolet radiation and skin cancer: are physiotherapists at risk? *Physiotherapy* **75**: 615–616.

Diffey, BL (1990) Ultraviolet radiation safety. In: Pal, SB (ed) *Handbook of Laboratory Health and Safety Measures*, 2nd edn. Kluwer Academic Publishers, London, pp 349–396.

Diffey, BL, Farr, PM (1987) An appraisal of ultraviolet radiation lamps used in the phototherapy of psoriasis. *British Journal of Dermatology* **117**: 49–56.

Diffey, BL, Harrington, TR, Challoner, AVJ (1978) A comparison of the anatomical uniformity of irradiation in two different photochemotherapy units. *British Journal of Dermatology* **99**: 361–363.

Diffey, BL, de Berker, DAR, Saunders, PJ, Farr, PM (1993) A device for phototesting patients before PUVA therapy. *British Journal of Dermatology* **129**: 700–703.

Dootson, G, Norris, PG, Gibson, CJ, Diffey, BL (1994) The practice of UVB phototherapy in the United Kingdom. *British Journal of Dermatology* **131**: 873–877.

Farr, PM, Diffey, BL (1991) PUVA treatment of psoriasis in the United Kingdom. *British Journal of Dermatology* **124**: 365–367.

Farr, PM, Diffey, BL, Marks, JM (1987) Phototherapy and anthralin treatment of psoriasis: new lamps for old. *British Medical Journal* **294**: 205–207.

Farr, PM, Diffey, BL (1988) Augmentation of ultraviolet erythema by indomethacin in actinic prurigo: evidence of mechanism of photosensitivity. *Photochemistry and Photobiology* **47**: 413–417.

Farr, PM, Diffey, BL, Higgins, EM, Matthews, JNS (1991) The action spectrum between 320 and 400 nm for clearance of psoriasis by psoralen photochemotherapy. *British Journal of Dermatology* **124**: 443–448.

Halpern, SM, Anstey, AV, Dawe, RS, *et al.* (2000) Guidelines for topical PUVA: a report of a workshop of the British Photodermatology Group. *British Journal of Dermatology* **142**: 22–31.

Hawk, JLM (ed) (1999) *Photodermatology*. Arnold, London.

Hudson-Peacock, MJ, Diffey, BL, Farr, PM (1994) Photoprotective action of emollients in ultraviolet therapy of psoriasis. *British Journal of Dermatology* **130**: 361–365.

Ibbotson, SH, Farr, PM (1999) The time-course of psoralen ultraviolet A (PUVA) erythema. *Journal of Investigative Dermatology* **113**: 346–349.

Johnson, BE (1984) The photobiology of the skin. In: Jarrett, A (ed) *The Physiology and Pathophysiology of the Skin*. Academic Press, London, pp 2434–2437.

Lever, LR, Farr, PM (1994) Skin cancers or premalignant lesions occur in half of high-dose PUVA patients. *British Journal of Dermatology* **131**: 215–219.

Medical Devices Agency 1998. *Medical Device and Equipment Management for Hospital and Community-based Organisations*. MDA DB9801. January. MDA.

Medical Devices Agency 1999. *Checks and Tests for Newly Delivered Medical Devices*. MDA DB9801, Suppl 1, December. MDA.

Norris, PG, Hawk, JLM, Baker, C *et al.* (1994) British Photodermatology Group Guidelines for PUVA. *British Journal of Dermatology* **130**: 246–255.

Parrish, JA, Jaenicke, KF (1981) Action spectrum for phototherapy of psoriasis. *Journal of Investigations in Dermatology* **76**: 359–362.

Sakuntabhai, A, Sharpe, GR, Farr, PM (1993) Response of psoriasis to twice weekly PUVA. *British Journal of Dermatology* **128**: 166–171.

Sollux Publishing Company (1933). Actinotherapy Technique. Sollux Publishing Company, Slough.

Stern, RS, Laird, N (1994) The carcinogenic risk of treatments for severe psoriasis: photochemotherapy follow-up study. *Cancer* **73**: 2759–2764.

Stern, RS, Nichols, KT, Vakeva, LH (1997) Malignant melanoma in patients treated for psoriasis with methoxalen (psoralen) and ultraviolet B radiation (PUVA). *New England Journal of Medicine* **336**: 1041–1045.

Stevenson, IH, Kenicer, KJA, Johnson, BE, Frain-Bell W (1981) Plasma 8-methoxypsoralen concentrations in photochemotherapy of psoriasis. *British Journal of Dermatology* **104**: 47–51.

Studniberg, HM, Weller, P (1993) PUVA, UVB, psoriasis, and nonmelanoma skin cancer. *Journal of the American Academy of Dermatology* **29**: 1013–1022.

SECTION CONTENT

14

Ultrasound therapy

Steve Young

INTRODUCTION

The aim of this chapter is to provide a detailed source of reference about ultrasound and its mechanisms of action on tissues, in both the physical and biological sense. Once clinicians know how a modality works they are then, in principle, in a position to predict with a high degree of accuracy what the correct treatment regimen should be for a particular injury, without having to rely solely on clinical experience and heresay. However, this is beset with problems as there is no general agreement in the clinical and laboratory research literature on how best to treat each individual type of injury. Also, no two injuries are identical. What may work for one lesion, for example, may not work for another. It is vital, therefore, that the clinician has as much knowledge as possible about the biology of healing and how electrotherapies interact with it in order to select and adapt the treatment regimen best to provide the much-needed repair stimulus. It must be understood, however, that some wounds will not repair irrespective of which electrotherapy modality is applied, because of the presence of some underlying deficiency in the wound environment.

History taking

Bearing this in mind, one of the first steps to be taken by the clinician before embarking on a course of therapy is to make sure that they have a full patient history so that any underlying complications are known (e.g. diabetes, venous insufficiency). These complications should be addressed before a course of therapy is undertaken. Failure to do this means that both clinician and patient waste time and money and, most importantly, there is a likelihood of compounding the problem and putting the patient at further risk.

Assessment of success

This leads on to another problem: once therapy has begun, how does the clinician then assess wound healing? It is important to have sensitive, quantitative diagnostic techniques which are easy to use and to interpret, and by which changes in a wound in response to therapy can be assessed. In an age of cost-guided medical care where the term 'clinical audit' is the buzzword (Department of Health, 1989), it is vital that the amount of time a patient is under care is cut to the absolute minimum. The costs for just one particular type of wound are enormous—£25 905 for a single patient with a pressure sore needing 12 weeks of inpatient treatment in 1988 (Hibbs, 1988, 1989)! The total cost for all such treatments becomes astronomical, and choosing the right treatment, based on strong clinical evidence can lead to enormous savings (Hibbs, 1989; Livesey and Simpson, 1989). This is highlighted in a study carried out in a recent cost-effectiveness study, which compared the relative savings that could be achieved using a range of alternative wound dressings (Harding, Cutting and Price, 2000). Savings of 50–500% were shown to be possible by using the right dressing on the right wound.

It is vital that we have objective and sensitive techniques by which we can assess wound healing. Only when we have this can the rate and quality of repair be optimised confidently. Chronic wounds present additional problems, because these wounds heal so slowly it is often difficult to obtain an early indication whether they are healing, remaining static or deteriorating. Often, much time is wasted using ineffective therapeutic modalities.

There are numerous methods for evaluating wound repair, and these will be discussed in Chapter 19 (Diagnostic and assessment applications).

Ultrasound usage

To say that ultrasound is a frequently used therapeutic modality in physiotherapy practice is a gross understatement. The results of a survey carried out in Britain in 1985 (ter Haar, Dyson and Oakley, 1985) showed that 20% of all physiotherapy treatments in NHS departments and 54% of all private treatments involved therapeutic ultrasound. It is obvious that if a modality is used so widely then it is vital that we understand fully its biological effects and mechanisms of action so that it can be used effectively and, more important, safely. In the 1985 survey, physiotherapists were asked to complete a questionnaire covering a range of topics including: technical details of their ultrasound machine, intensities and frequencies most commonly used, calibration procedures, and observed contraindications. The survey revealed that there existed large inconsistencies in the use of ultrasound and, therefore, signalled an urgent need for further education in the use of this modality. In summary, the survey highlighted the following:

1. intensities used varied by a factor of 300, from 0.1 to 3.0 W/cm^2
2. confusion existed over the choice of pulsed- or continuous-exposure mode
3. some of the inclusions in the list of contraindications were based on little or no scientific evidence
4. calibration was carried out, at best, once every 3–6 months in NHS departments and on average once a year in private practice. The availability of calibration equipment to physiotherapists was low, with only 20% of NHS and 6% of those in private practice having access to radiation balances.

Problems also appear to exist when it comes to making a choice of which type of electrotherapy to use when presented with the wide range of injuries that arrive at the clinic daily. A recent national survey (Kitchen, 1995) highlighted this uncertainty. The work pointed out that knowledge about electrotherapy's biological effects, clinical efficacy and safety are limited, and this compounds the decision-making process.

The purpose of this chapter is to present the relevant quantitative, clinical and laboratory data about therapeutic ultrasound. This should provide the clinician with the capacity to choose when and when not to use the modality and how to use it effectively and safely.

PHYSICAL EFFECTS OF ULTRASOUND

When ultrasound enters the body it can exert an effect on the cells and tissues via two physical mechanisms: thermal and non-thermal. It is important that we understand these mechanisms fully as some are stimulatory in their effect on the wound-healing process, whereas others are potentially dangerous. (For further details of the physical principles that underlie the behaviour of ultrasound, see Ch. 1.)

Thermal effects

When ultrasound travels through tissue a percentage of it is absorbed, and this leads to the generation of heat within that tissue. The amount of absorption depends upon the nature of the tissue, its degree of vascularisation, and the frequency of the ultrasound. Tissues with a high protein content absorb ultrasound more readily than those with a higher fat content, and the higher the frequency the greater is the absorption. A biologically significant thermal effect can be achieved if the temperature of the tissue is raised to between 40 and 45°C for at least 5 minutes. Controlled heating can produce desirable effects (Lehmann and De Lateur, 1982), which include pain relief, decrease in joint stiffness and increased blood flow.

The advantage of using ultrasound to deliver this heating effect is that the therapist has control over the depth at which the heating occurs. To do this, it is important that the therapist has

knowledge of half-value depth measurements (i.e. the depth of penetration of the ultrasound energy at which its intensity has decreased by a half) and of the selective heating of tissues. For example, the half-value depth for soft, irregular connective tissue is approximately 4 mm at 3 MHz, but is about 11 mm at 1 MHz. Structures which will be heated preferentially include periosteum, superficial cortical bone, joint menisci, fibrotic muscle, tendon sheaths and major nerve roots (Lehmann and Guy, 1972), and intermuscular interfaces (ter Haar and Hopewell, 1982). It is therefore important that the therapist has knowledge of the structures which lie between the ultrasound source and the injured tissue, and also beyond it.

Once delivered, the heat is then dissipated by both thermal diffusion and local blood flow, which can present a problem when treating injuries where the blood supply has been restricted by either the nature of the injury or the relatively avascular nature of the tissue itself (e.g. tendon). Another complication can occur when the ultrasound beam hits bone or a metal prosthesis. Because of the great acoustic impedance difference between these structures and the surrounding soft tissues there will be a reflection of about 30% of the incident energy back through the soft tissue. This means that further energy is deposited as heat during the beam's return journey. Therefore, heat rise in soft tissue will be higher when it is situated in front of a reflector. To complicate matters further, an interaction termed *mode conversion* also occurs at the interface of the soft tissue and the reflector (e.g. bone or metal prosthesis). During mode conversion, a percentage of the reflected incident energy is converted from a longitudinal waveform into a transverse or shear waveform which cannot propagate on the soft tissue side of the interface and is therefore absorbed rapidly, causing heat rise (and frequently pain) at the bone–soft tissue interface (periosteum).

Non-thermal effects

There are many situations where ultrasound produces bioeffects and yet significant temperature change is not involved (e.g. low spatial-average temporal-average (SATA) intensity). There is some evidence indicating where non-thermal mechanisms are thought to play a primary role in producing a therapeutically significant effect: stimulation of tissue regeneration (Dyson *et al.*, 1968), soft tissue repair (Dyson, Franks and Suckling, 1976; Paul *et al.*, 1960), blood flow in chronically ischaemic tissues (Hogan, Burke and Franklin, 1982), protein synthesis (Webster *et al.*, 1978) and bone repair (Dyson and Brookes, 1983).

The physical mechanisms thought to be involved in producing these non-thermal effects are one or more of the following: cavitation, acoustic streaming and standing waves.

Cavitation

Ultrasound can cause the formation of micrometer-sized bubbles or cavities in gas-containing fluids. Depending upon the pressure amplitude of the energy, the resultant bubbles can be either useful or dangerous. Low-pressure amplitudes result in the formation of bubbles which vibrate to a degree where reversible permeability changes are produced in cell membranes near to the cavitational event (Mortimer and Dyson, 1988). Changes in cell permeability to various ions such as calcium can have a profound effect upon the activity of the cell (Sutherland and Rall, 1968). High-pressure amplitudes can result in a more violent cavitational event (often called transient or collapse cavitation). During this event, the bubbles collapse during the positive pressure part of the cycle with such a ferocity that pressures in excess of 1000 MPa and temperatures in excess of 10 000 K are generated. This violent behaviour can lead to the formation of highly reactive free radicals. Although free radicals are produced by cells naturally (e.g. during cellular respiration), they are removed by free-radical scavengers. Production in excess of the natural free-radical scavenger system could, however, be damaging. Avoidance of a standing-wave field and use of low intensities during therapy make it unlikely that transient cavitation will occur.

Acoustic streaming

This refers to the unidirectional movement of a fluid in an ultrasound field. High-velocity gradients develop next to boundaries between fluids and structures such as cells, bubbles and tissue fibres. Acoustic streaming can stimulate cell activity if it occurs at the boundary of the cell membrane and the surrounding fluid. The resultant viscous stress on the membrane, providing it is not too severe, can alter the membrane's permeability and second-messenger activity (Dyson, 1982, 1985). This could result in therapeutically advantageous changes such as increased protein synthesis (Webster *et al.*, 1978), increased secretion from mast cells (Fyfe and Chahl, 1982), fibroblast mobility changes (Mummery, 1978), increased uptake of the second messenger calcium (Mortimer and Dyson, 1988; Mummery, 1978), and increased production of growth factors by macrophages (Young and Dyson, 1990a). All these effects could account for the acceleration of repair following ultrasound therapy.

Standing waves

When an ultrasound wave hits the interface between two tissues of different acoustic impedances (e.g. bone and muscle), reflection of a percentage of the wave will occur. The reflected waves can interact with oncoming incident waves to form a standing-wave field in which the peaks of intensity (*antinodes*) (see Ch. 1) of the waves are stationary and are separated by half a wavelength. Because the standing wave consists of two superimposed waves in addition to a travelling component, the peak intensities and pressures are higher than the normal incident wave. Between the antinodes, which are points of maximum and minimum pressure, there are *nodes*, which are points of fixed pressure. Gas bubbles collect at the antinodes, and cells (if in suspension) collect at the nodes (NCRP, 1983). Fixed cells, such as endothelial cells which line the blood vessels, can be damaged by microstreaming forces around bubbles if they are situated at the pressure antinodes. Erythrocytes can be lysed if they are swept through the arrays of bubbles situated at the pressure antinodes. Reversible blood cell stasis has been demonstrated, the cells forming bands half a wavelength apart centred on the pressure nodes (Dyson *et al.*, 1974). The increased pressure produced in standing-wave fields can cause transient cavitation and consequently the formation of free radicals (Nyborg, 1977). It is therefore important that therapists move the applicator continuously throughout treatment, and also use the lowest intensity required to cause an effect, to minimise the hazards involved in standing-wave field production (Dyson *et al.*, 1974).

Having discovered how ultrasound imparts its energy to the tissue we will now look at how this energy is utilised by cells and tissues in the wound-healing process.

TISSUE REPAIR

Following injury, a number of cellular and chemical events occur in soft tissues. Although these events are explained in detail in an earlier section of this book (Ch. 3), it is worth summarising them here in the context of ultrasound therapy.

Underlying repair process

The major cellular components of the repair process include platelets, mast cells, polymorphonuclear leucocytes (PMNLs), macrophages, T lymphocytes, fibroblasts and endothelial cells. These cells migrate as a module into the injury site in a well-defined sequence which is controlled by numerous soluble wound factors. These wound factors originate from a number of sources such as inflammatory cells (e.g. macrophages and PMNLs), inflammatory cascade systems (e.g. coagulation and complement), or from the products of damaged tissue breakdown.

The whole repair process, for convenience, can be divided into three phases (Clark, 1990), although it must be stated that these phases overlap considerably, lacking any distinct border between each other. The three phases are:

1. inflammation
2. proliferation/granulation tissue formation
3. remodelling.

There is now overwhelming evidence showing that the effectiveness of therapeutic ultrasound is dependent upon the phase of repair in which it is used. This will be discussed in more detail later in this chapter.

Inflammation

This early, dynamic phase of repair is characterised initially by clot formation. The blood platelet is a major constituent of the blood clot and, in addition to its activities associated with clotting, platelets also contain numerous biologically active substances, including prostaglandins, and serotonin and platelet-derived growth factor (PDGF). These substances have a profound effect upon the local environment of the wound and its subsequent repair (Clark, 1990). Mast cells present another source of biologically active substances, or wound factors, which help orchestrate the early repair sequences.

Neutrophils are the first PMNLs to enter the wound bed, attracted by an array of wound factors present at the wound site. The neutrophils' function is to clear the wound site of foreign particles such as bacteria and damaged tissue debris.

Macrophages enter the wound bed soon after the neutrophils, where they phagocytose bacteria and wound tissue debris. They also produce wound factors which direct granulation tissue formation (Leibovich and Ross, 1975).

Evidence will be presented later in this chapter which shows that, when used at the right time during wound repair and at the right levels of output, ultrasound can influence the release of these wound factors from the cells in and around the wound bed.

Proliferation/granulation tissue formation

During normal acute injury repair, the inflammatory phase is followed within several days by granulation tissue formation. This stage is often referred to as the *proliferative phase*. During this phase the wound void is filled with cells (mainly macrophages and fibroblasts), numerous blood vessels (angiogenesis) and a connective tissue matrix (composed of fibronectin, hyaluronic acid and collagen types I and III).

A new epidermis also forms during this phase of repair. The new epidermal cells migrate from the edge of the wound (and also from around hair follicles within the injury site in the case of partial-thickness wounds) towards the centre of the wound.

Wound contraction occurs during this phase of repair and can be defined as the process by which the size of a wound decreases by the centripetal movement of the whole thickness of surrounding skin (Peacock, 1984). In humans, skin is relatively immobile owing to its attachment to underlying structures. Therefore, in some instances where wounds occur over joints, any wound contraction may lead to immobilisation because of the tension developed through attachment of the skin to underlying structures. Thus excessive contraction is often seen as a serious complication to healing.

The stimulus controlling all of these events comes from numerous sources, of which macrophages constitute a main one. The release of active factors from macrophages is thought to be controlled, in part, by the relatively hypoxic environment of the wound (Knighton et al., 1983). The effect of ultrasound on the macrophage will be discussed in detail later.

Remodelling

Remodelling can continue for many months or years after the proliferative phase of repair. During remodelling, granulation tissue is gradually replaced by a scar which is composed of relatively acellular and avascular tissue. As the wound matures, the composition of the extracellular matrix changes. Initially, the extracellular matrix is composed of hyaluronic acid, fibronectin and collagens types I, III and V. The ratio of type I to III collagen then changes during remodelling until type I is dominant. Scar tissue is a poor substitute for unwounded skin. The rate at which wounds gain tensile strength is slow (Levenson et al., 1965), and they are at only 20 to 25% of their maximum strength 3 weeks after injury. The increase in wound strength depends upon two main factors: first, the rate of collagen deposition, remodelling and alignment, with the gradual formation of larger collagen bundles (Kischer and Shetlar, 1974), and secondly, alteration in the intermolecular cross-links (Bailey et al., 1975). It will be shown later in this chapter that, if used at the correct time after injury, ultrasound can improve both the cosmetic appearance and the mechanical properties of the resulting scar tissue.

The effect of ultrasound on body tissues

This section deals with the effect of ultrasound on soft tissues and bone, as well as its possible effects on pain and through phonophoresis. Low-frequency ultrasound is also noted.

The effect of ultrasound on the inflammatory phase of repair

As indicated previously, the inflammatory phase is extremely dynamic and, during it, numerous cell types (e.g. platelets, mast cells, macrophages and neutrophils) enter and leave the wound site. There is evidence to show that therapeutic ultrasound can interact with the above cells, influencing their activity and leading to the acceleration of repair.

Acoustic streaming forces have been shown to produce changes in platelet membrane permeability leading to the release of serotonin (Williams, 1974; Williams, Sykes and O'Brien, 1976). In addition to serotonin, platelets contain wound factors essential for successful repair (Ginsberg, 1981). If streaming can stimulate the release of serotonin, it may also influence the release of these other factors.

One of the major chemicals that modifies the wound environment at this time after injury is histamine. The mast cell is the major source of this factor, which is normally released by a process known as mast cell degranulation. In this process, the membrane of the cell, in response to increased levels of intracellular calcium (Yurt, 1981), ruptures and releases histamine and other products into the wound site. It has been shown that a single treatment of therapeutic ultrasound, if given soon after injury (i.e. during the early inflammatory phase), can stimulate mast cells to degranulate, thereby releasing histamine into the surrounding tissues (Fyfe and Chahl, 1982; Hashish, 1986). It is possible that ultrasound is stimulating the mast cell to degranulate by increasing its permeability to calcium. Increased calcium ion permeability has been demonstrated by a number of researchers. Calcium ions can act as intracellular messengers; when their distribution and concentration change in response to environmental modifications of the plasma membrane they act as an intracellular signal for the appropriate metabolic response. There is much evidence that ultrasound can produce membrane changes in a number of cell types. These range from gross destructive changes to more subtle reversible changes. Gross changes can be achieved if levels of ultrasound are high enough. Even when using therapeutic levels of ultrasound it is possible to achieve the necessary conditions for destruction if a standing-wave field is allowed to form because of bad clinical practice (i.e. failing to keep the applicator head moving). Dyson *et al.* (1974) demonstrated that if this phenomena occurs in the region of fine blood vessels it is possible to damage the endothelial cells lining the luminal side of the vessels.

Reversible membrane permeability changes to calcium have been demonstrated using therapeutic levels of ultrasound (Dinno *et al.*, 1989; Mortimer and Dyson, 1988; Mummery, 1978). The fact that this effect can be suppressed by irradiation under pressure suggests that cavitation is the physical mechanism responsible. Changes in permeability to other ions such as potassium have also been demonstrated (Chapman, Macnally and Tucker, 1979). Work by Dinno *et al.* (1989) demonstrated, in a frog-skin model, that ultrasound can modify the electrophysiological properties of the tissue; this research study reported an ultrasound-induced reduction in the sodium–potassium ATPase pump activity. A decrease in pump activity, if it occurs in neuronal plasma membranes, may inhibit the transduction of noxious stimuli

and subsequent neural transmission, which may account in part for the pain relief which is often experienced following clinical exposure to therapeutic ultrasound. It should be noted, however, that the mechanism of pain relief is still not understood fully, and much of it can be attributed to placebo effects.

As discussed above, the evidence is clear: therapeutic ultrasound can alter membrane permeability to various ions. The ability to affect calcium transport through cell membranes is of considerable clinical significance since calcium, in its role as an intracellular or second messenger, can have a profound effect on cell activity, for instance by increasing synthesis and secretion of wound factors by cells involved in the healing process. This has been shown to occur in macrophages in response to therapeutic levels of ultrasound (Young and Dyson, 1990a); as discussed earlier, these are one of the key cells in the wound-healing system, being a source of numerous wound factors. This in vitro study demonstrated that the ultrasound-induced change in wound factor secretion is frequency dependent. Ultrasound at an intensity of $0.5 W/cm^2$ (SATA) and a frequency of 0.75 MHz appeared to be most effective in encouraging the immediate release of factors already present in the cell cytoplasm, whereas the higher frequency 3.0 MHz appeared to be most effective in stimulating the production of new factors, which were then released some time later by the cells' normal secretory processes. Therefore, there appeared to be a delayed effect when treating with the higher frequency; however, the resulting liberated factors, when compared with those liberated using 0.75 MHz, were more potent in their effect on the stimulation of fibroblast population growth. One possible reason why these two frequencies induce different effects relates to the physical mechanisms involved. At each frequency the peak pressure generated by the ultrasound was that necessary for cavitation to occur (Williams, 1987). Cavitation is more likely to occur at the lower frequency, whereas heating is more likely to occur at the higher one. Therefore, the differing proportions of non-thermal to thermal mechanisms present in each of the two treatments may explain the difference seen in the resulting biological effects.

Hart (1993) also found that following the in vitro exposure of macrophages to ultrasound, a wound factor was released into the surrounding medium that was mitogenic for fibroblasts.

It has often been thought that ultrasound is an anti-inflammatory agent (Reid, 1981; Snow and Johnson, 1988). When viewed from a clinical standpoint—that is, rapid resolution of oedema (El Hag et al., 1985)—this conclusion is understandable. However, research has shown that ultrasound is not anti-inflammatory in its action (Goddard et al., 1983); rather, it encourages oedema formation to occur more rapidly (Fyfe and Chahl, 1985; Hustler, Zarod and Williams, 1978) and then to subside more rapidly than control sham-irradiated groups, so accelerating the whole process and driving the wound into the proliferative phase of repair sooner.

Further confirmation of this has been shown experimentally in acute surgical wounds (Young and Dyson, 1990b). In this study, full-thickness excised skin lesions in rats were exposed to therapeutic ultrasound (0.1 W/cm^2 SATA, 0.75 MHz or 3.0 MHz) daily for 7 days (5 minutes per day per wound). By 5 days after injury, the ultrasound-treated groups had significantly fewer inflammatory cells in the wound bed and more extensive granulation tissue than the sham-irradiated controls. Also, the alignment of the fibroblasts—parallel to the wound surface— in the wound beds of the ultrasound-treated groups was indicative of a more advanced stage of tissue organisation than the random alignment of fibroblasts seen in the sham-irradiated control wounds. The results obtained suggest that there had been an acceleration of the wounds through the inflammatory phase repair in response to ultrasound therapy. It was also noted that there were no abnormalities such as hypertrophy of the wound tissue seen in response to ultrasound therapy. Therefore, ultrasound therapy appears to accelerate the process without the risk of interfering with the control mechanisms which limit the development of granulation.

The effect of ultrasound on the proliferative phase of repair

The main events occurring during this phase of repair include cell infiltration into the wound bed, angiogenesis, matrix deposition, wound contraction and re-epithelialisation.

Cells such as fibroblasts and endothelial cells are recruited to the wound site by a combination of migration and proliferation. Mummery (1978) showed in vitro that fibroblast motility could be increased when they were exposed to therapeutic levels of ultrasound. With regard to cell proliferation, there is little evidence in the literature to suggest that ultrasound has a direct stimulatory effect on fibroblast stimulation. Most of the in vitro studies report either no effect or even an inhibitory effect on cell proliferation when exposed to therapeutic levels of ultrasound (Kaufman et al., 1977; Loch, Fisher and Kuwert, 1971). However, the literature shows that when tissues are exposed to ultrasound in vivo, a marked increase in wound bed cell number can be demonstrated (Dyson et al., 1970; Young and Dyson, 1990b). This anomaly may be explained if we examine the cellular interactions which occur during healing.

It was illustrated earlier that during wound repair much of the stimulus which controls the cellular events is derived from the macrophage. Therefore, it is highly likely that any increase in, for example, fibroblast proliferation, may be due in part to an indirect effect of ultrasound via the macrophage. Work by Young and Dyson (1990a) showed that if one exposes macrophages to therapeutic levels of ultrasound in vitro, then removes the surrounding culture medium and places it on fibroblast cultures, there is a large stimulatory effect on the proliferation of the fibroblasts. It therefore appears that macrophages are sensitive to ultrasound and, in response to therapeutic levels of it (0.5 W/cm^2 SATA), they release a factor or factors which stimulate fibroblasts to proliferate.

Ultrasound can also effect the rate of angiogenesis. Hogan, Burke and Franklin (1982) showed that capillaries develop more rapidly in chronically ischaemic muscle when exposed to ultrasound. Other work has shown that the exposure of skin lesions to ultrasound can stimulate the growth of blood capillaries into the wound site (Hosseinpour, 1988; Young and Dyson, 1990c).

When fibroblasts are exposed to ultrasound in vitro a marked stimulation in collagen secretion can be detected (Harvey *et al.*, 1975). It should be added that the degree of response is intensity dependent. When the fibroblasts were exposed to continuous ultrasound (0.5 W/cm^2 SA) a 20% increase in collagen secretion was recorded; however, when the ultrasound was pulsed (0.5 W/cm^2 SATA), a 30% increase was recorded. Webster *et al.* (1978) demonstrated an increase in protein synthesis when fibroblasts were exposed to ultrasound.

Wound contraction can be accelerated with ultrasound. Work by Dyson and Smalley (1983) showed that pulsed ultrasound (3 MHz, 0.5 W/cm^2 SATA) could stimulate the contraction of cryosurgical lesions. More recently, Hart (1993) showed that exposure of full-thickness excised skin lesions to low levels of pulsed ultrasound stimulated contraction, leading to a significantly smaller scar. Interestingly, he also found that the same degree of contraction he induced using an intensity of 0.5 W/cm^2 (SATA) could also be achieved by using the much lower intensity of 0.1 W/cm^2 (SATA). This is a significant finding which implies that clinicians can reduce their ultrasound treatment intensities by a significant degree and still achieve the desired results, via non-thermal effects. It is vital when treating tissues which have a compromised blood system, and hence no effective mechanism of dispersing excess heat, that the lowest possible ultrasound intensity is used.

In humans, wound closure is due mainly to granulation tissue formation and re-epithelialisation, whereas in animals, where the skin is more loosely connected to the underlying tissues, wound closure is due mainly to contraction. Dyson, Franks and Suckling (1976) found that ultrasound therapy (3 MHz, pulsed, 0.2 W/cm^2 SATA), accelerated the reduction in varicose ulcer area significantly (Fig. 14.1).

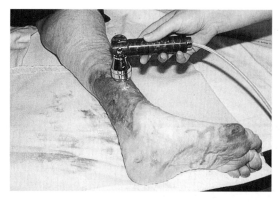

Figure 14.1 Ultrasound treatment to the edge of a varicose ulcer using a sterile gel medium.

Similar findings were reported by Roche and West (1984).

Callam *et al.* (1987) studied the effect of weekly ultrasound therapy (1 MHz, pulsed, 0.5 W/cm^2 SATA) on the healing of chronic leg ulcers. They found that there was a 20% increase in the healing rate of the ultrasound-treated ulcers. There have been negative reports as to the use of ultrasound treatment on these chronic conditions. Lundeberg *et al.* (1990) did not demonstrate any statistically significant difference between ultrasound-treated and sham-treated venous ulcers. However, a trend was noted by the investigators that suggested ultrasound was more effective than placebo treatment. Interestingly, they stated that their experimental design, particularly their sample size ($n = 44$), was such that an improvement of less than 30% could not be detected.

Accelerated wound closure has also been recorded in other chronic wounds such as pressure sores (McDiarmid *et al.*, 1985; Paul *et al.*, 1960). McDiarmid *et al.* also reported an interesting finding that microbiologically infected sores were more responsive to ultrasound therapy than uninfected sores. It is likely that the low-grade infection had in some way primed or further activated the healing system (e.g. recruiting more macrophages to the area), which in turn would produce an amplified signal to herald an early start to the other phases of repair.

The effect of ultrasound on the remodelling phase of repair

During remodelling the wound becomes relatively acellular and avascular, collagen content increases, and the tensile strength of the wound increases. The remodelling phase can last from months to years, depending upon the tissue involved and the nature of the injury. The mechanical properties of the scar are related to both the amount of collagen present and also the arrangement or alignment of the collagen fibres within the wound bed.

The effect of ultrasound on the properties of the scar depend very much upon the time at which the therapy was first instigated. By far the most effective regimens are those that are started soon after injury (i.e. during the inflammatory phase of repair). Webster (1980) found that when wounds were treated three times per week for 2 weeks after injury (0.1 W/cm² SATA) the resulting tensile strength and elasticity of the scar were significantly higher than that of the control group. Byl *et al.* (1992, 1993) demonstrated an increase in tensile strength and collagen content in incised lesions whose treatment was commenced during the inflammatory phase. They also compared different ultrasound intensities and found that the lower intensity (1 MHz, pulsed, 0.5 W/cm² SATA) was the most effective. Treatment with ultrasound during the inflammatory phase of repair not only increases the amount of collagen deposited in the wound but also encourages the deposition of that collagen in a pattern whose three-dimensional architecture more resembles that of uninjured skin than the untreated controls (Dyson, 1981). Jackson, Schwane and Starcher (1991) showed that the mechanical properties of injured tendon can be improved with ultrasound if treatment starts early enough; however, the levels used were relatively high, at 1.5 W/cm². Enwemeka, Rodriguez and Mendosa (1990) reported that increased tensile strength and elasticity can be achieved in injured tendons using much lower intensities (0.5 W/cm² SA). Figure 14.2 shows application of ultrasound to the elbow to treat tennis elbow.

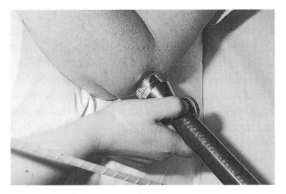

Figure 14.2 Ultrasound treatment for tennis elbow using gel as the transfer medium.

The effect of ultrasound on bone repair

Bone repairs in much the same way as soft tissues. Both repair processes consist of three overlapping phases: inflammation, proliferation and remodelling. However, in bone repair, the proliferative phase is subdivided into soft and hard callus formation. The soft callus is an equivalent to granulation tissue in soft tissue injuries, and it is within this tissue that new bone regenerates to form the hard callus. Much work has been carried out investigating the effects of ultrasound therapy on this process. Dyson and Brookes (1983) showed that it was possible to accelerate the repair of fibular fractures using therapeutic levels of ultrasound (1.5 or 3 MHz, pulsed, 0.5 W/cm² SATA). The treatments were for 5 minutes, four times per week. Treatments were carried out at different combinations of weeks after injury (e.g. during the first two weeks only, or during the third and fourth week only). The most effective treatments were found to be those which were carried out during the first 2 weeks of repair (i.e. during the inflammatory phase of repair). It was found that if treatment was delayed (i.e. started on weeks 3 to 4 after injury) the ultrasound appeared to stimulate cartilage growth, postponing bony union. Of the two frequencies used, 1.5 MHz was the more effective.

There have been many other reports of the effectiveness of ultrasound in the treatment of bone fractures. Pilla *et al.* (1990) showed that low-intensity ultrasound (1.5 or 3 MHz, pulsed, 0.3 W/cm^2) could stimulate fracture repair to such a degree that maximum strength was gained in the treated limbs by 17 days after injury, compared with 28 days in the controls. Tsai, Chang and Liu (1992a) demonstrated an increase in femoral fracture repair when using low intensities of ultrasound (1.5 MHz, pulsed, 0.5 W/cm^2); however, when they tried 1.5 W/cm^2 they found that treatments inhibited repair. The same team (Tsai, Chang and Liu, 1992b) found that, in the most effective output levels for stimulating repair, the production of endogenous PGE$_2$ was highest. They suggested that bone healing stimulated by ultrasound may be mediated via the production of PGE$_2$. More recent work (Heckman *et al.*, 1994) has investigated the effectiveness of low-intensity ultrasound on the healing of tibial fractures. The fractures were examined in a prospective, randomised, double-blind evaluation of low-intensity ultrasound. The treated group showed a significant decrease in the time to healing (86 days) when compared with the control group (114 days).

As with soft tissue repair, the evidence suggests that the best results are achieved when treatment is started as soon after injury as possible.

The effect of ultrasound on pain relief

A number of studies have attempted to evaluate the use of ultrasound in the treatment of pain. However, analysis of available data shows that there is a lack of evidence from large controlled studies, which would indicate what effect ultrasound is having on pain relief, and by what mechanism (Gam and Johannsen, 1995).

Ultrasound has been used by many clinicians for the treatment of carpal tunnel syndrome (Ebenbichler *et al.*, 1998) and stress fractures (Brand *et al.*, 1999). Although not large trials, these studies do indicate that ultrasound may be an option worth trying when treating pain. It is known that ultrasound can accelerate the inflammatory phase of wound healing, leading to a rapid resolution of oedema (El Hag *et al.*, 1985), so it is possible that many of the reports of pain relief with ultrasound could be due to

this—that is, get rid of swelling and you get rid of pain. A large, randomised, controlled clinical trial is necessary to establish the efficacy and mechanism of ultrasound in the treatment of pain.

Phonophoresis

Phonophoresis is defined as the migration of drug molecules through the skin under the influence of ultrasound. Theoretically phonophoresis is possible utilising the acoustic streaming forces, which exist in the ultrasound field. However, it is debatable whether these forces are strong enough to produce a net forward movement capable of pushing all drugs through the skin to their target tissue. In addition, it is often difficult to determine whether a biological effect of a topically applied drug is a result of its direct action on the underlying target tissue or of a systemic effect. This could be one reason why there have been many mixed reports on the effectiveness of this modality for pushing drugs into the skin. It is likely that phonophoresis will be dependent not only on the frequency, intensity, duty cycle and treatment duration of the ultrasound (Mitragotri *et al.*, 2000), but also on the nature of the drug molecule itself.

Research is needed to clarify what parameters of ultrasound are most efficient for facilitating topical drug diffusion, and also which drugs can be most effectively used.

Low-frequency ultrasound

Since the early 1990s there has been an interest in the use of low-frequency therapeutic ultrasound for the treatment of a variety of tissue injuries (Bradnock, Law and Roscoe, 1996). Typically this modality operates at a frequency of around 44–48 kHz, which is significantly lower than the usual therapy range of 1–3 MHz. One benefit of using such a low frequency is that the depth of penetration is greatly enhanced and the risks of standing waves are minimised. As with traditional ultrasound therapy there is a need for large controlled trials to establish where this relatively new modality can be used most effectively.

ULTRASOUND APPLICATION

A number of factors must be considered before using ultrasound:

- choice of ultrasound machine
- calibration
- choice of coupling medium
- frequency
- intensity
- pulsed or continuous mode
- treatment intervals
- duration of treatment
- potential hazards to both therapist and patient.

Choice of ultrasound machine

Most ultrasound machines have the same basic design, consisting of an ultrasound generator, which may be mains or battery-powered (or have dual capability). The generator comprises an oscillator circuit, transformer and microcomputer, and is linked via a coaxial cable to the treatment applicator. The applicator houses the transducer, which produces ultrasound when stimulated by the oscillating voltage from the generator. Machines generally come with a number of treatment applicators, each capable of producing a different output frequency. Intensity can be varied, and also the choice of output can be varied from pulsed mode (a range of pulses is usually available) to continuous mode.

The choice of machine purchase should be made using the following guidelines.

- **Safety.** Use only machine's that carry the British Standard mark BS 5724: part 1. This guarantees that the machine's design has been checked for electrical safety.
- **Beam non-uniformity ratio (BNR).** Use machines that have transducers with low BNRs (5–6). This means that the ultrasound field is relatively uniform across the transducer face and lacks high-intensity hotspots.
- **Frequency.** Depth of penetration and the choice of desired physical mechanism (thermal or nonthermal) are frequency dependent; it

makes sense to buy a machine that offers the greatest variety of frequencies (e.g. 0.75–3.0 MHz), thereby giving you greater flexibility in your therapy range.

- **Digital controls/displays.** These controls are easy to use and are more precise than the dated analogue meters and manual dials.
- **Self-diagnostics.** Many machines now have inbuilt diagnostic circuits which check the generator output each time the machine is turned on. If a fault occurs in the machine this system ensures rapid diagnosis of the fault and allows maintenance to be carried out more effectively.
- **Automatic timer.** Preset treatment times reduces the risk of overexposure to ultrasound.

Calibration

The machine must be calibrated on a regular basis, ideally once a week. The constant heavy usage that this type of equipment gets and the busy environment of the typical physiotherapy clinic (where items of equipment are sometimes dropped) mean it is likely that settings which corresponded to $1 \, W/cm^2$ last month may not give that output this month. It is very important to note that the reading on the machine power-output meter is not an accurate guide as to what is actually coming out of the treatment head; the machine must be calibrated against a dedicated calibration device such as a radiation balance. Such a device is inexpensive, accurate and simple to use, and it takes only minutes to carry out the calibration.

Choice of coupling medium

By the very nature of ultrasound it cannot travel through air and so, without an adequate exit path, the sound generated by the transducer would reflect back from the interface between the air and the applicator treatment surface, which could damage the delicate transducer. In order to provide the generated ultrasound with an 'escape route' from the treatment head into the body, some form of coupling agent needs to be placed between the applicator face and the body. The best coupling agent in terms of acoustic properties is water. The difference in acoustic impedance between water and soft tissue is small, which means that there is approximately only 0.2% reflection at the interface between the two.

The ideal coupling agent would have not only the acoustic properties of water, but would also satisfy the following (Dyson, 1990):

- no gas bubbles or other reflective objects
- gel-like viscosity, allowing ease of use
- sterile
- hypoallergenic
- chemically inert
- perform also as a wound dressing
- transparent
- inexpensive.

Unfortunately, the ideal agent does not exist. However, there are a number of agents that are adequate and, as long as the user is aware of each agent's limitations, we can make the necessary allowances for them during the treatment session.

Degassed water. Freedom from gas bubbles and other inclusions, together with the close acoustic impedance match of water with soft connective tissues when compared with air (water—1.52×10^6; fat—1.35×10^6; muscle—1.65–1.74×10^6; air—429), make water the ideal agent acoustically. However, the nature of water in terms of its viscosity limits its use and it can therefore be used only if it is in a container; this does not present a problem when treating the extremities of the body such as the hand, wrist, ankle and foot, which can easily be placed in a bowl of water (Fig. 14.3).

The ideal treatment bowl should be lined with ultrasound-absorbing material to prevent unwanted reflections from the side of the dish. The therapist can adapt a regular washing-up bowl easily by lining its entire submerged surface with the type of dimpled rubber matting used in cars as foot mats. The degassed water (distilled water will suffice) should be maintained at a sterile 37°C if an open wound is being treated. The injured area and treatment head are then submerged in the bowl. It is not necessary to make contact between the treatment

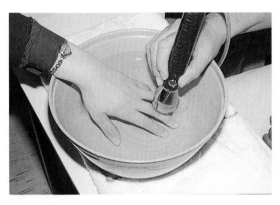

Figure 14.3 Ultrasound to the middle phalanges using degassed water as the transfer medium.

head and the injury because of the good transmission of ultrasound through water. If there is any risk of the operator's hand being submerged in the water during treatment, a rubber surgical glove over a thin cotton glove should be worn (Fig. 14.4); this reduces the possibility of ultrasound reflections being absorbed by the operator (the air trapped by the surgical glove makes a good reflective layer between the glove and the skin of the operator) and also reduces the possibility of cross-infection in the case of open wounds.

This form of ultrasound application has the advantages that the treatment head does not need to touch painful injury sites, and that irregular areas such as the finger can be treated easily.

As with all ultrasound treatments, the treatment head must be kept moving at all times in a circular motion to avoid standing-wave formation.

Aqueous gels, oils and emulsions. These materials have similar acoustic properties to water with the advantage that their higher viscosities make them more user friendly. Examples of commonly used gels are Sonogel (Enraf-Nonius) and Camcare (Electro-Medical Supplies Ltd). They can be applied directly to the skin, but care should be taken to ensure that no air bubbles become trapped in them. If used on broken skin then only sterile materials should be used; if these are not available then treatment should be limited to the surrounding intact skin. This can still be an effective form of treatment as many of

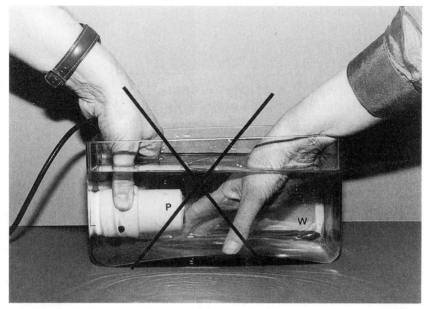

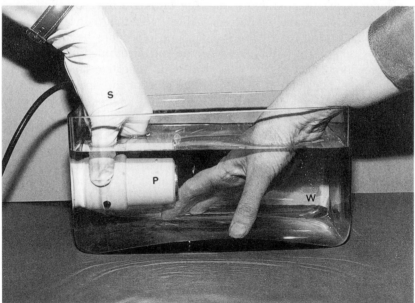

Figure 14.4 The incorrect and correct way to apply ultrasound therapy using the water immersion methods (P = ultrasound probe, S = surgical rubber glove, W = degassed water).

the reparative cells originate in this surrounding area and ultrasound will still have a stimulatory effect on their activity.

Wound dressings. There are now a number of wound dressings that can be used in conjunction with ultrasound therapy owing to their low sound-attenuation properties (Pringle, personal communication, 1993). They fall into two main categories:

1. polyurethane film dressings (e.g. OpSite, Smith and Nephew)

2. polyacrylamide agar gel dressings (e.g. Geliperm, Geistlich Pharmaceuticals).

Both dressing types attenuate little of the ultrasound energy (less than 5%). The dressings are used in the following way (Fig. 14.5):

1. if there is a wound cavity it must be filled with sterile saline until the surface of the saline is continuous with the surface of the surrounding edge of the wound
2. the dressing is then placed over the wound site, ensuring that no air becomes trapped underneath it
3. ultrasound coupling gel is then placed on the dressing surface, covering the wound site
4. the ultrasound treatment head is then placed on the gel and treatment started
5. after treatment, the excess gel can be wiped off the dressing and the dressing left in place to confer all the benefits of a moist environment to the healing wound (Dyson et al., 1988).

This form of treatment allows therapists whose treatment has been restricted previously to the edge of the wound to treat directly over the wound bed. This area is a rich source of new cells and tissue, thus making ultrasound therapy even more effective.

Frequency

Having control over the frequency of the ultrasound output gives the therapist control over the depth at which the energy can be targeted, and also over which physical mechanism is active. The basic rule is that the higher the frequency, the more superficial is the depth of penetration, leading to rapid attenuation of the ultrasound causing a biological effect mainly via

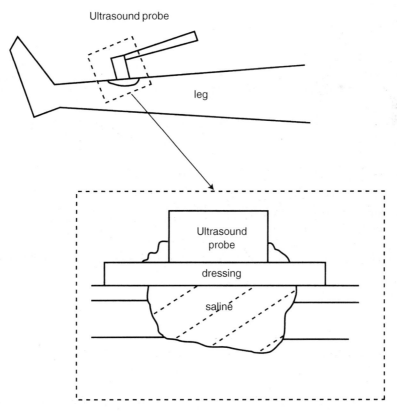

Figure 14.5 The correct procedure for applying ultrasound therapy to a cavity wound.

thermal mechanisms (cavitation is more likely to occur at lower frequencies). It must be noted in addition that the amount of attenuation is also dependent upon the nature of the tissue through which the ultrasound travels. Tissues with high protein content absorb energy more readily than those with a high fat or water content. Table 14.1 shows a guide to tissue absorption properties based upon half-value-depth data. Putting this information into practice, the therapist confronted with a superficial skin lesion would choose a 3 MHz applicator; a deeper muscular injury would require a 1 MHz applicator.

Intensity

Once the choice of frequency has been made so that the required depth of penetration can be achieved, the therapist has to make the decision as to what intensity level to use—that is, the damaged area can be reached, so now how much ultrasound do we apply?

There is no quantitative scientific or clinical information that indicates we must use high levels of ultrasound—that is, greater than 1 W/cm^2 (SATA)—to cause a significant biological effect in injured tissues. On the contrary, the data presented earlier in this chapter supported the use of intensities of 0.5 W/cm^2 (SATA) and less to achieve maximum healing rates in tissues such as skin, tendons and bone. The evidence also showed that levels of ultrasound in excess

of 1.5 W/cm^2 (SATA) have an adverse effect on healing tissues. Significant thermal effects can be achieved using intensities of between 0.5 and 1 W/cm^2 (SATA). Treatment below 0.5 W/cm^2 (SATA) should be used to invoke primarily non-thermal mechanisms.

Fortunately, there has been a trend over recent years towards the use of lower-intensity treatments. The advice to the therapist is **always use the lowest intensity that produces the required therapeutic effect, since higher intensities may be damaging** (Dyson, 1990). Generally, with acute conditions the intensity used should be no higher than 0.5 W/cm^2 (SATA), and for chronic conditions the levels should be no higher than 1 W/cm^2 (SATA).

Pulsed or continuous mode?

Pulsing ultrasound has a major effect on reducing the amount of heat generated in the tissues. A controversy exists as to what the major mechanisms are by which ultrasound stimulates injuries to heal. It is unlikely that a specific bio-effect occurs as a result of the exclusive action of either thermal or non-thermal mechanisms; it is more likely to be as a mixture of both. Therefore, the area is rather a grey one. However, based on the literature available, the flow diagram in Figure 14.6 gives an indication as to how the decision may be made.

Thermal effects are not desirable where the injury site has a compromised or low blood supply (e.g. tendon). In this case, healing should be achieved using non-thermal mechanisms—that is, pulse the ultrasound to reduce the temporal average (reduced heating) whilst maintaining the pulse average at a level high enough to achieve a biological effect.

Treatment intervals

The interval between successive treatments depends upon the nature of the injury.

Acute

The weight of the evidence with regards to the effectiveness of ultrasound therapy indicates

Table 14.1 The half value depth for 1 MHz ultrasound in a range of different media*

Medium	1 MHz (mm)	3 MHz (mm)
Water	11500.0	3833.0
Adipose tissue	50.0	16.5
Skeletal muscle (fibres parallel to sound beam)	24.6	8.0
Tendon	6.2	2.0
Skin	11.1	4.0
Skeletal muscle (fibres at right angles to sound beam)	9.0	3.0
Cartilage	6.0	2.0
Air	2.5	0.8
Compact bone	2.1	—

*From Hoogland, 1986.

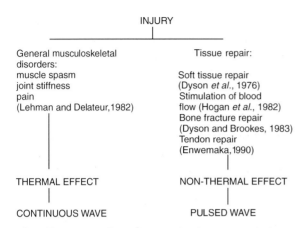

Figure 14.6 Flow diagram showing some criteria on which the decision to use pulsed or continuous ultrasound can be based.

that the earlier it is used after injury, the more effective it is; that is, it is best applied during the early inflammatory phase of repair (Oakley, 1978; Patrick, 1978). During this phase, macrophages and mast cells occupy the wound site and it has been shown that these cells are responsive to therapeutic ultrasound (Fyfe and Chahl, 1985; Young and Dyson, 1990a). Therapeutic ultrasound accelerates the inflammatory phase, resulting in a more rapid entry into the proliferative phase (Dyson, 1990; Young and Dyson, 1990b). During the inflammatory phase of repair, treatments should be once a day for approximately a week, or until swelling and pain have subsided. Treatments through the subsequent proliferative phase of repair can then be reduced to three times a week (McDiarmid and Burns, 1987). This should be maintained until the condition is resolved.

Chronic

The literature with regards to the treatment of chronic wounds is sparse, and also mixed in respect to the efficacy of ultrasound treatments and also the treatment intervals. In the case of venous leg ulcers, the positive reviews variously state a treatment regimen of once per week (Callam *et al.*, 1987) and three times per week (Dyson, Franks and Suckling, 1976). It is advisable to maintain treatment of chronic wounds beyond the inflammatory phase of repair into the proliferative phase as it has been shown that ultrasound can affect many of the processes that occur during this time, such as angiogenesis (Young and Dyson, 1990c), fibroblast activity (Dyson, 1987; Webster, 1980) and wound contraction (Hart, 1993). These effects have been achieved using low intensity (maximum of $0.5\,\mathrm{W/cm^2}$), which utilises primarily non-thermal mechanisms.

Duration of treatment

The duration of treatment depends upon the area of the injury. Typically, the area should be divided into zones which are approximately 1.5 times the area of the ultrasound treatment head, and then each zone should be treated for 1 or 2 minutes (Oakley, 1978). Subsequent treatment times should then be increased by 30 seconds per zone up to a maximum of 3 minutes (Oakley, 1978). Hoogland (1986) recommends that a total maximal treatment time of 15 minutes and that at least 1 minute should be spent in treating an area of 1 centimetre.

Potential hazards

Ultrasound can be an effective therapy or a potential hazard depending upon how it is applied. There exists a number of extensive lists of contraindications and precautions (Dyson, 1988; Hoogland, 1986; Reid, 1981). These include irradiation of the following:

- uterus during pregnancy
- gonads
- malignancies and precancerous lesions
- tissues previously treated by deep X-ray or other radiation
- vascular abnormalities, e.g. deep vein thrombosis, emboli, severe atherosclerosis
- acute infections
- cardiac area in advanced heart disease
- eye
- stellate ganglion

- haemophiliacs not covered by factor replacement
- areas over subcutaneous bony prominences
- epiphyseal plates
- spinal cord after laminectomy
- subcutaneous major nerves
- cranium
- anaesthetic areas.

Many of these contraindications have been included in the list even though they are not based on any hard scientific evidence. However, even if there is a remote chance that damage may occur then ultrasound should not be used.

Dyson (1988) lists the following basic precautions to be taken to ensure that ultrasound is used effectively and safely:

1. use ultrasound only if adequately trained to do so
2. use ultrasound to treat only those patients with conditions known to respond favourably to this treatment (unless it is being used experimentally)
3. use the lowest intensity that produces the required effect, because higher intensities may be damaging
4. move the applicator constantly throughout the treatment, to avoid the damaging effects of standing waves
5. if the patient feels any additional pain during treatment, either reduce the intensity to a pain-free level or abandon the treatment
6. use properly calibrated and maintained equipment
7. if there is any doubt, do not irradiate.

SUMMARY

In summary, it can be said that, if used correctly and at the right time after injury, ultrasound can be a very potent therapeutic force. 'Correctly' means using the lowest possible intensity to achieve the desired result (intensities above $1\,W/cm^2$ should not be necessary), and the 'right time after injury' means during the inflammatory phase of repair. Bearing in mind clinical audit, clinicians should take advantage of the numerous wound assessment techniques which now exist to test the effectiveness of their therapies. Finally, ultrasound can be dangerous if used incorrectly, so users must understand fully the mechanisms by which it works.

REFERENCES

Bailey, AJ, Bazin, S, Sims, TJ, LeLeus, M, Nicholetis, C, Delaunay, A (1975) Characterisation of the collagen of human hypertrophic and normal scars. *Biochemistry and Biophysics Acta* **405**: 412–421.

Bradnock, B, Law, HT, Roscoe, KA (1996) A quantitative comparative assessment of the immediate response to high frequency ultrasound and low frequency ultrasound (longwave therapy) in the treatment of acute ankle sprains. *Physiotherapy* **82**: 78–84.

Brand, JC, Brindle, T, Nyland, J, Caborn, DN, Johnson, DL (1999) Does pulsed low intensity ultrasound allow an early return to normal activities when treating stress fractures? A review of one tarsal navicular and eight stress fractures. *Iowa Orthopaedic Journal* **19**: 26–30.

Byl, NN, McKenzie, AL, West, JM, Whitney, JD, Hunt, TK, Scheuenstuhl, HA (1992). Low-dose ultrasound effects on wound healing: a controlled study with Yucatan pigs. *Archives of Physical Medicine in Rehabilitation* **73**: 656–664.

Byl, NN, McKenzie, AL, Wong, T, West, JM, Hunt, TK (1993) Incisional wound healing: a controlled study of low and high dose ultrasound. *Journal of Orthopaedic and Sports Physical Therapy* **18**: 619–628.

Callam, MJ, Harper, DR, Dale, JJ, Ruckley, CV, Prescott, RJ (1987) A controlled trial of weekly ultrasound therapy in chronic leg ulceration. *Lancet* **July 25**: 204–206.

Chapman, IV, Macnally, NA, Tucker, S (1979) Ultrasound induced changes in the rates of influx and efflux of potassium ions in rat thymocytes *in vitro*. *British Journal of Radiology* **47**: 411–415.

Clark, RAF (1990) Cutaneous wound repair. In: Goldsmith, LE (ed) *Biochemistry and Physiology of the Skin*. Oxford University Press, Oxford, pp 576–601.

Department of Health (1989) *Working for Patients. Medical Audit. Working Paper 6.* HMSO, London.

Dinno, MA, Dyson, M, Young, SR, Mortimer, AJ, Hart, J, Crum, LA (1989) The significance of membrane changes in the safe and effective use of therapeutic and diagnostic ultrasound. *Physics in Medicine and Biology* **34**: 1543–1552.

Dyson, M (1981) The effect of ultrasound on the rate of wound healing and the quality of scar tissue. In: Mortimer, AJ, Lee, N (eds) *Proceedings of the International*

Symposium on Therapeutic Ultrasound, Manitoba. Canadian Physiotherapy Association, Winnipeg, pp 110–123.

Dyson, M (1982) Nonthermal cellular effects of ultrasound. *British Journal of Cancer* 45(suppl. V): 165–171.

Dyson, M (1985) Therapeutic applications of ultrasound. In: Nyborg, WL, Ziskin, MC (eds) *Biological Effects of Ultrasound. Clinics in Diagnostic Ultrasound*. Churchill Livingstone, New York, pp 121–133.

Dyson, M (1987) Mechanisms involved in therapeutic ultrasound. *Physiotherapy* 73: 116–120.

Dyson, M (1988) The use of ultrasound in sports physiotherapy. In: Grisogono, V (ed) *Sports Injuries*, Bromley, I, Wattseries, N (series eds). *International Perspectives in Physical Therapy*, 25. Churchill Livingstone, New York, pp 213–232.

Dyson, M (1990) Role of ultrasound in wound healing. In: Kloth, LC, McCulloch, JM, Feedar, JA (ed) *Wound Healing: Alternatives in Management*. FA Davis, Philadelphia, pp 259–285.

Dyson, M, Brookes, M (1983) Stimulation of bone repair by ultrasound. In: Lerski, RA, Morley, P (eds) *Ultrasound 82, Proceedings 3rd Meeting World Federation of Ultrasound in Medicine and Biology*. Pergamon Press, Oxford.

Dyson, M, Pond, JB, Joseph, J, Warwick, R (1968) Stimulation of tissue repair by pulsed wave ultrasound. *IEEE Transactions on Sonics and Ultrasonics* **SU-17**: 133–140.

Dyson, M, Pond, JB, Joseph, J, Warwick, R (1970) The stimulation of tissue regeneration by means of ultrasound. *Clinical Science* 35: 273–285.

Dyson, M, Pond, JB, Woodward, J, Broadbent, J (1974) The production of blood cell stasis and endothelial cell damage in the blood vessels of chick embryos treated with ultrasound in a stationary wave field. *Ultrasound and Medical Biology* 1: 133–148.

Dyson, M, Franks, C, Suckling, J (1976) Stimulation of healing varicose ulcers by ultrasound. *Ultrasonics* 14: 232–236.

Dyson, M, Smalley, DS (1983) Effects of ultrasound on wound contraction. In: Millner, R, Rosenfeld, E, Cobet, U (eds) *Ultrasound Interactions in Biology and Medicine*. Plenum, New York, p 151.

Dyson, M, Young, SR, Pendle, CL, Webster, DF, Lang, SM (1988) Comparison of the effects of moist and dry conditions of tissue repair. *Journal of Investigations in Dermatology* 91: 434–439.

Ebenbichler, GR, Resch, KL, Nicolakis, P, *et al.* (1998) Ultrasound treatment for treating the carpel tunnel syndrome: randomised 'sham' controlled trial. *British Medical Journal* 316(7133): 731–735.

El Hag, M, Coghlan, K, Christmas, P, Harvey, W, Harris, M (1985) The anti-inflammatory effects of dexamethasone and therapeutic ultrasound in oral surgery. *British Journal of Oral Maxillofacial Surgery* 23: 17–23.

Enwemeka, CS, Rodriguez, O, Mendosa, S (1990) The biomechanical effects of low-intensity ultrasound on healing tendons. *Ultrasound in Medicine and Biology* 16: 801–807.

Fyfe, MC, Chahl, LA (1982) Mast cell degranulation: A possible mechanism of action of therapeutic ultrasound. *Ultrasound in Medicine and Biology* 8(suppl 1): 62.

Fyfe, MC, Chahl, LA (1985) The effect of single or repeated applications of 'therapeutic' ultrasound on plasma extravasation during silver nitrate induced inflammation of the rat hindpaw ankle joint *in vivo*. *Ultrasound in Medicine and Biology* 11: 273–283.

Gam, AN, Johannsen, F (1995) Ultrasound therapy in musculoskeletal disorders: a meta-analysis. *Pain* 63: 85–91.

Ginsberg, M (1981) Role of platelets in inflammation and rheumatic disease. *Advances in Inflammation Research* 2: 53.

Goddard, DH, Revell, PA, Cason, J, Gallagher, S, Currey, HLF (1983) Ultrasound has no anti-inflammatory effect. *Annals of Rheumatic Diseases* 42: 582–584.

ter Haar, G, Hopewell, JW (1982) Ultrasonic heating of mammalian tissue *in vivo*. *British Journal of Cancer* 45(suppl V): 65–67.

ter Haar, G, Dyson, M, Oakley, EM (1985) The use of ultrasound by physiotherapists in Britain, 1985. *Ultrasound in Medicine and Biology* 13: 659–663.

Harding, K, Cutting, K, Price, P (2000) The cost-effectiveness of wound management protocols of care. *British Journal of Nursing* 9: S6–S24.

Hart, J (1993) *The Effect of Therapeutic Ultrasound on Dermal Repair with Emphasis on Fibroblast Activity*. PhD Thesis, University of London.

Harvey, W, Dyson, M, Pond, JB, Grahame, R (1975) The stimulation of protein synthesis in human fibroblasts by therapeutic ultrasound. *Rheumatic Rehabilitation* 14: 237.

Hashish, I (1986) *The Effects of Ultrasound Therapy on Post Operative Inflammation*. PhD Thesis, University of London.

Heckman, JD, Ryaby, JP, McCabe, J, Frey, JJ, Kilcoyne, RF (1994) Acceleration of tibial fracture-healing by non-invasive, low-intensity pulsed ultrasound. *Journal of Bone and Joint Surgery (American volume)* 76: 26–34.

Hibbs, P (1988) *Pressure Area Care for the City and Hackney Health Authority*. St Bartholomew's Hospital, London.

Hibbs, P (1989) The economics of pressure sores. *Care of the Critically Ill* 5(6): 247–250.

Hogan, RDB, Burke, KM, Franklin, TD (1982) The effect of ultrasound on the microvascular hemodynamics in skeletal muscle: effects during ischemia. *Microvascular Research* 23: 370–379.

Hoogland, R (1986) *Ultrasound Therapy*. Enraf Nonius, Delft, Holland.

Hosseinpour, AR (1988) The effects of ultrasound on angiogenesis and wound healing. BSc Thesis, University of London.

Hustler, JE, Zarod, AP, Williams, AR (1978) Ultrasonic modification of experimental bruising in the guinea pig pinna. *Ultrasonics* 16(5): 223–228.

Jackson, BA, Schwane, JA, Starcher, BC (1991) Effect of ultrasound therapy on the repair of achilles tendon injuries in rats. *Medicine and Science in Sports and Exercise* 23: 171–176.

Kaufman, GE, Miller, MW, Griffiths, TD, Ciaravino, V, Carstenson, EL (1977) Lysis and viability of cultured mammalian cells exposed to 1 MHz ultrasound. *Ultrasound in Medicine and Biology* 3: 21–25.

Kischer, CW, Schetlar, MR (1974) Collagen and mucopolysaccharides in the hypertrophic scar. *Connective Tissue Research* 2: 205–213.

Kitchen, S (1995) *Electrophysical Agents: Their Nature and Therapeutic Usage*. PhD Thesis, University of London, p 2.

Knighton, DR, Hunt, TK, Scheuenstuhl, H, Halliday, BJ (1983) Oxygen tension regulates the expression of angiogenesis factor by macrophages. *Science* 221: 1283–1285.

Lehmann, JF, Guy, AW (1972) Ultrasound therapy. In: Reid, J, Sikov, M (eds) *Interaction of Ultrasound and Biological Tissues*. DHEW Publication, (FDA) 73–8008, USA. Government Printing Office, Washington DC, pp 141–152.

Lehmann, JF, DeLateur, BJ (1982) Therapeutic heat. In: Lehmann, JF (ed) *Therapeutic Heat and Cold,* 3rd edn. Williams and Wilkins, Baltimore, MD, p 404.

Leibovich, SJ, Ross, R (1975) The role of the macrophage in wound repair. *American Journal of Pathology* **78**: 71–92.

Levenson, SM, Geever, EG, Crowley, LV, Oates, JF, Berard, CW, Rosen, H (1965) The healing of rat skin wounds. *Annals of Surgery* **161**: 293–308.

Livesey, B, Simpson, G (1989) The hard cost of soft sores. *Health Service Journal* **99**: 5143, p 231.

Loch, EG, Fisher, AB, Kuwert, E (1971) Effect of diagnostic and therapeutic intensities of ultrasonics on normal and malignant human cells *in vitro. American Journal of Obstetrics and Gynecology* **110**: 457–460.

Lundeberg, T, Nordstrom, F, Brodda-Jansen, Eriksson, SV, Kjartansson, J, Samuelson, UE (1990) Pulsed ultrasound does not improve healing of venous ulcers. *Scandanavian Journal of Rehabilitation Medicine* **22**: 195–197.

McDiarmid, T, Burns, PN (1987) Clinical applications of therapeutic ultrasound. *Physiotherapy* **73**: 155.

McDiarmid, T, Burns, PN, Lewith, GT, Machin, D (1985) Ultrasound and the treatment of pressure sores. *Physiotherapy* **71**: 66–70.

Mitragotri, S, Farrell, J, Tang, H, Terahara, T, Kost, J, Langer, R (2000) Determination of threshold energy dose for ultrasound-induced transdermal drug transport. *Journal of Controlled Release* **63**: 41–52.

Mortimer, AJ, Dyson, M (1988) The effect of therapeutic ultrasound on calcium uptake in fibroblasts. *Ultrasound in Medicine and Biology* **14**: 499–506.

Mummery, CL (1978) *The Effect of Ultrasound on Fibroblasts in Vitro.* PhD Thesis, University of London.

NCRP (1983) *Biological Effects of Ultrasound: Mechanisms and Implications.* Report No. 74, p 82.

Nyborg, WL (1977) *Physical Mechanisms for Biological Effects of Ultrasound.* DHEW 78-8062. US Government Printing Office, Washington DC.

Oakley, EM (1978) Applications of continuous beam ultrasound at therapeutic levels. *Physiotherapy* **64**: 169–172.

Patrick, MK (1978) Applications of therapeutic pulsed ultrasound. *Physiotherapy* **64**: 103–104.

Paul, BJ, Lafratta, CW, Dawson, AR, Baab, E, Bullock, F (1960) Use of ultrasound in the treatment of pressure sores in patients with spinal cord injuries. *Archives of Physical Medicine in Rehabilitation* **41**: 438–440.

Peacock, EE (1984) Contraction. In: Peacock, EE (ed) *Wound Repair,* 3rd edn. WB Saunders, New York, pp 39–55.

Pilla, AA, Mont, MA, Nasser, PR, *et al.* (1990) Non-invasive low-intensity pulsed ultrasound accelerates bone healing in the rabbit. *Journal of Orthopaedic Trauma* **4**: 246–253.

Reid, DC (1981) Possible contraindications and precautions associated with ultrasound therapy. In: Mortimer, AJ, Lee, N (eds) *Proceedings of the International Symposium on Therapeutic Ultrasound.* Canadian Physiotherapy Association, Winnipeg, p 274.

Roche, C, West, J (1984) A controlled trial investigating the effect of ultrasound on venous ulcers referred from general practitioners. *Physiotherapy* **70**: 475–477.

Snow, CJ, Johnson, KJ (1988) Effect of therapeutic ultrasound on acute inflammation. *Physiotherapy Canada* **40**: 162–167.

Sutherland, EW, Rall, EW (1968) Formation of cyclic adenine ribonucleotide by tissue particles. *Journal of Biological Chemistry* **232**: 1065–1076.

Tsai, CL, Chang, WH, Liu, TK (1992a) Preliminary studies of duration and intensity of ultrasonic treatments on fracture repair. *Chinese Journal of Physiology* **35**: 21–26.

Tsai, CL, Chang, WH, Liu, TK (1992b) Ultrasonic effect on fracture repair and prostaglandin E2 production. *Chinese Journal of Physiology* **35**: 168.

Webster, DF (1980) *The Effect of Ultrasound on Wound Healing.* PhD Thesis, University of London.

Webster, DF, Pond, JB, Dyson, M, Harvey, W (1978) The role of cavitation in the *in vitro* stimulation of protein synthesis in human fibroblasts by ultrasound. *Ultrasound in Medicine and Biology* **4**: 343–351.

Williams, AR (1974) Release of serotonin from platelets by acoustic streaming. *Journal of the Acoustic Society of America* **56**: 1640.

Williams, AR (1987) Production and transmission of ultrasound. *Physiotherapy* **73**(3): 113–116.

Williams, AR, Sykes, SM, O'Brien, WD (1976) Ultrasonic exposure modifies platelet morphology and function *in vitro. Ultrasound in Medicine and Biology* **2**: 311–317.

Young, SR, Dyson M (1990a) Macrophage responsiveness to therapeutic ultrasound. *Ultrasound in Medicine and Biology* **16**: 809–816.

Young, SR, Dyson, M (1990b) The effect of therapeutic ultrasound on the healing of full-thickness excised skin lesions. *Ultrasonics* **28**: 175–180.

Young, SR, Dyson, M (1990c). The effect of therapeutic ultrasound on angiogenesis. *Ultrasound in Medicine and Biology* **16**: 261–269.

Yurt, RW (1981) Role of the mast cell in trauma. In: Dineen, P, Hildick-Smith, G (eds) *The Surgical Wound.* Lea and Febiger, Philadelphia, p 62.

Low-frequency currents

SECTION CONTENTS

15

Low-frequency currents—an introduction

Tracey Howe
Margaret Trevor

INTRODUCTION

Recent advances in miniaturised electronics have created increased interest in electrical stimulation. Neuromuscular electrical stimulation (NMES) and electrical muscle stimulation (EMS) are practised by increasing numbers of physiotherapists and others to achieve many effects including strengthening and re-education of muscle, reduction of oedema, relief of pain and wound repair. A number of different types of named currents are used but it is important to remember that the underlying principles remain similar; either muscle or nerve is stimulated either directly or indirectly.

The following text will outline the characteristics and parameters used during neuromuscular stimulation; waveforms commonly used will then be described and the importance of different parameters discussed. The following chapters will then consider in more detail a number of 'types' of stimulation which are recognised by practitioners.

Neuromuscular stimulators produce electrical pulse trains that cause excitation of peripheral nerves and subsequently muscle tissue (Hultman *et al.*, 1983). These electrical pulses enter the body tissues via surface electrodes and hence all types of stimulators may correctly be called transcutaneous neuromuscular stimulators. The characteristics and parameters of the pulse trains produced by different neuromuscular stimulators vary, and the electrical output they produce may be either constant current or constant voltage in nature. The electrical output, current or voltage, remains constant even with alterations in skin resistance or impedance caused by alterations in temperature or sweating, etc.

As the use of neuromuscular stimulators has increased in popularity this has led to an increase in the types of stimulator on the market. The parameters are fixed on some stimulators whereas others allow the parameters to be modified, within limits, by the operator. The nomenclature used by the manufacturers of these stimulators, and many commonly used terms, are either misleading or inadequate when used to describe complex stimuli. It is important that any stimuli whether rectangular or complex can be adequately described.

Standardised format

For a pulsatile stimulation to be successfully reproduced by another operator or at a subsequent session the following information must be recorded: the type of output and its amplitude value (e.g. constant current at 20 mA), the shape or the waveform (e.g. asymmetrical biphasic), either the duration of the pulse or the mark : space ratio of the pulse train (e.g. 10 μs or 1 : 90) and the repetition frequency of the pulses (e.g. 100 Hz). If the stimulation is to be produced on a stimulator other than the original device then graphical or pictorial information of the waveform will be required.

Many research papers do not state information regarding the parameters used. This makes it difficult to reproduce work or indeed to translate the results of published work into clinical practice. Singer, De Domenico and Strauss (1987) suggested that there is a need for standardisation on the reporting of methodology.

Definition of terms

Some terms such as galvanic current and faradic stimulation are unique to physiotherapy. Their definitions, given in the literature, are far from universal and so the authors will describe them using the standardised format where possible.

To assist the reader with this chapter any historically used physiotherapy terms will be underlined.

PULSE CHARACTERISTICS AND PARAMETERS USED DURING NEUROMUSCULAR STIMULATION

Currents

There are two types of current: direct current (DC) and alternating current (AC). A direct current is one in which the flow of electrons is in one direction only (Fig. 15.1A) This current may be constant or continuous but varying. An alternating current is one in which the current flows first one way and then another (Fig. 15.1B). The tendency is to think that AC is symmetrical and continuous because we are used to handling sine wave signals. The shape and duration of the AC waveform (faradic current) will be discussed later. AC is often delivered at high frequencies, which lowers skin impedance and thus delivers more current to the motor nerves (Savage, 1984).

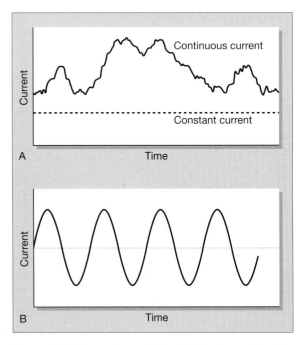

Figure 15.1 Types of current flow. A: Direct current: continuous and constant. B: Alternating current.

Amplitude

The output values for the pulse are expressed in milliamps (mA) or volts (V) depending on whether the stimulator produces a constant-current or a constant-voltage output. These values recorded as amplitude can be described in several ways (Fig. 15.2). *Instantaneous amplitude* is the magnitude of the current or voltage deviation from its zero value at a given instant in time. *Maximum amplitude* (peak amplitude), is the largest deviation from the zero value. High-voltage stimulators deliver peak outputs of around 150 V and low voltage stimulators deliver 100 V or less.

Waveform

A waveform is the shape obtained by plotting the instantaneous amplitude of a varying quantity against time in rectangular coordinates, which for AC signals includes the deviation across the resting (zero) value. The difference between a pulse and a waveform is demonstrated in Figure 15.3. Figure 15.3A shows two unidirectional pulses while Figure 15.3B gives two symmetrical biphasic waveforms and Figure 15.3C shows two asymmetrical biphasic waveforms.

Pulse

A stimulus may be either discrete, a single pulse; or a pulse train, a series of pulses. A pulse (impulse) is a sudden departure of short duration of voltage or current from a steady value

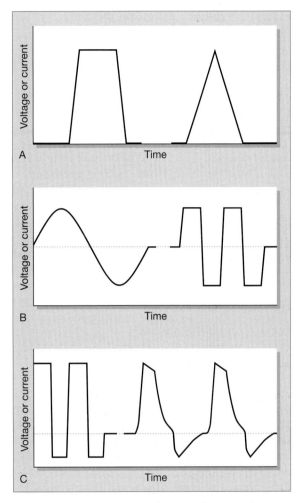

Figure 15.3   Pulses and waveforms. A: Square and triangular pulses. B: Symmetrical waveforms C: Asymmetrical waveforms.

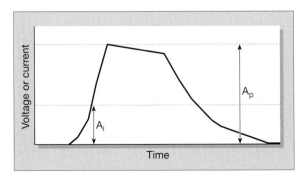

Figure 15.2   Amplitude measurement of a pulse: peak (A$_p$) and instantaneous (A$_i$).

(Amos, 1981). The pulses may vary in their shape and duration (short, <1 ms or long, >1 ms). If a monophasic pulse train were to be delivered to tissue a net charge would build up in the body, which could be harmful. This charge must either be allowed to discharge naturally or be removed by applying a consecutive reverse pulse. The reverse pulse, which is sometimes called a recovery pulse, has to balance the delivered charge. This is achieved by using either a symmetrical pulse of opposite phase or a pulse of the same area as the delivered pulse and once again of opposite phase. These two consecutive pulses, the delivery pulse and the reverse pulse, make up the stimulator waveform.

Pulse duration

Pulse duration, sometimes known as <u>pulse width</u>, is defined as the time taken for the instantaneous value of a pulse to rise and fall to a specified fraction of the peak value—that is, the duration of the output pulse at 50% of the maximum amplitude (BSI, 1990) (Fig. 15.4). Pulse width is expressed in microseconds (μs). For a symmetrical square wave the pulse duration is that of the delivery pulse and additionally the waveform has a mark:space ratio of 1:1. We need to be aware that when manufacturers give the pulse duration they are only considering the delivery part of the waveform as described above. They class the reverse phase or recovery time and any quiescent time to be the space in the mark:space ratio (i.e. the 'off' part of the duty cycle).

Frequency

The frequency of the stimulus train, the inter-pulse interval, is the time between the start of one pulse and the start of the next pulse (Fig. 15.5). This is usually given in Hz and is actually the pulse repetition frequency (PRF) when the mark:space ratio is constant. The *mean frequency* value is used for non-uniform stimulus trains where pulses are produced at irregular intervals—with variable mark:space ratios, or for mixed frequency stimulation where more than one frequency is produced throughout a period of stimulation.

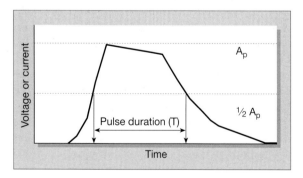

Figure 15.4 Duration of a pulse.

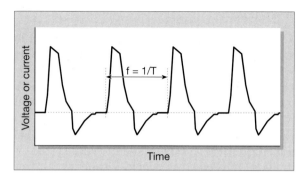

Figure 15.5 Frequency of a pulse train.

Continuous signal

A continuous signal is actually one where there is no quiescent time between waveforms; that is, a sine wave is a continuous symmetrical biphasic signal. Manufacturers of neuromuscular simulators use the term <u>continuous signal</u> (sometimes called a <u>normal signal</u>) to describe a pulse train where the pulses are delivered with a fixed mark:space ratio for the duration of stimulation. We need to make sure that a second delivery pulse cannot arrive before the end of the reverse pulse, or the resultant DC off-set could produce tissue damage. Sometimes the parameters given for neuromuscular stimulators do not make it possible to calculate the conditions under which a DC off-set will result. Remember the pulse duration looks only at the delivery time of the waveform, so a DC off-set will result with a symmetrical biphasic waveform if the pulse duration exceeds half the interpulse interval.

Duration of stimulus

The duration of stimulation may be defined as the time for which stimulation was applied—that is, the time for which the device was energised (switched on), usually hours or minutes.

Duty cycle

The duty cycle of the stimulator is comprised of an 'on-time' reflecting the duration of pulse delivery and an 'off-time', the duration of recovery and quiescence. The total duty-cycle time is the sum of the 'on- and off-times'.

Charge density

The amount of energy applied to the stimulated tissue per pulse is related to the charge density where charge density is the pulse duration multiplied by the current. Charge density is expressed in microcoulombs (µC). Electrical energy, which is measured in joules (J), is calculated from the product of the voltage and charge density. In neuromuscular stimulators either the current or the voltage is kept constant, not both, and therefore a simple calculation of the energy deposited is not possible.

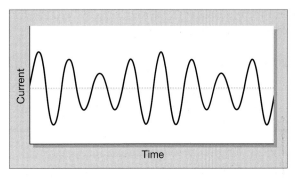

Figure 15.6   Interference-modulated current.

TYPES OF STIMULATION CURRENTS AND WAVEFORMS

Faradic stimulation consists of pulses which have a biphasic waveform and a pulse duration which is typically 0.3 ms. The pulse duration is always below 1 ms and the PRF is less than 100 Hz. This means that the largest duty cycle is 10% and the corresponding mark : space ratio would be 1 : 9.

Galvanic stimulation, which is described as interrupted DC, has no reverse pulse; the authors can only say that it conventionally has a pulse duration of about 100 ms.

There are two stimulation currents whose waveforms are produced from sinusoidal signals: *interference-modulated current*, or interferential current, and *tone-burst current*.

Interference-modulated current refers to the current produced by the interference pattern generated in the tissues by two slightly different high frequency (about 4000 Hz) sine waves (Fig. 15.6).

Tone-burst current is sometimes referred to as 'Russian stimulation' because Russian scientists were the first to utilise this sort of current. It was described as: a high-frequency (2500 Hz) carrier current interspersed with 10 ms periods when no current flows, producing 50 bursts per second. We could describe it more fully as bursts of a 2500 Hz sine wave, with a burst : space ratio

of 1 : 1 and a burst repetition frequency (BRF) of 50 Hz.

The pulse trains from some stimulators can be manipulated, with manufacturers usually offering pulse-burst mode and ramping or modulation mode.

In the pulse-burst mode the number of individual pulses per burst is fixed, as is their PRF (say 100 Hz), and only the pulse width remains adjustable. The actual shape of the individual pulse waveform needs to be described before we identify the signal parameters to be consistent with our standard convention. The parameters, depending on the actual settings of the device, are: bursts of a X Hz pulse train, with a burst duration of Y ms, a burst : space ratio of B : S and a burst repetition frequency of Z Hz.

In modulation mode or ramping there is a gradual increase in the charge applied to the tissue and hence an increase in the intensity of muscle contraction attained. In ramping mode this is achieved by a gradual increase in the amplitude or pulse width of the pulse train (Fig. 15.7). This allows for accommodation of the nervous tissue to pulse delivery. In modulation mode the amplitude of the pulses rises over a given time, remains constant for a given time and then falls once again for a set time. This rise, plateau and fall cycle continually repeats throughout the duration of stimulation.

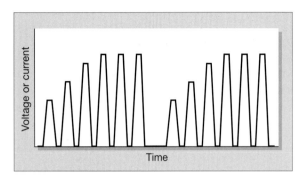

Figure 15.7 Ramping by slowly increasing the intensity of the current.

THE IMPORTANCE OF STIMULATION PARAMETERS

Waveform

Galvanic stimulation is useful only for stimulating denervated muscle whereas interrupted direct current, including faradic stimulation, is able to stimulate innervated muscle. However, both techniques create thermal and chemical reactions under the electrodes and are often painful and therefore should be used with caution.

Baker, Bowman and McNeal (1988) investigated the effects of six different waveforms on comfort during neuromuscular stimulation. An asymmetric balanced biphasic square waveform (35 Hz) was reported to be comfortable and effective in stimulating the extensor and flexor muscles of the wrist. However, in the quadriceps muscles a symmetric biphasic square waveform (50 Hz) was preferred by subjects. Delitto and Rose (1986) reported that subjects' perception of discomfort alters with changes in waveform (50 Hz) and that individual preferences exist for different waveforms.

Amplitude

When stimulating a muscle at a constant frequency the only way to increase the force produced is to recruit more motor units by increasing the intensity (amplitude of the waveform) of stimulation (Low and Reid, 1990).

Pulse duration

The most suitable pulse duration for motor stimulation of the triceps brachii was found to be between 20–200 μs, the most comfortable being 100 μs; pulse durations less than 100 μs were suitable for sensory stimulation (Alon, Allin and Inbar, 1983).

Electrodes

The size of electrodes may have an affect on the amount of muscle stimulated and hence the intensity of the contraction produced (Alon, 1989). Reversing the polarity of electrodes has little effect on the force generated during stimulation with biphasic waveforms; however, changes greater than 20% were seen with monophasic waveforms (McNeal and Baker, 1988).

Percutaneous stimulation of healthy muscle selectively activates nerve endings and not the muscle fibres directly (Hultman *et al.*, 1983). It is postulated that slow rising pulses of long duration selectively stimulate denervated muscle, as opposed to fast rising pulses of short duration, which stimulate innervated muscle. There is no scientific evidence to show that denervated muscle can be stimulated directly; however, neither is there any evidence to refute it (Belanger, 1991).

PRINCIPLES OF CLINICAL APPLICATION

The principles identified here are applicable to the safe application of all muscle and nerve electrical stimulation. (Additional details are available in each individual chapter, following.)

Application

- Conduct general safety checks with respect to the equipment. Check the subject with respect to contraindications listed in each chapter.
- **Explain the treatment fully to the patient.**

- Collect the necessary equipment, e.g.:
  — electrical stimulator, appropriate electrodes, wiring
  — soap and water for cleaning the skin
  — contact gel/sponge, electrodes, covers, etc.
  — means of attaching electrodes, e.g. tape/straps/Velcro®.
- Position the patient so he or she is comfortable and can remain in the given position for the duration of the treatment. Ensure that the position allows the electrode to be placed over the necessary treatment points. Should the person be undergoing prolonged treatment (e.g. TENS) ensure that normal movement is possible with the electrodes and equipment in place.
- The skin should be uncovered and examined for any contraindications to treatment.
- Test the equipment as appropriate; demonstrate the technique to the patient.
- Wash the skin over the region of electrode contact. You may reduce skin resistance by soaking the skin for 3 to 4 minutes either in a bath or with a warm, damp pad.
- Select appropriate treatment parameters.
- Always turn all intensity dials to zero before beginning the treatment.
- Place the electrodes as appropriate for the treatment in question.
- Increase the intensity until the desired result is produced.
- **Never lift the active electrode from the skin or replace it without turning the intensity to zero**.
- Terminate the treatment; check the skin condition.
- Keep a full record of your treatment.

Safety checks

- Mechanical safety of equipment.
- Output of the machine.
- Check skin sensation for information only— lack of sensitivity is *not* a contraindication to treatment but you should take particular care to watch for any changes in skin colour due to chemical irritation of the skin under the electrodes.

Warnings

Ensure patients are clear about what to expect; they will experience some sensory stimulation which is exacerbated when the active electrode is not well placed or when there is poor contact between the skin/contact medium/electrode. They should be told to report any unexpected sensations or changes in their condition.

Dosage

See individual chapters for information with respect to this.

SUMMARY

All stimulators that produce electrical pulses, which enter the body tissues via surface electrodes, may be classified as percutaneous neuromuscular stimulators. The type of output produced by such stimulators varies considerably. It is important to be aware of the differences in pulse characteristics and parameters and the relative effects that they may have. Accurate reporting of such information in the scientific literature will facilitate the transference of research work into clinical practice.

REFERENCES

Alon, G (1989) Electro-orthopedics: A review of present electrophysiological responses and clinical efficacy of transcutaneous stimulation. *Advances in Sports Medicine and Fitness* **2**: 295–324.

Alon, G, Allin, J, Inbar, GF (1983) Optimisation of pulse duration and pulse charge during transcutaneous electrical nerve stimulation. *Australian Journal of Physiotherapy* **29**(5): 195–201.

Amos, SW (1981) *Dictionary of Electronics,* Butterworths, London.

Baker, LL, Bowman, BR, McNeal, DR (1988) Effects of waveform on comfort during neuromuscular electrical stimulation. *Clinical Orthopaedics and Related Research* **233**: 75–85.

Belanger, AY (1991) Neuromuscular electrostimulation in physiotherapy: a critical appraisal of controversial issues. *Physiotherapy Theory and Practice* **7**: 83–89.

British Standards Institution (1990) *Medical Electrical Equipment: Specification* for *Nerve and Muscle Stimulators.* BS 5724: Section 2.10. British Standards Institution.

Delitto, A, Rose, SJ (1986) Comparative comfort of three waveforms used in electrically eliciting quadriceps femoris muscle contractions. *Physical Therapy* **66**: 1704–1707.

Hultman, E, Sjoholm, H, Jaderholm, EKJ, Krynicki, J (1983) Evaluation of methods for electrical stimulation of human skeletal muscle in situ. *Pflugers Archives* **398**: 139–141.

Low, J, Reid, A (1990) *Electrotherapy Explained.* Butterworth-Heinemann, London.

McNeal, DR, Baker, LL (1988) Effects of joint angle, electrodes and waveform on electrical stimulation of the quadriceps and hamstrings. *Annals of Biomedical Engineering* **16**: 299–310.

Savage, B (1984) *Interferential Therapy.* Faber & Faber, London.

Singer, KP, De Domenico, G, Strauss, G (1987) Electro-motor stimulation for research methodology and reporting: a need for standardisation. *Australian Journal of Physiotherapy* **33**(1): 43–47.

16

Neuromuscular and muscular electrical stimulation

Suzanne McDonough
Sheila Kitchen

INTRODUCTION

In order to apply electrical stimulation effectively it is important to revise some basic principles of how nerves are activated by electrical signals and how muscle contracts in response to these signals (see Ch. 4). It is also important to understand types of muscle fibre, patterns of normal recruitment of muscle fibres and how this is reversed when electrical stimulation is used. This is covered in Chapter 8, which also identified the differences between electrical stimulation and voluntary exercise and discussed the mechanisms underlying increases in strength with electrical stimulation. The previous chapter, Chapter 15 discussed the types of current which may be used to produce an electrical response in muscle and nerve (and links to Ch. 4) and the parameters that may be varied to produce different responses.

This chapter will examine the clinical areas in which electrical stimulation has been used, and review the relevant literature to identify what is known about the clinical effects of treatment and why these may occur. The practical application of neuromuscular electrical stimulation (NMES) for innervated muscle and electrical muscular stimulation (EMS) for denervated muscle will be discussed.

TYPES OF UNIT

There are a multitude of commercially available electrical stimulation units (using a variety of current types) which are marketed under a variety of names. Units can either be portable (battery operated) or line powered and there has been some debate as to which type of unit is better for muscle strengthening. Some investigators have argued that line-powered units can produce greater strength gains as these units may cause higher training contraction force levels, particularly when used for larger muscle groups such as quadriceps (Snyder-Mackler *et al.*, 1995). However, there is no clear evidence for the greater efficacy of either type of machine. It is essential that the user checks that the machine to be used has available the parameters required for treatment—though this chapter will show that there is some lack of clarity about the most effective to use on all occasions.

NOMENCLATURE AND TYPES OF ELECTRICAL STIMULATION IN NERVE AND MUSCLE

The Clinical Electrophysiology Section of the American Physical Therapy Association established a unified terminology for clinical electrical currents—that is, (a) direct current, (b) alternating current and (c) pulsed current (Kloth and Cummings, 1991). Use of this terminology should make the task of classifying commercial stimulators and interpreting the results of research studies more simple. However, this terminology does not appear to have been widely adopted and inconsistencies remain in the literature with regard to nomenclature. Investigators have used the following terms interchangeably and sometimes the precise form of electrical stimulation is gleaned only by careful review of the particular paper.

Neuromuscular electrical stimulation (NMES)

This form of electrical stimulation is commonly used at sufficiently high intensities to produce muscular contraction and may be applied to the muscle during movement or without functional movement occurring.

Functional electrical or neuromuscular stimulation (FES/FNS)

This term is used when the aim of treatment is to enhance or produce functional movement. The level of complexity of FES may range from its use (with dual-channel stimulators) to enhance dorsiflexion during gait in children with cerebral palsy (Atwater *et al.*, 1991) to multichannel FES to activate many muscles to restore stance and gait in patients with paraplegia (Hömberg, 1997).

Therapeutic electrical stimulation (TES)

This term has been used specifically to describe a form of electrical stimulation that produces sensory effects only (Beck, 1997; Pape, 1997; Steinbok, Reiner and Kestle, 1997). Unfortunately the term 'therapeutic electrical stimulation' has also been used by some investigators to differentiate between electrical stimulation applied to promote function (FES) and that applied for some other therapeutic function, for example NMES for children with cerebral palsy (Hazlewood *et al.*, 1994) and adults with spasticity and spinal cord injury (Chae *et al.*, 2000; Pease, 1998).

Electrical stimulation (ES)

The meaning of the generic term, ES, is further complicated by the expanding use of electrical stimulation. Some investigators may not simply be applying it to strengthen weakened muscles but may also be investigating its role in promoting functional recovery (Pandyan, Granat and Stott, 1997; Powell *et al.*, 1999; Steinbok, Reiner and Kestle, 1997) and decrease spasticity in neurological conditions (Alfieri, 1982; Hesse *et al.*, 1998; Vodovnik, Bowman and Hufford, 1984).

EVIDENCE OF CLINICAL EFFICACY

Although there is an abundance of literature in this area, reviews reveal inconsistent findings on what effects can be produced with electrical stimulation, the specific parameters to produce these effects and what the underlying principle of these effects may be. This may be due to certain underlying problems with the literature, rather than an intrinsic lack of efficacy. Shortcomings in the literature include the following.

- Some early studies did not include a comparison group and therefore have not identified the benefit of electrical stimulation over other forms of intervention. For example, electrical stimulation has been shown to strengthen atrophied muscle significantly (Singer *et al.*, 1983; William and Street, 1976) but has no additional benefit over some studies with a matched voluntary exercise group (Grove-Lainey, Walmsley and Andrew, 1983).
- The subject numbers in some studies are too small; small studies can produce findings both for (Delitto *et al.*, 1988; Snyder-Mackler *et al.*, 1991) and against (Grove-Lainey, Walmsley and Andrew, 1983; Sisk *et al.*, 1987) a modality, neither of which provide reliable evidence.
- Even some well-designed randomised controlled trials make interpretation of the findings difficult as there is no consistency between electrical stimulation, or exercise protocols, or both. An example is differences in the 'intensity' used for NMES ('intensity' here applies to several parameters, i.e. not only the intensity of the applied current, but also the frequency and duty cycle), which may account for the conflicting findings about the effectiveness of NMES to strengthen muscle. NMES has been found by Snyder-Mackler *et al.* (1995) to be significantly more effective for strengthening quadriceps than voluntary exercise, whereas Lieber, Silva and Daniel (1996) and Paternostro-Sluga *et al.* (1999) showed that NMES was no more effective than voluntary exercise. However, the parameters used in the latter two studies were considered 'low intensity' by Snyder-Mackler *et al.* (1995), and so possibly not suitable for strengthening.
- Even within studies, in which the aim has been to compare different types of electrical stimulation, there have been a number of varying factors, which makes it very difficult to establish which factor may be the important variable which leads to strengthening in a trial.

Snyder-Mackler *et al.* (1995) showed that 'high-intensity' NMES (as defined above) caused significantly more strengthening than both 'low-intensity' NMES and voluntary exercise. Snyder-Mackler *et al.* (1995) argue that the difference in results can be accounted for by the fact that the 'high-intensity' group trained harder than the 'low-intensity' group. There is evidence that the higher the training contraction force the greater is the improvement in quadriceps strength (Snyder-Mackler *et al.*, 1995) and these authors concluded that these results supported the use of line-powered units. However, it is important to note that the protocols for battery-operated and line-powered units were very different in this study. Some of the differences may be explained by the placebo effect of a bigger line-powered unit or the therapist–patient interaction, which was absent when patients used a portable unit at home.

Nevertheless, there does appear to be evidence for the clinical effectiveness of electrical stimulation for strengthening muscle, improving function and reducing tone in patient populations. The shortcomings in the research base, however, mean it is not possible to assign particular effects to certain interactions of parameters, and only broad guidelines can be given. The following section will examine the evidence for clinical efficacy in a number of areas; possible treatment parameters to achieve these effects will be presented in the section on application.

Strengthening in non-neurological conditions

Two mechanisms for strengthening muscle with NMES have been proposed. First, strength gains may be achieved in the same manner as standard voluntary strengthening programmes which use low number of repetitions with high external loads and a high intensity of muscle contraction (at least 75% of maximum). The second mechanism by which strengthening may occur is the preferential recruitment of type II phasic muscle fibres which have a lower threshold for NMES (Delitto and Snyder-Mackler, 1990; Lake, 1992).

Electrical stimulation of healthy muscle

In general, the research evidence does not support the use of electrical stimulation for increasing either strength or endurance in healthy muscle. It has been clearly shown that the combination of electrical stimulation and exercise is no more effective than exercise alone (Currier and Mann, 1983; Wolf et al., 1986). It is worth noting that in general the effects seen with NMES were produced at much lower training strengths than those used for voluntary exercise.

There is, however, some controversy over whether NMES is more effective for strengthening abdominal muscles than voluntary exercise. Although multiple muscle group NMES (which includes stimulation of the abdominal muscles) as used in muscle-toning clinics has proven totally ineffective in muscle strengthening (Lake, 1988; Lake and Gillespie, 1988), there is some evidence that NMES combined with voluntary exercise can be more effective than exercise alone for abdominal training in healthy subjects (Alon et al., 1987). This may be explained by the fact that in many healthy adults the abdominal muscles are atrophic or that use of NMES makes it easier to learn the correct activation of the abdominal muscles. A similar argument could be put forward for the fact that one study has shown that NMES is more effective than exercise for strengthening of the back musculature (Kahanovitz et al., 1987).

Electrical stimulation of atrophied muscle

Electrical stimulation for strengthening is useful clinically in cases involving immobilisation or contraindications to dynamic exercise to prevent disuse atrophy (Selkowitz, 1989), in early rehabilitation by facilitating muscle contraction, in selective muscle strengthening or muscle re-education (Lake, 1992).

There are many studies that have examined the effects of electrical stimulation on strength in patient populations, for example following anterior cruciate ligament repair (Delitto et al., 1988; Lieber, Silva and Daniel, 1996; Paternostro-Sluga et al., 1999; Sisk et al., 1987; Snyder-Mackler et al., 1991; Wigerstad-Lossing et al., 1997) or in

patellofemoral disorders (Horodyski and Sharp, 1985). Some of these studies have shown that NMES (with or without voluntary exercise) causes greater strength improvement than voluntary exercise alone (Delitto et al., 1988; Horodyski and Sharp, 1985; Snyder-Mackler et al., 1991, 1995; Wigerstad-Lossing et al., 1997), whereas other studies have shown that NMES is only as effective as voluntary exercise when the intensity of the voluntary exercise programme is greater (Lieber, Silva and Daniel, 1996; Paternostro-Sluga et al., 1999). In a review by Lake (1992) the evidence for selective strengthening of vastus medialis and abductor hallucis are discussed.

Although studies examining the effect of NMES have focused largely on rehabilitation of knee injuries (see O'Callaghan and Oldham, 1997 for a recent review), it has also been shown to be useful in rehabilitation of patients with pelvic floor dysfunction, which can lead to faecal (Fynes et al., 1999) and urinary incontinence (Sand et al., 1995). In the study by Fynes et al. (1999), electrical stimulation was performed via an endoanal probe using low-frequency 20 Hz and high-frequency 50 Hz settings to target static (slow-twitch) and dynamic (fast-twitch) fibre activity with a 20% ramp modulation time. Over 12 weeks of treatment (one session per week), electrical stimulation combined with audiovisual biofeedback of muscle activity significantly improved continence scores (Fynes et al., 1999). Significant improvements in urinary incontinence were found after 15 weeks of pelvic floor muscle stimulation (see Sand et al., 1995 for a detailed description of the parameters used).

Electrical stimulation of denervated muscle

Despite more than a century of use of EMS to stimulate denervated muscle, controversy over its use and efficacy still continues (Davies, 1983; Delitto et al., 1995). This is primarily due to the variety of treatment protocols which have been used to assess care. Though there is no current consensus about the duty cycle which should be used, the frequency of stimulation or the number of contractions which should be employed, Snyder-Mackler and Robinson (1995) suggest that EMS can delay atrophy and its associated changes. However, they also note that there is no evidence to suggest that such a delay is significant in terms of final recovery.

Use of electrical stimulation in adults with neurological conditions

The effects of electrical stimulation in neurological rehabilitation can be divided into improved motor function (Chae *et al.*, 1998; Fransisco *et al.*, 1998; Hesse *et al.*, 1998; Pandyan and Granat, 1997; Powell *et al.*, 1999; Weingarden, Zeilig and Heruti, 1998), reduction in spasticity (Alfieri 1982; Hesse *et al.*, 1998; Vodovnik, Bowman and Hufford, 1984; Weingarden, Zeilig and Heruti, 1998), increase in muscle strength (Glanz *et al.*, 1996; Powell *et al.*, 1999), increase in range of movement of the wrist (Pandyan, Granat and Stott, 1997; Powell *et al.*, 1999) and reduction of shoulder subluxation in stroke patients (Chantraine *et al.*, 1999; Faghri *et al.*, 1994; Wang, Chan and Tsai, 2000).

Motor recovery

Several studies have reported enhancement in motor recovery or function, or both, after use of NMES to the upper limb (Chae *et al.*, 1998; Fransisco *et al.*, 1998; Hesse *et al.*, 1998; Pandyan, Granat and Stott, 1997; Powell *et al.*, 1999; Weingarden, Zeilig and Heruti, 1998). Three of the studies applied NMES to acute stroke patients (Chae *et al.*, 1998; Fransisco *et al.*, 1998; Powell *et al.*, 1999), two to chronic stroke patients (Hesse *et al.*, 1998; Weingarden, Zeilig and Heruti, 1998) and one to a mixture of chronic and acute stroke patients (Pandyan, Granat and Stott, 1997). The subject numbers in these studies ranged from small ($n = 9$, 11 and 10 respectively: Fransisco *et al.*, 1998; Pandyan, Granat and Stott, 1997; Weingarden, Zeilig and Heruti, 1998) to medium ($n = 28$ and 24: Chae *et al.*, 1998; Hesse *et al.*, 1998) and large ($n = 60$: Powell *et al.*, 1999). There were a number of study designs used, from pilot studies (Fransisco

et al., 1998; Weingarden, Zeilig and Heruti, 1998) to controlled studies (Chae *et al.*, 1998; Hesse *et al.*, 1998; Powell *et al.*, 1999).

Strength

A meta-analysis of studies which used various forms of electrical stimulation in stroke patients showed that strength of wrist, knee and ankle extensors was significantly increased after 3–4 weeks of treatment (Glanz *et al.*, 1996). A more recent randomised controlled trial confirmed this finding of increased strength in wrist extensors after 8 weeks of treatment (Powell *et al.*, 1999).

Shoulder subluxation after stroke

There is some evidence (from small studies and one large controlled trial*) that early use, within 28 days of onset of stroke, of electrical stimulation may reduce the degree of shoulder subluxation and prevent further capsular stretch in acute stroke patients (Chantraine *et al.*, 1999*; Faghri *et al.*, 1994; Wang, Chan and Tsai, 2000). These studies applied NMES to the posterior deltoid (active electrode) and supraspinatus muscles (passive electrode) at an intensity level sufficient to produce muscular contraction. (Only one study specified the movement, i.e. humeral elevation and some abduction and extension—Faghri *et al.*, 1994.)

Reducing spasticity in adults with neurological conditions

The term spasticity is used in a variety of circumstances describing impaired movement execution, enhanced muscular resistance against passive movement or abnormal limb postures (Hummelsheim and Mauritz, 1997). Spasticity has been explained by enhanced motoneuron excitability to the muscle (Artieda, Quesada and Obeso, 1991) and altered mechanical properties of the muscle (Dietz, Quintern and Berger, 1981). Hömberg (1997) reviewed some evidence for the effectiveness of electrical stimulation in reducing spasticity (of spinal or cerebral origin). He discussed both FES and NMES interchangeably under the heading of FES. There is evidence for reduction in spasticity of the agonist when NMES was applied to the antagonist muscle (Alfieri, 1982) or to both agonist and antagonist muscles (Hesse et al., 1998; Vodovnik, Bowman and Hufford, 1984; Weingarden, Zeilig and Heruti, 1998), however the mechanisms underpinning these effects are still unclear. In one randomised controlled trial NMES had no effect on spasticity when it was applied to the agonist only (Powell et al., 1999).

It has been proposed that stimulation of the antagonist reduces spasticity in the agonist via the group Ia reciprocal inhibitory pathway (Hömberg, 1997; Levine, Knott and Kabot, 1952) or via polysynaptic pathways mediated by flexion reflex afferents (Apkarian and Naumann, 1991). Whereas stimulation of the spastic agonist may lead to a reduction in activity via recurrent inhibition of its own α motoneuron (Granit, Pascoe and Steg, 1957; Ryall et al., 1972). It is also possible that, by stretching the agonist or the antagonist muscles through their available range of movement, mechanical factors are altered so leading to a reduction in spasticity (Botte, Nickel and Akeson, 1988). Indeed electrical stimulation for motor relearning after stroke may produce its desired effects by virtue of the fact it produces a desired muscle contraction in muscles that are otherwise not activated at all, abnormally activated, or abnormally responding (Daly and Ruff, 2000).

Regardless of the method used there is evidence of positive effects, although further controlled studies are required to confirm these findings. The evidence also suggests that use of NMES in a nonfunctional way can produce effects so that if the clinician only has access to a very simple battery-operated NMES device it is possible to use this to reduce spasticity (Alfieri, 1982).

Children: strengthening atrophied muscle in neurological conditions

Investigators have assessed the effects of applying electrical stimulation to the trunk, and upper and lower limb muscles in children with cerebral palsy. Although the findings have generally been encouraging, only two of the study designs included a control group (Hazlewood et al., 1994; Steinbok, Reiner and Kestle, 1997) and none included a placebo group. It is also difficult to summarise the results as a plethora of different outcome measures were used. However, the main positive findings (the most powerful findings are identified with an asterisk) were that electrical stimulation significantly improved function (Pape et al., 1993; Steinbok, Reiner and Kestle, 1997*), and ankle dorsiflexion range of movement in sitting (Hazlewood et al., 1994*) or heel strike (Comeaux et al., 1997). There was also some evidence that muscle strength improved (Beck, 1997; Carmick, 1997b; Hazlewood et al., 1994) but further controlled research with larger subject numbers is required to answer this question definitively.

Two main forms of electrical stimulation were used in the former studies: either TES or NMES. TES is electrical stimulation applied at a low intensity (subcontraction) level, thus producing sensory stimulation only. It was generally applied for up to 8 hours during sleep and is tenuously proposed to cause increased blood flow during a time of trophic hormone stimulation, causing an increase in muscle bulk. Observable changes in muscle bulk take 6–8 weeks (Beck, 1997; Pape, 1997), although Pape argues that additional activity is required to produce strength gains (Pape, 1997).

Pape (1997) states that her approach is based on similar chronic low-level electrical stimulation used by basic scientists quoting the work of Lieber (1986). However, there is no reference to the wealth of literature in both animals and humans, which shows that chronic electrical stimulation can modify muscle properties. Chapter 8 of this textbook provides a review of the underlying mechanisms.

As previously discussed NMES is thought to strengthen muscle by the overload principle or by preferentially recruiting the type II phasic muscle fibres (Lake, 1992), thereby improving strength and decreasing sensitivity to stretch (Rose and McGill, 1988).

PRACTICAL APPLICATION

Though both innervated and denervated muscle may be caused to contract through the use of current applied to the skin, most studies today focus on the use of electrical currents to stimulate innervated muscle. The method of application of treatment for both is, however, identical. Chapter 15 provides basic details of practical application; additional details follow.

Skin preparation

Prior to treatment the skin should either be washed with soap and water or cleaned with a proprietary, alcohol-based wipe. This is in order to remove skin debris (including dead epithelial cells and sebum), sweat and dirt. It is necessary to do this in order to facilitate good contact between the electrode and the skin and thus reduce the electrical resistance of the interface.

Electrodes

Types and attachment

Electrodes are principally of two types.

1. Polymer-based electrodes: carbon–rubber electrodes have been introduced on to the market in recent years and are currently the most popular type owing to their ease of use. They consist of carbon-impregnated silicone rubber (Fig. 16.1). Such electrodes are reusable, can be cut to size and can be moulded to the skin surface provided the surface is not too irregular. They are normally coupled to the skin through the use of an electrically conductive gel and must be taped into place securely. Other polymer-based electrodes are also available but are generally less efficient at transmitting electrical stimuli to the tissue (Nolan, 1991). Recent advances in electrode design have further increased the ease with which they can be applied and improved their electrical contact with the skin. Such electrodes are considerably more malleable than those previously available and have an even layer of conductive material already in place; it is these particular qualities

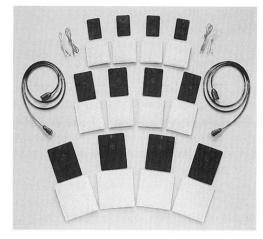

Figure 16.1 Carbon–rubber electrodes. (Photograph courtesy of Electro-Medical Supplies (Greenham) Ltd, Wantage.)

that allow them to make more effective contact with the skin. In addition, they are self-adhesive and reusable, factors which make them quick, easy and economical to use.

2. More traditional tin-plate or aluminium electrodes may also be used. These are coupled to the skin with saline water, which is normally retained within a cotton pad or sponge, and are securely located against the tissue. In addition, coupling may be achieved by placing both the body part to be stimulated and the electrodes in a water bath. These electrodes may be cut to the required size and are reusable; they are, however, less malleable than many of their commercial counterparts.

A number of authors, including Nelson et al. (1980) and Nolan (1991), have compared the efficiency with which various electrodes conduct stimuli to the tissues. Nelson et al. (1980) demonstrated that metal electrodes are most efficient whilst Nolan (1991) showed that carbon–rubber electrodes are generally more efficient than many other polymer-based types. However, the final choice is determined by assessing all the factors mentioned above.

Both hand-held and pad electrodes are available. The first facilitates rapid movement of the electrode, which may be particularly useful when searching for the optimal stimulation point. The second is more useful for a prolonged period of stimulation.

Electrode size

Fundamentally, choice of electrode size depends on the size of the muscle to be stimulated and the intensity of the contraction to be elicited. Small electrodes may be used to localise stimulation to small muscles or to apply a stimulus over a nerve which supplies a muscle. Larger electrodes are needed to stimulate larger muscles and muscle groups and to act as dispersive terminals (see below).

Though the spread of the electrical current over the surface of electrodes may be irregular (e.g. the intensity is often greater at the point where the current enters the electrode), it is generally true to say that the larger the electrode the lower is the intensity of current per unit area. Thus, small electrodes tend to lead to stronger muscle contractions. However, it should be remembered that the final stimulus received by the tissue is also dependent on other factors such as the point at which the current enters the electrode and the nature and efficiency of the contact medium.

Electrode placement

Electrodes may be sited on muscles in a number of ways. First, a primary electrode may be placed over the 'motor point' of a muscle. This may be defined as the point on the surface of the skin that allows a contraction to occur using the least energy. In general, the motor point of a muscle is located over the belly of a muscle, often but not always at the junction between the upper and middle thirds of the belly. Figures 16.2–16.9 show the approximate positions of these points. It is important to remember, however, that these points act only as a guide; alternative placements may be both more effective and more comfortable in certain individuals. When using this technique, a second dispersive or indifferent electrode must be placed elsewhere on the body part, at a convenient location near to the muscle being treated. This electrode should be larger, so that the current density across it is lower and it is therefore unlikely to elicit either motor or sensory responses. This method is suitable for innervated muscle and is sometimes called a *unipolar* technique.

Secondly, electrodes of a similar size may be placed at either end of a muscle belly. This method is suitable for both innervated and denervated muscle and may be termed *bipolar*. Two hand-held electrodes may be used or, if the treatment is to be for a longer period of time, two electrodes may be taped or adhered to the tissue.

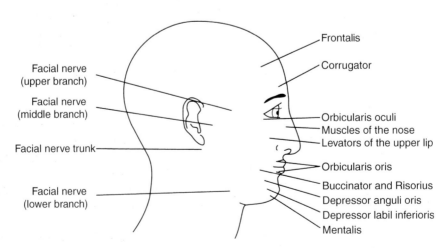

Figure 16.2 Motor points of some of the muscles supplied by the facial nerve.

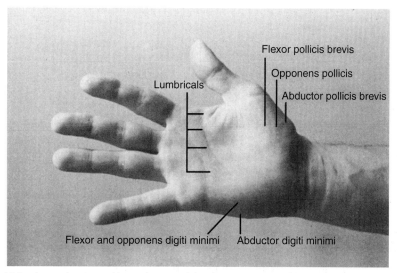

Figure 16.3 Approximate positions of some of the motor points on the anterior aspect of the hand.

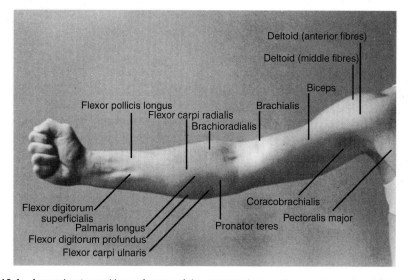

Figure 16.4 Approximate positions of some of the motor points on the anterior aspect of the right arm.

Treatment parameters

The treatment parameters affecting muscle and nerve response have been described in the last chapter. These include current waveform, pulse amplitude and duration, pulse frequency, duty cycle, ramp modulation and duration of treatment.

Patient preference must also be borne in mind, though it is not clear from the literature which waveforms are most acceptable. Bowman and Barker (1985) suggest that symmetrical, biphasic waves are generally preferred, whereas Delitto and Rose (1986) reported there to be no significant differences between sinusoidal, rectangular and triangular waves. The therapist should therefore adjust the waveform in order to produce a satisfactory contraction in as comfortable a fashion as possible. In order to produce a contraction of a designated intensity, it should

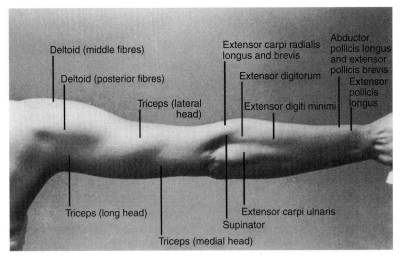

Figure 16.5 Approximate positions of some of the motor points on the posterior aspect of the right arm.

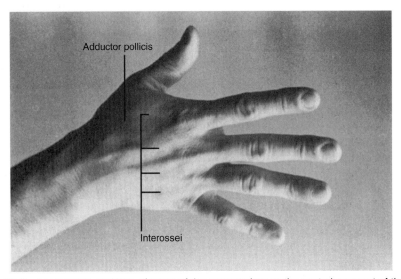

Figure 16.6 Approximate positions of some of the motor points on the posterior aspect of the hand.

be remembered that the shorter the pulse duration, the greater is the pulse amplitude needed; this is demonstrated in the strength—duration curve shown in Figure 16.10A. Figure 16.10B shows that the same relationship between pulse duration and amplitude exists for denervated muscle; however, the figure also shows that the whole curve is shifted to the right, such muscle requiring pulses of longer duration and greater amplitude than innervated tissue.

Force of contraction is determined by the amplitude, frequency, duration and shape of the stimulating waveform, and these factors are discussed in Chapter 15. A considerable number of researchers have examined the ways in which these parameters may be combined to produce optimal contractions, though to date no single combination of parameters has been shown to be most effective; these are discussed below.

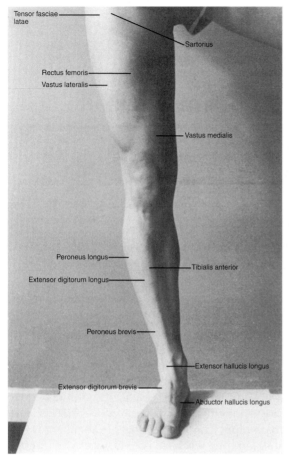

Figure 16.7 Approximate positions of some of the motor points on the anterior aspect of the right leg.

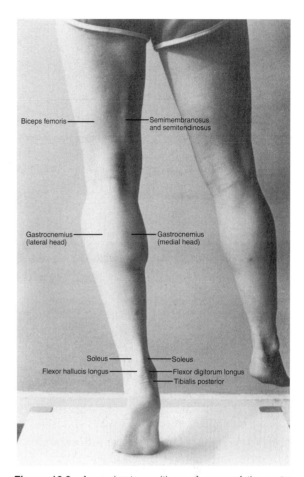

Figure 16.8 Approximate positions of some of the motor points on the posterior aspect of the left leg.

However, in summary, regardless of the reason for using electrical stimulation Table 16.1 provides a guide to the range of parameters that can be used.

Strengthening/re-education

There is a comprehensive review of the parameters that should be used for strengthening muscle in Lake (1992). Some of the details are identified here. The same parameters can be used for re-education as for strengthening, but there is no evidence that high stimulus intensities are required (Lake, 1992). If the aim of treatment is facilitation of muscle contraction, for example in the case of painful inhibition of the quadriceps complex, it is important to progress treatment by instructing the patient to 'feel' the muscle action and then try to contract along with the electrical stimulation. Once the patient starts to contract the muscle voluntarily the intensity of NMES can be gradually reduced.

Frequency of current. Initially low frequencies (20 Hz) and short contraction/long relaxation times can be used in order to minimise muscle fatigue (Jones, Bigland-Ritchie and Edwards, 1979). It is worth noting that the rate of muscle fatigue during NMES is greater than that seen during voluntary contraction (Binder-Macleod and Snyder-Mackler, 1993). Lake (1992) suggests 60 Hz as a starting frequency with an on : off ratio of 1 : 3. However, comparison of strength gains

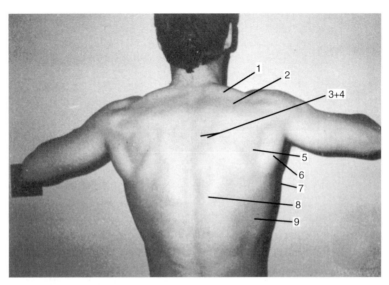

Figure 16.9 Approximate positions of some of the motor points of the back. 1 = trapezius (upper fibres); 2 = supraspinatus; 3 = rhomboids; 4 = trapezius (middle fibres); 5 = infraspinatus; 6 = teres major and minor; 7 = serratus anterior; 8 = trapezius (lower fibres); 9 = latissimus dorsi.

produced at 20 Hz, 45 Hz and 80 Hz in normal quadriceps femoris showed no significant difference (Balogun *et al.*, 1993).

Duty cycles/ramp times. The on:off ratio should be modified to match the fatigue characteristics of the muscle being stimulated. A moderate ramp of 2–3 seconds should be used, except in cases of high current intensities where longer ramp-up and ramp-down times (5 seconds) may be more appropriate (Lake, 1992). There is evidence that if the on-time is 10 seconds then the off-time must be at least 60 seconds to avoid fatigue (Binder-Macleod and Snyder-Mackler, 1993). If the aim of treatment is to strengthen muscle then treatment can be progressed over a number of sessions by increasing the frequency up to 100 Hz (Binder-Macleod and Guerin, 1990) and altering the duty cycle so that the contraction time is lengthened and the relaxation time reduced. Evidence suggests that the stronger the induced contraction force in the muscle the greater are the strength gains (Snyder-Mackler *et al.*, 1995). In addition, inducing fatigue is an important component of any strengthening regimen (by altering the duty cycle), although in early treatment sessions of weakened muscle the parameters are chosen to minimise fatigue (Lake, 1992).

Frequency of treatment. The frequency of sessions and the number of contractions can also be increased over time and generally follow the same principles used in voluntary exercise strengthening programmes—that is, 8–15 maximum contractions per session, for 3–5 sessions per week, over 3–5 weeks of training (Lake, 1992).

Motor recovery following neurological damage

Comparison of parameters used between studies reveals a wide range (Chae *et al.*, 1998; Fransisco *et al.*, 1998; Hesse *et al.*, 1998; Pandyan, Granat and Stott, 1997; Powell *et al.*, 1999; Weingarden, Zeilig and Heruti, 1998). However, in general the parameter ranges were: frequency 20–100 Hz, pulse duration 200–300 µs, short ramp-up and ramp-down and intensities set to produce a maximum range of movement. NMES was most commonly applied for 30 minutes two to three times daily, though in one study this was increased to several hours a day (Weingarden, Zeilig and Heruti, 1998). Treatment was applied for varying periods of time, for instance 8 weeks (Powell *et al.*, 1999) to 6 months (Weingarden, Zeilig and Heruti, 1998). A reasonable guide

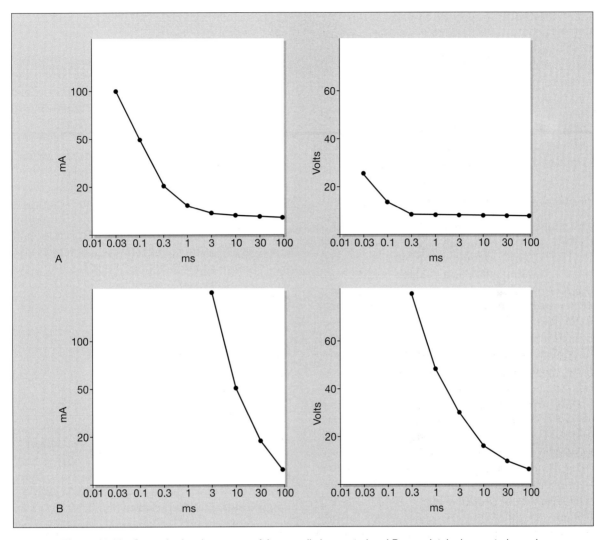

Figure 16.10 Strength–duration curves of A: normally innervated and B: completely denervated muscle.

Table 16.1 Parameters used for electrical stimulation

Type of current	Pulsatile or burst-modulated AC
Amplitude of stimulation	Maximum tolerable/to produce maximum range of movement
Pulse duration	100–300 μs
Waveform	Subject preference
Frequency of stimulation	20–100 pulses or bursts/s
Duty cycle	start with on : off of 2 s : 10 s or 5 s : 15 s
Type of contractions	Isometric
Number of contractions per session	10–20 at maximum tolerable intensity or 15 minutes per session 2–3 times daily
Frequency of sessions	3–7 times/week

for treatment time may be Powell *et al.* (1999), which was a well-designed randomised controlled trial—frequency 20 Hz, pulse duration 300 μs, contraction–relaxation times of 5 s : 20 s initially, progressing to 5 s : 5 s, ramp-up of 1 s and ramp-down of 1.5 s. Intensity was set to produce maximum wrist extension (Powell *et al.*, 1999). However, no studies have been carried out in this group of subjects to identify if an optimum range of parameters exists.

Shoulder subluxation after stroke

The studies discussed in the previous section used a range of parameters (with no rationale for choice), with frequencies of less than 30 Hz, pulse duration of 350 μs, duty cycle ratios initially of 1 : 3 and 1 : 5 with very brief contraction times of 2 seconds; these were gradually increased up to 12–24 seconds and the relaxation time was reduced to 2 seconds. The length of application changed over the 5–6 week period from 90 minutes to 6 hours and was applied for 5–7 days per week. Two studies showed maintenance of effect at follow-up of 6 weeks (Faghri *et al.*, 1994) and at 24 months (Chantraine *et al.*, 1999). In contrast, Wang, Chan and Tsai (2000) in a smaller study showed no follow-up at 6 weeks. This difference may be explained by adjuvant therapy and maintenance exercise programmes in the former two studies (Chantraine *et al.*, 1999; Faghri *et al.*, 1994).

Reduction of spasticity

Based on the studies cited in the last section, the following parameters have been used most often to produce a reduction in spasticity: frequency of 20–50 Hz; pulse duration 200–500 μs; ramp of 0.1–0.5 ms; on : off time with equal short contraction and rest times (i.e. 2 s : 2 s or 5 s : 5 s); intensity with just minimal movement to full available range of movement; session time of 30 minutes for 3–5 days up to 2–6 months; and frequency of session two to three times daily.

Children: strengthening atrophied muscle in neurological conditions

Regardless of the type of electrical stimulation used, most authors in the studies discussed above used similar parameters (i.e. frequencies of 30–45 Hz, pulse durations of 100 μs–300 ms, ramp pulse shapes with rise times of 0.5–2 s). There was some variation in on : off times, but most studies used equal on : off times (Carmick 1993a, 1993b, 1995 and 1997; Comeaux *et al.*, 1997; Pape *et al.*, 1993; Steinbok, Reiner and Kestle, 1997). Intensity and the total treatment time depended on the type of stimulation required. TES tended to be applied for at least 48 hours per week for 6–14 months whereas NMES was most commonly applied for a 1–3 hours per week in short daily sessions over a 2 month period.

HAZARDS

A number of hazards should be guarded against when using NMES. These include:

- chemical damage due to inadequate skin protection when direct or interrupted direct current is used
- disruption of stimulating devices due to the proximity of diathermy equipment, which can result in altered output

CONTRAINDICATIONS

NMES should not be used, or should be used with caution, in patients with the following:

- pacemakers
- peripheral vascular disease, especially when there is the possibility of loosening thrombi
- hypertensive and hypotensive subjects, as NMES may affect the autonomic responses of these patients
- areas of excess adipose tissue in obese subjects, as these subjects may require high

levels of stimuli, which may lead to autonomic changes
- neoplastic tissue
- areas of active tissue infection
- devitalised skin—for example, after treatment with deep X-ray therapy
- patients who are unable to understand the nature of the intervention or provide feedback about the treatment.

In addition, treatment should not be applied over the following areas:

- carotid sinus

- thoracic region—it has been suggested that NMES may interfere with the function of the heart
- phrenic nerve
- trunk, in a pregnant subject.

Electrical stimulation of innervated muscle continues to be a popular form of treatment, though stimulation of denervated muscle is less popular. However, as with many other electro-physical agents, there are still major gaps in our knowledge about the effects it has, the most effective parameters to use and its long-term efficacy.

REFERENCES

Alfieri, V (1982) Electrical treatments of spasticity: reflex tonic activity in hemiplegic patients and selected specific electrostimulation. *Scandinavian Journal of Rehabilitation Medicine* **14**: 177–182.

Alon, G, McCombe, SA, Koutsantonis, S et al. (1987) Comparison of the effects of electrical stimulation and exercise on abdominal musculature. *Journal of Orthopaedic Sports Physical Therapy* **8**: 567–573.

Apkarian, JA, Naumann, S (1991) Stretch reflex inhibition using electrical stimulation in normal subjects and subjects with spasticity. *Journal of Biomedical Engineering* **13**: 67–73.

Artieda, J, Quesada, P, Obeso, J (1991) Reciprocal inhibition between forearm muscles in spastic hemiplegia. *Neurology* **41**: 286–289.

Atwater, SW, Tatarka, ME, Kathrein, JE et al. (1991) Electromyography-triggered electrical stimulation for children with cerebral palsy: a pilot study. *Pediatric Physical Therapy* **3**: 190–199.

Balogun, JA, Onilari, OO, Akeju, OA et al. (1993) High voltage electrical stimulation in the augmentation of muscle strength: effects of pulse frequency. *Archives of Physical Medicine and Rehabilitation* **74**: 910–916.

Beck, S (1997) Use of sensory level electrical stimulation in the physical therapy management of a child with cerebral palsy. *Pediatric Physical Therapy* **9**: 137–138.

Binder-Macleod, SA, Guerin, T (1990) Preservation of force output through progressive reduction of stimulation frequency in human quadriceps femoris muscle. *Physical Therapy* **70**: 619–625.

Binder-Macleod, SA, Snyder-Mackler, L (1993) Muscle fatigue: clinical implications for fatigue assessment and neuromuscular electrical stimulation. *Physical Therapy* **73**(12): 902–910.

Botte, MJ, Nickel, VL, Akeson, WH (1988) Spasticity and contractures. Physiologic aspects of formation. *Clinical Orthopaedics* **233**: 7–18.

Bowman, BR, Barker, LL (1985) Effects of waveform parameters on comfort during transcutaneous neuromuscular electrical stimulation. *Annals of Biomedical Engineering* **13**: 59–74.

Carmick, J (1993a) Clinical use of neuromuscular electrical stimulation for children with cerebral palsy, part 1: lower extremity. *Physical Therapy* **73**: 505–513.

Carmick, J (1993b) Clinical use of neuromuscular electrical stimulation for children with cerebral palsy, part 2: upper extremity. *Physical Therapy* **73**: 514–520.

Carmick, J (1995) Managing equinus in children with cerebral palsy: electrical stimulation to strengthen the triceps surae muscle. *Developmental Medicine and Child Neurology* **37**: 965–975.

Carmick, J (1997) Use of neuromuscular electrical stimulation and a dorsal wrist splint to improve the hand function of a child with spastic hemiparesis. *Physical Therapy* **77**: 661–671.

Chae, J, Bethoux, F, Bohinc, T et al. (1998) Neuromuscular stimulation for upper extremity motor and functional recovery in acute hemiplegia. *Stroke* **19**: 975–979.

Chae, J, Kilgore, K, Triolo, R et al. (2000) Neuromuscular stimulation for motor neuroprosthesis in hemiplegia. *Critical Reviews in Physical and Rehabilitation Medicine* **12**: 1–23.

Chantraine, A, Baribeault, A, Uebelhart, D et al. (1999) Shoulder pain and dysfunction in hemiplegia: effects of functional electrical stimulation. *Archives of Physical Medicine and Rehabilitation* **80**: 328–331.

Comeaux, P, Patterson, N, Rubin, M et al. (1997) Effect of neuromuscular electrical stimulation during gait in children with cerebral palsy. *Pediatric Physical Therapy* **9**: 103–109.

Currier, DP, Mann, R (1983) Muscular strength development by electrical stimulation in normal subjects. *Physical Therapy* **63**: 915–921.

Daly, JJ, Ruff, RL (2000) Electrically induced recovery of gait components for older patients with chronic stroke. *American Journal of Physical Medicine and Rehabilitation* **79**(4): 349–360.

Davies, HL (1983) Is electrostimulation beneficial to denervated nerve? A review of results from basic research. *Physiotherapy* (Canada) **35**: 306–310.

Delitto, A, Rose, SJ (1986) Comparative comfort of three wave forms used in electrically elicited quadriceps femoris contractions. *Physical Therapy* **66**: 1704–1707.

Delitto, A, Snyder-Mackler, L, Robinson, AJ (1995) Electrical stimulation of muscle: techniques and applications. In: Robinson, AJ, Snyder-Mackler, L (eds) *Clinical Electrophysiology: Electrotherapy and Electrophysiological Testing.* Williams and Wilkins, Baltimore, MD.

Delitto, A, Snyder-Mackler, L (1990) Two theories of muscle strength augmentation using percutaneous electrical stimulation. *Physical Therapy* **70**: 158–164.

Delitto, A, Rose, SJ, McKowen, JM *et al.* (1988) Electrical stimulation versus voluntary exercise in strengthening thigh musculature after anterior cruciate ligament surgery. *Physical Therapy* **68**: 660–663.

Dietz, V, Quintern, J, Berger, W (1981) Electrophysiological studies of gait in spasticity and rigidity. Evidence that altered mechanical properties of muscle contribute to hypertonia. *Brain* **104**: 431–449.

Faghri, D, Rodgers, M, Glaser, R *et al.* (1994) The effects of functional electrical stimulation on shoulder subluxation, arm function recovery, and shoulder pain in hemiplegic stroke patients. *Archives of Physical Medicine and Rehabilitation* **75**: 73–79.

Fransisco, G, Chae, J, Chawla, H *et al.* (1998) Electromyogram-triggered neuromuscular stimulation for improving the arm function of acute stroke survivors: a randomised pilot study. *Archives of Physical Medicine and Rehabilitation* **79**: 571–575.

Fynes, M, Marshall, K, Cassidy, M *et al.* (1999) A prospective, randomised study comparing the effect of augmented biofeedback with sensory biofeedback alone on fecal incontinence after obstetric trauma. *Diseases of the Colon and Rectum* **42**(6): 753–758.

Glanz, M, Klawansky, S, Stason, W *et al.* (1996) Functional electrostimulation in poststroke rehabilitation: a meta-analysis of the randomised controlled trials. *Archives of Physical Medicine and Rehabilitation* **77**: 549–553.

Granit, R, Pascoe, JE, Steg, G (1957) The behaviour of tonic alpha and gamma motoneurones during stimulation of recurrent collaterals. *Journal of Physiology* **13**(8): 381–400.

Grove-Lainey, C, Walmsley RP, Andrew, GM (1983) Effectiveness of exercise alone versus exercise plus electrical stimulation in strengthening the quadriceps muscle. *Physiotherapy Canada* **35**: 5–11.

Hazlewood, ME, Brown, JK, Rowe, PJ *et al.* (1994) The use of therapeutic electrical stimulation in the treatment of hemiplegic cerebral palsy. *Developmental Medicine and Child Neurology* **36**: 661–673.

Hesse, S, Reiter, F, Konrad, M *et al.* (1998) Botulinum toxin type A and short term electrical stimulation in the treatment of upper limb flexor spasticity after stroke: a randomised, double-blind, placebo-controlled trial. *Clinical Rehabilitation* **12**: 381–388.

Hömberg, V (1997) Is rehabilitation effective in spastic syndromes? In: Thilmann, F *et al.* (eds), *Spasticity Mechanisms and Management.* Springer-Verlag, Berlin, pp 439–450.

Horodyski, MB, Sharp, RL (1985) Effects of electrical stimulation on subjects with patellofemoral pain syndrome. *Medicine and Science in Sports and Exercise* **17**(2): 225–255.

Hummelsheim, H, Mauritz, KH (1993) Neurological mechanisms of spasticity. Modification by physiotherapy. In: Thilmann, F *et al.* (eds), *Spasticity Mechanisms and Management.* Springer-Verlag, Berlin, pp 427–437.

Jones, DA, Bigland-Ritchie, B, Edwards, RHT (1979) Excitation frequency and muscle fatigue: mechanical responses during voluntary and stimulated contractions. *Experimental Neurology* **64**: 401–413.

Kahanovitz, N, Nordin, M, Verderame, R *et al.* (1987) Normal trunk muscle strength and endurance in woman and the effects of exercises and electrical stimulation, part 2: comparative analysis of electrical stimulation and exercises to increase trunk muscle strength and endurance. *Spine* **12**: 112–118.

Kloth, LC, Cummings, JP (1991) *Electrotherapeutic Terminology in Physical Therapy,* section on clinical electrophysiology. American Physical Therapy Association, Alexandria, VA.

Lake, DA (1988) The effects of neuromuscular stimulation as applied by 'toning salons' on muscle strength and body shape. *Physical Therapy* **68**: 789. Abstract RO77.

Lake, DA (1992) Neuromuscular electrical stimulation. An overview of its application in the treatment of sports injuries. *Sports Medicine* **15**(5): 320–336.

Lake, DA, Gillespie, WJ (1988) Electrical stimulation (NMES) does not decrease body fat. *Medicine and Science in Sports and Exercise* **20** (suppl): S22. Abstract 131.

Levine, MG, Knott, M, Kabot, H (1952) Relaxation of spasticity by electrical stimulation of antagonist muscles. *Archives of Physical Medicine* **33**: 668–673.

Lieber, RL (1986) Skeletal muscle adaptability III. Muscle properties following chronic electrical stimulation. *Developmental Medicine and Child Neurology* **28**: 662–670.

Lieber, RL, Silva, PD, Daniel, DM (1996) Equal effectiveness of electrical and volitional strength training for quadriceps femoris muscles after anterior cruciate ligament surgery. *Journal of Orthopaedic Research* **14**: 131–138.

Nelson, H, Smith, M, Bowman, B *et al.* (1980) Electrode effectiveness during transcutaneous motor stimulation. *Archives of Physical Medicine and Rehabilitation* **61**: 73–77.

Nolan, MF (1991) Conductive differences in electrodes used with transcutaneous electrical nerve stimulation devices. *Physical Therapy* **71**: 746–751.

O'Callaghan, MJ, Oldham, J (1997) A critical review of electrical stimulation of the quadriceps muscles. *Critical Reviews in Physical and Rehabilitation Medicine* **9**: 301–314.

Pandyan, AD, Granat, MH, Stott, DJ (1997) Effects of electrical stimulation on flexion contractures in hemiplegic wrist. *Clinical Rehabilitation* **11**: 123–130.

Pape, K (1997) Therapeutic electrical stimulation (TES) for the treatment of disuse muscle atrophy in cerebral palsy. *Pediatric Physical Therapy* **9**: 110–112.

Pape, KE, Kirsch, SE, Galil, A *et al.* (1993) Neuromuscular approach to the motor deficits of cerebral palsy: a pilot study. *Journal of Orthopaedics* **13**: 628–633.

Paternostro-Sluga, T, Fialka, C, Alacamliogliu, Y *et al.* (1999) Neuromuscular electrical stimulation after anterior cruciate ligament surgery. *Clinical Orthopaedics and Related Research* **368**: 166–175.

Pease, W (1998) Therapeutic electrical stimulation for spasticity. Quantitative gait analysis. *American Journal of Physical Medicine and Rehabilitation* **77**: 351–355.

Powell, J, Pandyan, D, Granat, M *et al.* (1999) Electrical stimulation of wrist extensors in poststroke hemiplegia. *Stroke* **30**: 1384–1389.

Rose, J, McGill, KC (1998) The motor unit in cerebral palsy. *Developmental Medicine and Child Neurology* **40**: 270–277.

Ryall, RW, Piercy, MF, Polosa, C *et al.* (1972) Excitation of Renshaw cells in relation to orthodromic and antidromic excitation of motoneurons. *Journal of Neurophysiology* **35**: 137–148.

Sand, PK, Richardson, DA, Staskin, DR *et al.* (1995) Pelvic floor electrical stimulation in the treatment of genuine stress incontinence: a multicenter, placebo-controlled trial. *American Journal of Obstetrics and Gynecology* **173**: 72–79.

Selkowitz, DM (1989) High frequency electrical stimulation in muscle strengthening. A review and discussion. *American Journal of Sports Medicine* **17**(1): 103–111.

Singer, KP, Gow, PJ, Otway, WF *et al.* (1983) A comparison of electrical muscle stimulation isometric, isotonic and isokinetic strength training programmes. *New Zealand Journal of Sports Medicine* **11**: 61–63.

Sisk, TD, Stralka, SW, Deering, MB *et al.* (1987) Effects of electrical stimulation on quadriceps strength after reconstructive surgery of the anterior cruciate ligament. *American Journal of Sports Medicine* **15**: 215–219.

Steinbok, P, Reiner, A, Kestle, JR (1997) Therapeutic electrical stimulation following selective posterior rhizotomy in children with spastic diplegic cerebral palsy: a randomized clinical trial. *Developmental Medicine and Child Neurology* **39**: 515–520.

Snyder-Mackler, L, Ladin, Z, Schepsis, A *et al.* (1991) Electrical stimulation of the thigh muscles after reconstruction of the anterior cruciate ligament. Effect of electrically elicited contractions of the quadriceps femoris and hamstring muscles on gait and strength of the thigh muscles. *Journal of Bone and Joint Surgery* (Am), **73**: 1025–1036.

Snyder-Mackler, L, Delitto, A, Bailey, S *et al.* (1995) Strength of the quadriceps femoris muscle and functional recovery after reconstruction of the anterior cruciate ligament. A prospective, randomised clinical trial of electrical stimulation. *Journal of Bone and Joint Surgery* **77A**(8): 1166–1173.

Vodovnik, L, Bowman, BR, Hufford, P (1984) Effects of electrical stimulation on spinal spasticity. *Scandinavian Journal of Rehabilitation Medicine* **16**: 29–34.

Wang, RY, Chan, RC, Tsai, MW (2000) Functional electrical stimulation on chronic and acute hemiplegic subluxation. *American Journal of Physical Medicine and Rehabilitation* **79**(4): 385–390.

Weingarden, HP, Zeilig, G, Heruti, R (1998) Hybrid functional electrical stimulation orthosis system for the upper limb. Effects on spasticity in chronic stable hemiplegia. *American Journal of Physical Medicine and Rehabilitation* **77**(4): 276–281.

Wigerstad-Lossing, I, Grimby, G, Jonsson, T *et al.* (1997) Effects of electrical muscle stimulation combined with voluntary contraction after knee ligament surgery. *Medicine and Science in Sports and Exercise* **20**(1): 93.

William, JG, Street, M (1976) Sequential faradism in quadriceps rehabilitation. *Physiotherapy* **62**: 252–254.

Wolf, SL, Gideon, BA, Saar, D *et al.* (1986) The effect of muscle stimulation during resistive training on performance parameters. *American Journal of Sports Medicine* **14**: 18–23.

17

Transcutaneous electrical nerve stimulation (TENS)

Mark Johnson

INTRODUCTION

Transcutaneous electrical nerve stimulation (TENS) is a simple, non-invasive analgesic technique that is used extensively in health-care settings by physiotherapists, nurses and midwifes (Johnson, 1997; Pope, Mockett and Wright, 1995; Reeve, Menon and Corabian, 1996; Robertson and Spurritt, 1998). It can be administered in the clinic by health-care professionals or at home by patients who have purchased a TENS device directly from manufacturers. TENS is mainly used for the symptomatic management of acute and non-malignant chronic pain (Box 17.1, Walsh, 1997a; Woolf and Thompson, 1994). However, TENS is also used in palliative care to manage pain caused by metastatic bone disease and neoplasm (Thompson and Filshie, 1993). It is also claimed that TENS has antiemetic and tissue-healing effects although it is used less often for these actions (Box 17.1, Walsh, 1997b).

During TENS, pulsed currents are generated by a portable pulse generator and delivered across the intact surface of the skin via conducting pads called electrodes (Fig. 17.1). The conventional way of administering TENS is to use electrical characteristics that selectively activate large diameter 'touch' fibres (Aβ) without activating smaller diameter nociceptive fibres (Aδ and C). Evidence suggests that this will produce pain relief in a similar way to 'rubbing the pain better' (see Mechanisms of action). In practice, conventional TENS is delivered to generate a

Box 17.1   Common medical conditions that TENS has been used to treat

Analgesic effects of TENS
Relief of acute pain
- Postoperative pain
- Labour pain
- Dysmenorrhoea
- Musculoskeletal pain
- Bone fractures
- Dental procedures

Relief of chronic pain
- Low back
- Arthritis
- Stump and phantom
- Postherpetic neuralgia
- Trigeminal neuralgia
- Causalgia
- Peripheral nerve injuries
- Angina pectoris
- Facial pain
- Metastatic bone pain

Non-analgesic effects of TENS
Antiemetic effects
- Postoperative nausea associated with opioid medication
- Nausea associated with chemotherapy
- Morning sickness
- Motion/travel sickness

Improving blood flow
- Reduction in ischaemia due to reconstructive surgery
- Reduction of symptoms associated with Raynaud's disease and diabetic neuropathy
- Improved healing of wounds and ulcers

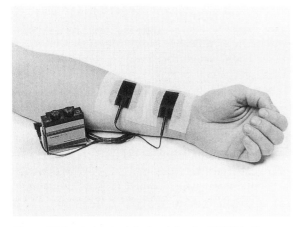

Figure 17.1   A standard device delivering TENS to the arm. There is increasing use of self-adhesive electrodes rather than black carbon-rubber electrodes that require conductive gel and tape as shown in the diagram.

strong but comfortable paraesthesia within the site of pain using frequencies between 1 and 250 pulses per second (p.p.s.) and pulse durations between 50 and 1000 μs.

In medicine, TENS is the most frequently used electrotherapy for producing pain relief. It is popular because it is non-invasive, easy to administer and has few side-effects or drug interactions. As there is no potential for toxicity or overdose, patients can administer TENS themselves and titrate the dosage of treatment as required. TENS effects are rapid in onset for most patients so benefit can be achieved almost immediately. TENS is cheap when compared with long-term drug therapy and some TENS devices are available for less than £30.00.

HISTORY

There is evidence that ancient Egyptians used electrogenic fish to treat ailments in 2500BC, although the Roman Physician Scribonius Largus is credited with the first documented report of the use of electrogenic fish in medicine in AD46 (Kane and Taub, 1975). The development of electrostatic generators in the eighteenth century increased the use of medical electricity, although its popularity declined in the nineteenth and early twentieth century due to variable clinical results and the development of alternative treatments (Stillings, 1975). Interest in the use of electricity to relieve pain was reawakened in 1965 by Melzack and Wall (1965) who provided a physiological rationale for electroanalgesic effects. They proposed that transmission of noxious information could be inhibited by activity in large diameter peripheral afferents or by activity in pain-inhibitory pathways descending from the brain (Fig. 17.2). Wall and Sweet (1967) used high-frequency percutaneous electrical stimulation to activate large diameter peripheral afferents artificially and found that this relieved chronic pain in patients. Pain relief was also demonstrated when electrical currents were used to stimulate the periaqueductal grey (PAG) region of the midbrain (Reynolds, 1969), which is part of the descending pain-inhibitory pathway. Shealy, Mortimer and Reswick (1967) found that electrical stimulation of the dorsal columns, which form the central transmission pathway of large diameter peripheral afferents, also produced pain relief. TENS was used to predict the success of dorsal column stimulation implants until it was realised that it could be used as a successful modality on its own (Long, 1973, 1974).

DEFINITION

By definition, any stimulating device which delivers electrical currents across the intact surface of the skin is TENS, although the technical characteristics of a standard TENS device are given in Table 17.1 and Figure 17.3. Developments in electronic technology have meant that

Table 17.1 Typical features of TENS devices

Weight dimensions	50–250 g 6 × 5 × 2 cm (small device) 12 × 9 × 4 cm (large device)
Cost	£30–150
Pulse waveform (fixed)	Monophasic Symmetrical biphasic Asymmetrical biphasic
Pulse amplitude (adjustable)	1–50 mA into a 1 kΩ load
Pulse duration (often fixed)	10–1000 µs
Pulse frequency (adjustable)	1–250 p.p.s.
Pulse pattern	Continuous, burst (random frequency, modulated amplitude, modulated frequency, modulated pulse duration)
Channels	1 or 2
Batteries	PP3 (9 V), rechargeable
Additional features	Timer Most devices deliver constant current output

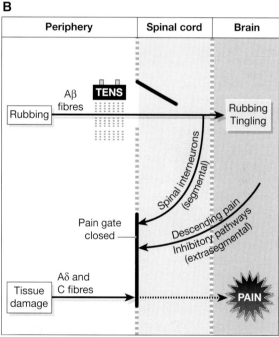

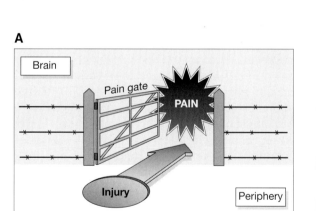

Figure 17.2 The 'Pain Gate'. A: Under normal physiological circumstances, the brain generates pain sensations by processing incoming noxious information arising from stimuli such as tissue damage. In order for noxious information to reach the brain it must pass through a metaphorical 'pain gate' located in lower levels of the central nervous system. In physiological terms, the gate is formed by excitatory and inhibitory synapses regulating the flow of neural information through the central nervous system. This 'pain gate' is opened by noxious events in the periphery. B: The pain gate can be closed by activation of mechanoreceptors through 'rubbing the skin'. This generates activity in large diameter Aβ afferents, which inhibits the onward transmission of noxious information. This closing of the 'pain gate' results in less noxious information reaching the brain reducing the sensation of pain. The neuronal circuitry involved is segmental in its organisation. The aim of conventional TENS is to activate Aβ fibres using electrical currents. The pain gate can also be closed by the activation of pain-inhibitory pathways which originate in the brain and descend to the spinal cord through the brainstem (extrasegmental circuitry). These pathways become active during psychological activities such as motivation and when small diameter peripheral fibres (Aδ) are excited physiologically. The aim of AL-TENS is to excite small diameter peripheral fibres to activate the descending pain-inhibitory pathways.

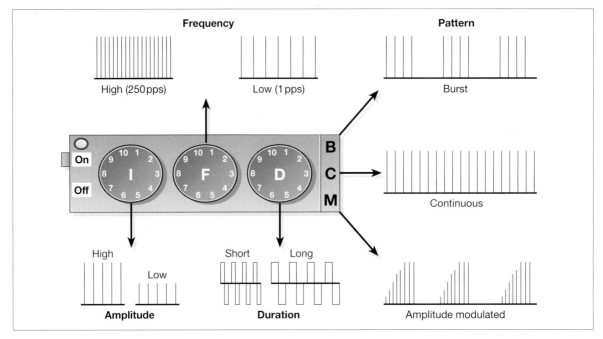

Figure 17.3 Schematic diagram of the output characteristics of a standard TENS device (topographic view, each vertical line represents one pulse). The intensity control dial (I) regulates the current amplitude of individual pulses, the frequency control dial (F) regulates the rate of pulse delivery (pulses per second = p.p.s.) and the pulse duration control dial (D) regulates the time duration of each pulse. Most TENS devices offer alternative patterns of pulse delivery such as burst, continuous and amplitude modulated.

a variety of TENS-like devices are available on the market (Table 17.2). However, the clinical effectiveness of these TENS-like devices is not known owing to a lack of randomised controlled clinical trials (RCTs). Unfortunately, the increasing number of TENS-like devices has created a literature littered with inconsistent and ambiguous terminology and this has led to confusion in nomenclature. Nevertheless, the main types of TENS described in the literature are conventional TENS, acupuncture-like TENS (AL-TENS) and intense TENS (Table 17.3, Walsh, 1997c; Woolf and Thompson, 1994). At present, conventional TENS remains the most commonly used method for delivering currents in clinical practice (Johnson, Ashton and Thompson 1991a).

PHYSICAL PRINCIPLES

The electrical characteristics of TENS are chosen with a view to selectively activate different populations of nerve fibres as this is believed to produce different analgesic outcomes (Table 17.3). A standard TENS device provides a range of possible ways that TENS currents could be delivered so it is important to review the principles of nerve fibre activation (Fig. 17.3). Large diameter nerve fibres such as Aβ and Aα have low thresholds of activation to electrical stimuli when compared with their small diameter counterparts (Aδ and C). The current amplitude needed to excite a nerve fibre declines with increasing pulse duration and increasing pulse frequency. Pulse durations of 10–1000 μs provide the greatest separation (and sensitivity) of pulse amplitudes required to selectively activate large diameter afferents, small diameter afferents and motor efferents (Fig. 17.4, Howson, 1978). Thus, to activate large diameter fibres (Aβ) without activating smaller diameter nociceptive fibres (Aδ and C) one would select low-intensity, high-frequency (10–250 p.p.s.) currents with pulse durations between 10 and 1000 μs (see Howson, 1978; Walsh, 1997d; Woolf and Thompson, 1994

Table 17.2 Characteristics of TENS-like devices

Device	Experimental work	Manufacturers claim	Typical stimulating characteristics
Action potential simulation (APS)	Odendaal and Joubert (1999)	Pain relief Improve mobility Improve circulation Reduce inflammation	Monophasic square pulse with exponential decay Delivered by two electrodes Pulse amplitude low (< 25 mA), duration long (800 μs–6.6 ms), frequency fixed at 150 p.p.s
Codetron	Pomeranz and Niznick (1987) Fargas-Babjak et al. (1989; 1992).	Pain relief Reduce habituation	Square wave Delivered randomly to one of six electrodes Pulse amplitude low, duration long (1 ms), frequency low (2 p.p.s.)
H wave stimulation	McDowell et al. (1995; 1999)	Pain relief Improve mobility Improve circulation Reduce inflammation Promote wound healing	'Unique' biphasic wave with exponential decay Delivered by two electrodes Pulse amplitude low (< 10 mA), duration long (fixed at 16 ms), frequency low (2–60 p.p.s.)
Interference currents	See Chapter 18	Pain relief Improve mobility Improve circulation Reduce inflammation Promote wound healing Muscle re-education	Two out-of-phase currents which interfere with each other to produce an amplitude-modulated wave Traditionally, delivered by four electrodes Pulse amplitude low, amplitude-modulated frequency 1–200 Hz (carrier wave frequencies approximately 2–4 kHz)
Microcurrent	Johannsen et al. (1993) Johnson et al. (1997)	Promote wound healing Pain relief Other indications often claimed	Modified square direct current with monophasic or biphasic pulses changing polarity at regular intervals (0.4 s) Delivered by two electrodes Pulse amplitude low (1–600 μA with no paraesthesia), frequency depends on manufacturer (1–5000 p.p.s.) Many variants exist (e.g. transcranial stimulation for migraine and insomnia)
Transcutaneous spinal electroanalgesia (TSE)	Macdonald and Coates (1995)	Pain relief, especially allodynia and hyperalgesia due to central sensitisation	Differentiated wave Delivered by two electrodes positioned on spinal cord at T1 and T12 or straddling C3–C5 Pulse amplitude high (although no paraesthesia), duration very short (1.5–4 μs, frequency high (600–10 000 p.p.s.)

for discussion). Increasing the pulse duration will lead to the activation of small diameter fibres at lower pulse amplitudes.

In practice, it is difficult to predict the exact nature and distribution of currents when they are passed across the intact surface of the skin due to the complex and non-homogeneous impedance of the tissue. However, as the skin offers high impedance at pulse frequencies used by TENS it is likely that currents will remain superficial stimulating cutaneous nerve fibres rather than deep-seated visceral and muscle nerve fibres. Moreover, different TENS devices use a variety of pulse waveforms. Generally, these can be divided into monophasic and biphasic waveforms (Fig. 17.5). It is the cathode

(usually the black lead) that excites the axon so in practice the cathode is placed proximal to the anode to prevent the blockade of nerve transmission due to hyperpolarisation (Fig. 17.6). Devices which use biphasic waveforms with zero net current flow will alternate the cathode and anode between the two electrodes. Zero net current flow may prevent the build-up of ion concentrations beneath electrodes, preventing adverse skin reactions due to polar concentrations (Kantor, Alon and Ho, 1994; Walsh, 1997d).

The introduction of novel features on devices, such as modulated amplitude, modulated frequency and modulated duration (Fig. 17.7), enable manufacturers to gain a competitive edge in the market-place but are rarely supported by

Table 17.3 The characteristics of different types of TENS

	Aim of currents	Main fibre-type responsible for effects	Desired outcome—patient experience	Optimal electrical characteristics	Electrode position	Analgesic profile	Duration of treatment	Main mechanism of analgesic action
Conventional TENS	Activate large diameter non-noxious cutaneous afferents	Aβ, mechano-receptors	Strong comfortable electrical paraesthesia with minimal muscle activity	High frequency/low intensity Amplitude = low Duration = 100–200 μs Frequency = 10–200 p.p.s. Pattern = continuous	Over site of pain Dermatomal	Rapid onset <30 min after switch-on Rapid offset <30 min after switch-off	Continuously when in pain	Segmental
AL-TENS	Activate motor efferents to produce phasic muscle twitch leading to activation of small diameter non-noxious muscle afferents (GIII)	GIII, Aδ ergoreceptors	Strong comfortable phasic muscle contraction	Low frequency/high intensity Amplitude = high Duration = 100–200 μs Frequency = ~100 p.p.s. within burst Pattern = burst	Over motor point/muscle at site of pain Myotomal	?Delayed onset >30 min after switch-on ?Delayed offset >1 h after switch-off	~30 min/session	Extrasegmental Segmental
Intense TENS	Activate small diameter 'pin-prick' cutaneous afferents	Aδ, nociceptors	Highest intensity tolerable with minimal muscle contraction	High frequency/high intensity Amplitude = highest tolerable Duration >1000 μs Frequency = ~200 p.p.s. Pattern = continuous	Over site of pain or proximal over main nerve bundle	Rapid onset <30 min after switch-on ?Delayed offset >1 h after switch-off May experience hypoaesthesia	~15 min/session	Peripheral Extrasegmental Segmental

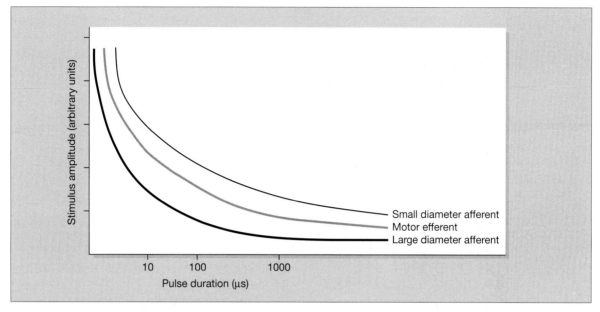

Figure 17.4 Strength–duration curve for fibre activation. As pulse duration increases less current amplitude is needed to excite an axon to generate an action potential. Small pulse durations are unable to excite nerve axons even at high current amplitudes. Large diameter axons require lower current amplitudes than small diameter fibres. Thus, passing pulsed currents across the surface of the skin excites large diameter non-noxious sensory nerves first (paraesthesia), followed by motor efferents (muscle contraction) and small diameter noxious afferents (pain). Alteration of pulse duration is one means of helping the selective recruitment of different types of nerve fibre. For example, intense TENS should use long pulse durations ($>1000\,\mu s$) as they activate small diameter afferents more readily. During conventional TENS pulse durations ~ 100–$200\,\mu s$ are used as there is a large separation (difference) in the amplitude needed to recruit different types of fibre. This enables greater sensitivity when using the intensity (amplitude) dial so that a strong but comfortable paraesthesia can be achieved without muscle contraction or pain.

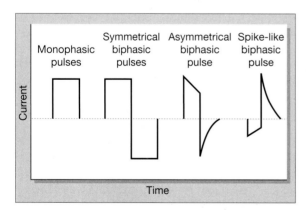

Figure 17.5 Common pulse waveforms used in TENS.

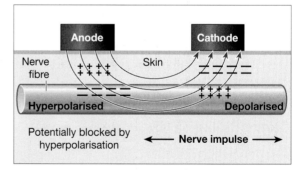

Figure 17.6 Fibre activation by TENS. When devices use waveforms which produce net DC outputs which are not zero, the cathode excites (depolarisation) the axon and the nerve impulse will travel in both directions down the axon. The anode tends to inhibit the axon (hyperpolarisation) and this could extinguish the nerve impulse. Thus, during conventional TENS the cathode should be positioned proximal to the anode so that the nerve impulse is transmitted to the central nervous system unimpeded. However, during AL-TENS the cathode should be placed distal, or over the motor point, as the purpose of AL-TENS currents is to activate a motor efferent.

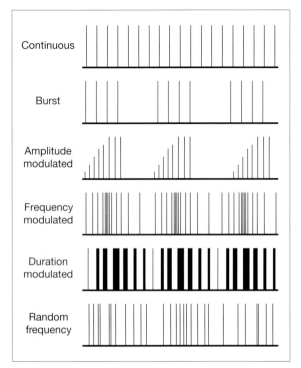

Figure 17.7 Novel pulse patterns available on TENS devices. Modulated patterns fluctuate between upper and lower limits over a fixed period of time and this is usually preset in the design of the TENS device.

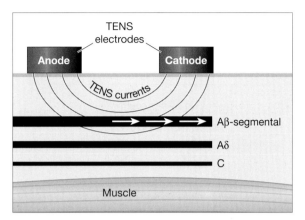

Figure 17.8 The aim of conventional TENS is to selectively activate Aβ afferents producing segmental analgesia.

proven improvements in clinical effectiveness. Unfortunately, the ever-increasing complexity of TENS devices has led to confusion about the most appropriate way to administer TENS. Therefore it is important to summarise the principles for the main types of TENS.

Conventional TENS

The aim of conventional TENS is to activate selectively large diameter Aβ fibres without concurrently activating small diameter Aδ and C (pain-related) fibres or muscle efferents (Fig. 17.8). Evidence from animal and human studies supports the hypothesis that conventional TENS produces segmental analgesia with a rapid onset and offset and which is localised to the dermatome (see Mechanisms of action). Theoretically, high-frequency, low-intensity pulsed currents would be most effective in selectively activating

large diameter fibres, although in practice this will be achieved whenever the TENS user reports that they experience a comfortable paraesthesia beneath the electrodes.

During conventional TENS currents are usually delivered between 10 and 200 p.p.s., and 100–200 μs with pulse amplitude titrated to produce a strong comfortable and non-painful paraesthesia (Table 17.3). As large diameter fibres have short refractory periods they can generate nerve impulses at high frequencies. This means that they are more able to generate high-frequency volleys of nerve impulses when high-frequency currents are delivered. Thus, greater afferent barrages will be produced in large diameter nerve fibres when high frequencies (10–200 p.p.s.) are used. The pattern of pulse delivery is usually continuous, although conventional TENS can also be achieved by delivering the pulses in 'bursts' or 'trains' and this has been described by some authors as pulsed or burst TENS (Walsh, 1997c; Woolf and Thompson, 1994). It is likely that continuous TENS and burst TENS produce similar effects when delivered at a strong but comfortable level without concurrent muscle twitches.

Acupuncture-like TENS (AL-TENS)

The majority of commentators believe that AL-TENS should be defined as the induction of forceful but non-painful phasic muscle contractions

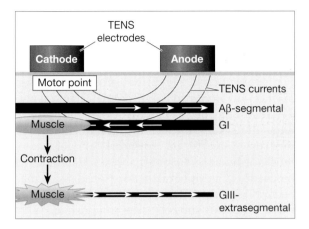

Figure 17.9 The aim of AL-TENS is to selectively activate group I (GI) efferents producing a muscle contraction, which results in activity in ergoreceptors and group III (GIII) afferents. GIII afferents are small in diameter and have been shown to produce extrasegmental analgesia through the activation of descending pain inhibitory pathways. Aβ afferents will also be activated during AL-TENS producing segmental analgesia. Note the position of the cathode.

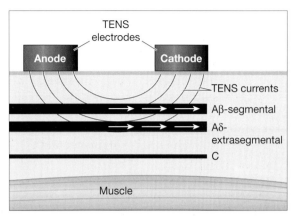

Figure 17.10 The aim of intense TENS is to selectively activate Aδ afferents leading to extrasegmental analgesia. Aβ afferents will also be activated producing segmental analgesia.

at myotomes related to the origin of the pain (Eriksson and Sjölund, 1976; Johnson, 1998; Meyerson, 1983; Sjölund, Eriksson and Loeser, 1990; Walsh, 1997c; Woolf and Thompson, 1994). The purpose of AL-TENS is to selectively activate small diameter fibres (Aδ or group III) arising from muscles (ergoreceptors) by the induction of phasic muscle twitches (Fig. 17.9). Thus, TENS is delivered over motor points to activate Aα efferents to generate a phasic muscle twitch resulting in ergoreceptor activity (Table 17.3). Patients report discomfort when low-frequency pulses are used to generate muscle twitches so bursts of pulses are used instead (Eriksson and Sjölund, 1976). Evidence suggests that AL-TENS produces extrasegmental analgesia in a manner similar to that suggested for acupuncture (see Mechanisms of action). However, there is inconsistency in the use of the term, 'AL-TENS', as some commentators describe AL-TENS as the delivery of TENS over acupuncture points irrespective of muscle activity (Lewers *et al.*, 1989; Lewis *et al.*, 1990; Longobardi *et al.*, 1989; Rieb and Pomeranz, 1992). A critical review of AL-TENS can be found in Johnson (1998).

Intense TENS

The aim of intense TENS is to activate small diameter Aδ cutaneous afferents by delivering TENS over peripheral nerves arising from the site of pain at an intensity which is just tolerable to the patient (Jeans, 1979; Melzack, Vetere and Finch, 1983, Fig. 17.10). Thus, TENS is delivered over the site of pain or main nerve bundle arising from the pain using high-frequency and high-intensity currents which are just bearable to the patient (Table 17.3). As intense TENS acts in part as a counterirritant it can be delivered for only a short time but it may prove useful for minor surgical procedures such as wound dressing and suture removal. Activity in cutaneous Aδ afferents induced by intense TENS has been shown to produce peripheral blockade of nociceptive afferent activity and segmental and extrasegmental analgesia (see Mechanisms of action).

Practical implications

The theoretical relationship between pulse frequency, duration and pattern may break down as currents follow the path of least resistance through the underlying tissue. So in clinical practice a trial and error approach is used whereby patients titrate current amplitude, frequency and duration to produce the appropriate outcome. The patients' report of the sensation produced by TENS is the easiest means of assessing the type of fibre active. A strong non-painful electrical paraesthesia is mediated by large diameter afferents and a mildly painful electrical paraesthesia is mediated by recruitment of small diameter afferents. The presence of a strong non-painful phasic muscle contraction is likely to excite muscle ergoreceptors.

KNOWN BIOLOGICAL EFFECTS

TENS effects can be subdivided into analgesic and non-analgesic effects (Box 17.1). In clinical practice, TENS is predominantly used for its symptomatic relief of pain although there is increasing use of TENS as an antiemetic and for restoration of blood flow to ischaemic tissue and wounds. There is, however, less published research on the non-analgesic effects of TENS and some of the experimental work in the field is contradictory. The reader is guided to Walsh (1997b) for a discussion of the non-analgesic effects of TENS. In contrast, the mechanism by which TENS produces pain relief has received much attention.

Mechanisms of action

Stimulation-induced analgesia can be categorised according to the anatomical site of action into peripheral, segmental and extrasegmental. In general, the main action of conventional TENS is segmental analgesia mediated by Aβ fibre activity. The main action of AL-TENS is extrasegmental analgesia mediated by ergoreceptor activity. The main action of intense TENS is extrasegmental analgesia via activity in small diameter cutaneous afferents. Conventional and intense TENS are also likely to produce peripheral blockade of afferent information in the fibre type that they activate.

Peripheral mechanisms

The delivery of electrical currents over a nerve fibre will elicit nerve impulses that travel in both directions along the nerve axon, termed

antidromic activation (Fig. 17.11). TENS-induced nerve impulses travelling away from the central nervous system will collide with and extinguish afferent impulses arising from tissue damage. For conventional TENS, antidromic activation is likely to occur in large diameter fibres and as tissue damage may produce some activity in large diameter fibres conventional TENS may mediate some of its analgesia by peripheral blockade in large diameter fibres. TENS-induced blockade of peripheral nerve transmission has been demonstrated by Walsh *et al.* (1998) in healthy human subjects. They found that TENS delivered at 110 p.p.s. significantly increased the negative peak latency of the compound action potential and this suggests that there was a slowing of transmission in the peripheral nerve. Nardone and Schieppati (1989) have also reported that the latency of early somatosensory evoked potentials (SEPs) was increased during TENS in healthy subjects and concluded that conventional TENS could produce a 'busy line-effect' in large afferent fibres.

The contribution of peripheral blockade on analgesia is likely to be greater during intense TENS. Impulses travelling in Aδ fibres induced

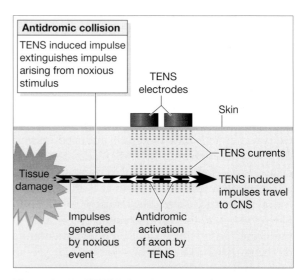

Figure 17.11 TENS-induced blockade of peripheral transmission. Impulses generated by TENS will travel in both directions down an axon (antidromic activation) leading to a collision with noxious impulses travelling toward the central nervous system (CNS).

by intense TENS will collide with nociceptive impulses, also travelling in Aδ fibres. Ignelzi and Nyquist (1976) demonstrated that electrical stimulation (at intensities likely to recruit Aδ fibres) can reduce the conduction velocity and amplitude of Aα, Aβ and Aδ components of the compound action potential recorded from isolated nerves in the cat. The greatest change was found in the Aδ component. However, Levin and Hui-Chan (1993) have shown that healthy subjects cannot tolerate direct activation of Aδ afferents by TENS and therefore intense TENS is administered for only brief periods of time in clinical practice.

Segmental mechanisms

Conventional TENS produces analgesia predominantly by a segmental mechanism whereby activity generated in Aβ fibres inhibits ongoing activity in second-order nociceptive (pain related) neurons in the dorsal horn of the spinal cord (Fig. 17.12). Workers have shown that activity in large diameter afferents will inhibit nociceptive reflexes in animals when the influence of pain-inhibitory pathways descending from the brain has been removed by spinal transection (Sjölund, 1985; Woolf, Mitchell and Barrett, 1980; Woolf, Thompson and King, 1988). Garrison and Foreman (1994) showed that TENS could significantly reduce ongoing nociceptor cell activity in the dorsal horn cell when it was applied to somatic receptive fields. Follow-up work after spinal cords had been transected at T12 demonstrated that spontaneously and noxiously evoked cell activities were still reduced during TENS. This demonstrates that the neuronal circuitry for conventional TENS analgesia is located in the spinal cord and it is likely that a combination of pre- and postsynaptic inhibition takes place (Garrison and Foreman, 1996).

Studies using the opioid receptor antagonist naloxone have failed to reverse analgesia from high-frequency TENS, suggesting that non-opioid transmitters may be involved in this synaptic inhibition (see Thompson (1989) for review). Studies by Duggan and Foong (1985) using anaesthetised cats suggest that the

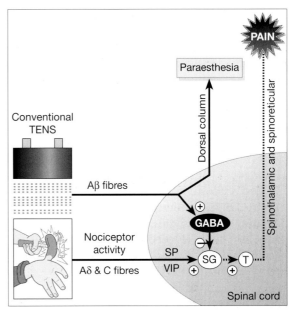

Figure 17.12 Neurophysiology of conventional TENS analgesia. Activity in Aδ and C fibres from nociceptors leads to excitation (+) of interneurons in the substantia gelatinosa (SG) of the spinal cord via neurotransmitters like substance P (SP, cutaneous nociceptors) or vasoactive intestinal peptide (VIP, visceral nociceptors). Central nociceptor transmission neurons (T) project to the brain via spinoreticular and spinothalamic tracts to produce a sensory experience of pain. TENS-induced activity in Aβ afferents leads to the inhibition (−) of SG and T cells (dotted line) via the release of gamma amino butyric acid (GABA, black interneuron). Paraesthesia associated with TENS is generated by information travelling to the brain via the dorsal columns.

inhibitory neurotransmitter gamma aminobutyric acid (GABA) may play a role. The clinical observation that conventional TENS produces analgesia that is short lasting and rapid in onset is consistent with synaptic inhibition at a segmental level.

A number of workers have shown that TENS-induced activity in Aδ fibres during intense TENS can lead to long-term depression (LTD) of central nociceptor cell activity for up to 2 hours. Low-frequency stimulation of Aδ-fibres (1 p.p.s., 0.1 ms) has been shown to produce LTD in animals which is not influenced by bicuculline, which is a GABA receptor antagonist, but is abolished by D-2-amino-5-phosphonovaleric acid, which is a N-methyl-D-aspartate (NMDA) receptor antagonist (Sandkühler, 2000; Sandkühler *et al.*, 1997). This suggests that glutamate rather than GABA may be involved in LTD induced by intense TENS. The time course of latency and amplitude changes in SEPs after high-frequency (200 p.p.s.) electrical stimulation of the digital nerves in healthy subjects supports the concept that TENS can produce LTD of central nociceptive cells (Macefield and Burke, 1991). One practical outcome of this work may be introduction of 'sequential TENS' where conventional TENS is administered at a strong but comfortable level in the first instance followed by a brief period of intense TENS leading to longer post-stimulation analgesia (Sandkühler, 2000).

Extrasegmental mechanisms

TENS-induced activity in small diameter afferents has also been shown to produce extrasegmental analgesia through the activation of structures which form the descending pain-inhibitory pathways, such as periaqueductal grey (PAG), nucleus raphe magnus and nucleus raphe gigantocellularis. Antinociception in animals produced by stimulation of cutaneous Aδ fibres is reduced by spinal transection, suggesting a role for extrasegmental structures (Chung *et al.*, 1984a, b; Woolf, Mitchell and Barrett, 1980). Phasic muscle contractions produced during AL-TENS generates activity in small diameter muscle afferents (ergoreceptors) leading to activation of the descending pain-inhibitory pathways (Fig. 17.13). The importance of muscle afferent activity in this effect has been shown in animal studies by Sjölund (1988) who found that greater antinociception occurred when muscle rather than skin afferents were activated by low-frequency (2 bursts per second) TENS. Duranti, Pantaleo and Bellini (1988) confirmed this in humans by demonstrating that there was no difference in analgesia produced by currents delivered through the skin (e.g. AL-TENS) compared to currents which by passed the skin (e.g. intramuscular electrical nerve stimulation; IENS).

There is growing evidence that AL-TENS but not conventional TENS is mediated by

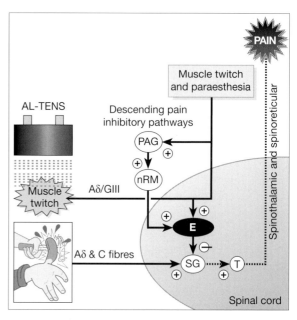

Figure 17.13 Neurophysiology of AL-TENS analgesia. Actvity in Aδ and C fibres from nociceptors leads to excitation (+) of central nociceptor transmission neurons (T) which project to the brain to produce a sensory experience of pain. TENS-induced activity in small diameter muscle afferents (Aδ, GIII) leads to the activation of brainstem nuclei such as the periaqueductal grey (PAG) and nucleus raphe magnus (nRM). These nuclei form the descending pain inhibitory pathways which excite interneurons which inhibit (–) SG and T cells (dotted line) via the release of met-enkephalin (E, black interneuron). It is likely that paraesthesia and sensations related to the muscle twitch are relayed to the brain via the dorsal columns.

endorphins. Sjölund, Terenius and Eriksson, (1977) reported that AL-TENS increased cerebrospinal (CSF) endorphin levels in nine patients suffering chronic pain and that AL-TENS analgesia was naloxone reversible (Sjölund and Eriksson, 1979). However, naloxone failed to reverse analgesia produced by conventional TENS in pain patients (Abram, Reyolds and Cusick, 1981; Hansson *et al.*, 1986; Woolf *et al*, 1978). Claims that conventional TENS can elevate plasma β-endorphin and β-lipotrophin in healthy subjects (Facchinetti *et al.*, 1986) have not been confirmed (Johnson *et al.*, 1992) and it seems unlikely that β-endorphin would cross the blood–brain barrier owing to its large size.

Analgesic effects

As different mechanisms contribute to analgesia produced by different types of TENS it is plausible that they will have different analgesic profiles. In fact this is the rationale for the use of different types of TENS. Evidence from laboratory and clinical studies show that TENS analgesia is maximal when the stimulator is switched on irrespective of the type of TENS used (Fishbain *et al.*, 1996; Johnson *et al.*, 1991a; Walsh, 1997c; Woolf and Thompson 1994). This explains the finding that long-term users of TENS administer conventional TENS continuously throughout the day to achieve adequate analgesia (Chabal *et al.*, 1998; Fishbain *et al.*, 1996; Johnson *et al.*, 1991a; Nash, Williams and Machin, 1990). Poststimulation analgesia has been reported to occur in some patients and this may be due to LTD and activation of descending pain inhibitory pathways. Reports of the duration of these poststimulation effects vary widely from 18 hours (Augustinsson, Carlsson and Pellettieri, 1976) to 2 hours (Johnson *et al.*, 1991a). It is possible that natural fluctuations in symptoms and the patient's expectation of treatment effects may have contributed to some extent to these observations.

There are remarkably few studies which have systematically investigated the analgesic profiles of a range of TENS pulse frequencies, pulse durations and pulse patterns when all other stimulating characteristics are fixed. There is an extensive literature of studies which have compared the analgesic effects of two pulse frequencies (usually high ~100 p.p.s. and low ~2 p.p.s.) in animals, healthy humans and patients in pain. However, the TENS characteristics used in many of these studies appear to have been chosen ad hoc, which makes synthesis of the findings between groups almost impossible (see tables in Walsh 1997a and e).

Sjölund (1985) delivered seven different stimulation frequencies (10, 40, 60, 80, 100, 120 and 160 p.p.s.) to a dissected skin nerve in lightly anaesthetised rats and reported that a stimulation frequency of 80 p.p.s. gave the most profound inhibition of the C-fibre-evoked flexion reflex.

In a follow-up study they reported that a pulse-train repetition rate of around 1 Hz was most effective in inhibition of the C-fibre-evoked flexion reflex. Johnson *et al.* (1989) assessed the analgesic effects of five stimulating frequencies (10, 20, 40, 80 and 160 p.p.s.) on cold-induced pain in healthy subjects. TENS frequencies between 20 and 80 p.p.s. produced greatest analgesia when delivered at a strong but comfortable intensity, with 80 p.p.s. producing the least intersubject variation in response (e.g. the most reliable effect among subjects). Thus, when trying out conventional TENS on a patient for the first time it seems sensible to start with frequencies around 80 p.p.s.

Johnson *et al.* (1991) systematically investigated the analgesic effects of burst, amplitude-modulated, random (frequency of pulse delivery) and continuous TENS delivered at a strong but comfortable level on cold-induced pain in healthy subjects. All pulse patterns elevated ice-pain threshold but there were no significant differences between the groups when all other stimulating characteristics were fixed. Tulgar *et al.* (1991a) demonstrated that a variety of patterns of pulse delivery were equally effective in managing patients' pain. However, patients preferred modulated patterns of TENS such as frequency modulation and burst rather than continuous (Tulgar *et al.*, 1991b). This seems to contrast with Johnson, Ashton and Thompson (1991a) who found that the majority of long-term users of TENS preferred continuous rather than burst mode. More systematic investigations which compare the analgesic effects of a range of (i.e. more than two) stimulating characteristics when all other variables are fixed are clearly needed.

KNOWN EFFICACY: THE CLINICAL EFFECTIVENESS OF TENS

There is an extensive literature on the clinical effectiveness of TENS although the majority of reports are anecdotal or of clinical trials lacking appropriate control groups. These reports are of limited use in determining the clinical effectiveness as they do not take account of normal fluctuations in the patient's symptoms, the treatment effects of concurrent interventions or the patient's expectation of treatment success. Placebo-controlled clinical trials should be used to determine the absolute effectiveness of treatments so that the effects due to the active ingredient (e.g. the electrical currents for TENS) can be isolated from the effects associated with the act of giving the treatment. Placebo or sham TENS is usually achieved by preventing TENS currents from reaching the patient, for example by cutting wires within the device. Failure to blind patients and investigators to the different treatment groups in placebo-controlled trials, as well as failure to randomise the sample population into treatment groups, will markedly overestimate treatment effects (see McQuay and Moore, 1998a; Schulz et al., 1995 for discussion). Unfortunately, there are many practical difficulties in designing and blinding treatment groups in studies which examine technique-based interventions like TENS (Bjordal and Greve, 1998; Deyo et al., 1990a; Thorsteinsson, 1990).

Carroll et al. (1996) demonstrated the impact of using non-randomised trials in determining TENS effectiveness; 17 of 19 non-randomised controlled trials (non-RCTs) reported that TENS had a positive analgesic effect whereas 15 of 17 randomised controlled trials (RCTs) reported that TENS had no effect for postoperative pain. Carroll et al. (1996) concluded that non-randomised studies on TENS, or any other treatment, will overestimate treatment effects. Therefore, in a climate of evidence-based medicine the findings of systematic reviews of randomised controlled clinical trials will be used to determine effectiveness (Table 17.4).

TENS and acute pain

Postoperative pain

Hymes et al. (1974) were the first to report the success of conventional TENS for acute pain resulting from surgery using sterile electrodes straddling the incision (Fig. 17.14). Potentially, TENS could relieve pain and reduce concurrent opioid consumption and associated adverse

Table 17.4 Outcomes of systematic reviews

Condition	Existing reviews
Acute pain	Reeve, Menon and Corabian (1996) Range of conditions (dysmenorrhea, dental, cervical, orofacial, sickle cell disease) TENS effective 7/14 RCTs Reviewers conclusion: evidence inconclusive—poor RCT methodology in field
Postoperative pain	Reeve, Menon and Corabian (1996) TENS effective 12/20 RCTs Reviewers conclusion: evidence inconclusive—poor RCT methodology in field
	Carroll et al. (1996) TENS effective in 2/17 RCTs Reviewers conclusion: limited evidence of effectiveness
Labour pain	Reeve, Menon and Corabian (1996) TENS effective 3/9 RCTs Reviewers conclusion: evidence inconclusive—poor RCT methodology in field
	Carroll et al. (1997a) TENS effective 3/8 RCTs Reviewers conclusion: limited evidence of effectiveness
	Carroll et al. (1997b—update of Carroll et al. (1997a) review) TENS effective 3/10 RCTs Reviewers conclusion: limited evidence of effectiveness
Chronic pain	Reeve, Menon and Corabian (1996) Range of conditions (low back, pancreatitis, arthritis, angina) TENS effective 9/20 RCTs Reviewers conclusion: evidence inconclusive—poor RCT methodology in field
	McQuay and Moore (1998b) Range of conditions (low back, pancreatitis, osteoarthritis, dysmenorrhea) TENS effective 10/24 RCTs Reviewers conclusion: evidence inconclusive—poor RCT methodology in field TENS dosage too low
	Flowerdew and Gadsby (1997)/ Gadsby and Flowerdew (1997) Low back pain (6 RCTs) Odds ratio vs. placebo, conventional TENS (1.62), AL-TENS (7.22) Reviewers conclusion: TENS effective—poor RCT methodology in field

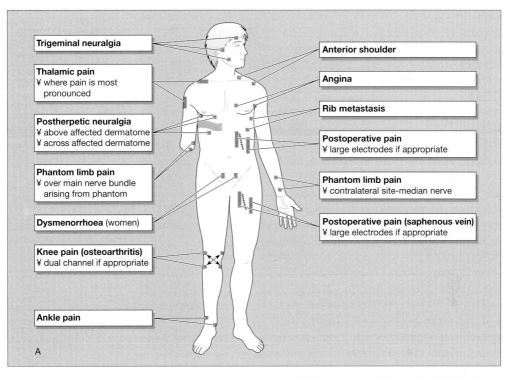

Trigeminal neuralgia

Thalamic pain
¥ where pain is most
  pronounced

Postherpetic neuralgia
¥ above affected dermatome
¥ across affected dermatome

Phantom limb pain
¥ over main nerve bundle
  arising from phantom

Dysmenorrhoea (women)

Knee pain (osteoarthritis)
¥ dual channel if appropriate

Ankle pain

A

Anterior shoulder

Angina

Rib metastasis

Postoperative pain
¥ large electrodes if appropriate

Phantom limb pain
¥ contralateral site-median nerve

Postoperative pain (saphenous vein)
¥ large electrodes if appropriate

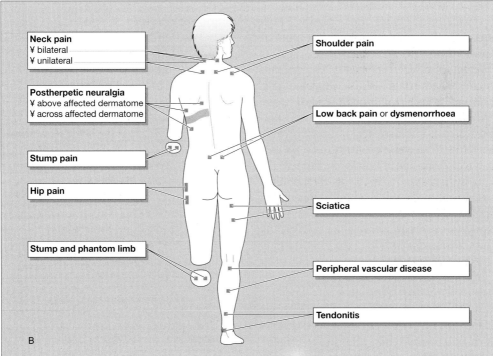

Neck pain
¥ bilateral
¥ unilateral

Postherpetic neuralgia
¥ above affected dermatome
¥ across affected dermatome

Stump pain

Hip pain

Stump and phantom limb

B

Shoulder pain

Low back pain or dysmenorrhoea

Sciatica

Peripheral vascular disease

Tendonitis

Figure 17.14   A: Electrode positions for common pain conditions—anterior view. B: Electrode positions for common pain conditions—posterior view.

events such as respiratory depression. Clinical trials have shown that TENS reduces pain and additional analgesic intake and improves respiratory function (Ali, Yaffe and Serrette, 1981; Bayindir *et al.*, 1991; Benedetti *et al.*, 1997; Chiu *et al.*, 1999; Schuster and Infante, 1980; Warfield, Stein and Frank, 1985). However, the existing literature has been reviewed systematically by Carroll *et al.* (1996) who found that 15 of 17 RCTs reported that TENS produced no significant benefit when compared with placebo; this group concluded that TENS was not effective for the management of postoperative pain. A systematic review on acute pain, including postoperative pain, by Reeve, Menon and Corabian (1996) reported that 12 of 20 RCTs found that TENS was beneficial in postoperative pain, suggesting that TENS may be of some benefit (Table 17.4).

Closer examination reveals discrepancies in the judgements of individual RCT outcome by the reviewers, which may undermine confidence in their findings. For example, the RCT by Conn *et al.* (1986) was judged as a negative outcome study by Carroll *et al.* (1996) and a positive outcome study by Reeve, Menon and Corabian (1996). Conn *et al.* (1986) concluded that *'its (TENS) use in this situation (postappendicectomy pain) cannot be recommended'*. Difficulties in making judgements about trial outcome may arise when multiple outcome measures have been used, leading to combinations of positive and negative effects. This makes summary judgements of effectiveness by reviewers difficult. In addition, Benedetti *et al.* (1997) has shown that TENS was effective for mild to moderate pain associated with thoracic surgical procedures but ineffective for severe pain. However, reductions in mild pain are harder to detect than reductions in severe pain, and studies which include only those patients with mild to moderate pain will lose sensitivity in the detection of outcome measure, while TENS trials attempting to optimise trial sensitivity by including only patients with severe pain would bias the study toward negative outcome. This may be overlooked in systematic reviews, so it would be hasty to accept the findings of the systematic reviews on TENS and postoperative pain without further scrutiny (Bjordal and Greve, 1998; Johnson, 2000).

Labour pain

The popularity of TENS for labour pain is due in part to published reports of patient satisfaction and trials demonstrating TENS success without appropriate control groups (Augustinsson *et al.*, 1977; Bundsen *et al.*, 1978; Grim and Morey, 1985; Kubista, Kucena and Riss, 1978; Miller-Jones, 1980; Stewart, 1979; Vincenti, Cervellin and Mega, 1982). Augustinsson *et al.* (1976) pioneered the use of TENS in obstetrics by applying TENS to areas of the spinal cord which correspond to the input of nociceptive afferents associated with the first and second stages of labour (e.g. T10–L1 and S2–S4 respectively, Fig. 17.15). They reported that 88% of 147 women obtained pain relief using this method although the study failed to include a placebo control group (Augustinsson *et al.*, 1977). Manufacturers market specially designed obstetric TENS devices which have dual channels and a 'boost' control button for contraction pain.

Two systematic reviews on TENS and labour pain concluded that evidence for TENS analgesia during labour is weak (Carroll *et al.*, 1997a; Reeve, Menon and Corabian, 1996; Table 17.4). Reeve, Menon and Corabian (1996) reported that seven of nine RCTs showed no differences between TENS and sham TENS or conventional pain management (Bundsen and Ericson, 1982; Chia *et al.*, 1990; Lee *et al.*, 1990; Nesheim, 1981; Thomas *et al.*, 1988). Carroll *et al.* (1997a) reported that five of eight RCTs showed no benefits from TENS and this was confirmed in an updated review that included two additional RCTs (Carroll *et al.*, 1997b). Interestingly, Carroll *et al.* (1997b) reported that the odds ratio for trials recording additional analgesic intervention was 0.57, suggesting that analgesic intervention may be less likely with TENS, although number-needed-to-treat was high (14, 95% confidence interval 7.3–11.9). RCTs that used analgesic intake as an outcome measure would have compromised the validity of pain relief scores as patients in both sham and active TENS groups

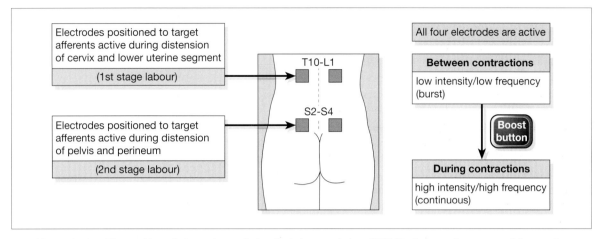

Figure 17.15 The position of electrodes and electrical characteristics of TENS when used to manage labour pain.

would consume analgesics to achieve maximal pain relief. Thus, differences in pain relief scores between TENS and sham are less likely, which will bias outcome towards no difference between groups.

In systematic reviews credence is given to trials with high methodological scores such as van der Ploeg *et al.* (1996), Harrison *et al.* (1986) and Thomas *et al.* (1988). Van der Ploeg *et al.* (1996) reported no significant differences between active and sham TENS in 94 women for additional analgesic intervention or pain relief scores. Harrison *et al.* (1986) conducted an RCT on 150 women and reported no differences between active and sham TENS users for pain relief or additional analgesic intervention. The RCT by Thomas *et al.* (1988) on 280 parturients found no significant differences between active and sham TENS for analgesic intervention or pain scores. Interestingly, under double-blind conditions women favoured active TENS when compared with sham TENS in studies by Harrison *et al.* (1986) and Thomas *et al.* (1988).

The evidence is weak for the continued use of TENS in the management of labour pain. However, this conflicts with the clinical experience of midwives and with patient satisfaction on the use of TENS (Johnson, 1997). It is possible that methodological problems associated with RCTs examining technique-based interventions may seriously bias the outcome of the systematic reviews (Bjordal and Greve, 1998). The self-report of pain relief may be unreliable when patients are experiencing fluctuating emotional and traumatic conditions as in the different stages of labour. Responses solicited at the end of childbirth, when women are relaxed and may be in a better position to judge and reflect on the effects of the intervention, may be more appropriate. Moreover, RCTs by Champagne *et al.* (1984) and Wattrisse *et al.* (1993) used transcranial TENS administered via electrodes placed on the temple. Transcranial TENS delivers electrical currents with markedly different characteristics to those of conventional obstetric TENS (Table 17.2) and it could be argued that these studies should not have been included in the review. Interestingly both of these studies demonstrated beneficial effects. Nevertheless, this raises questions about the appropriateness of the treatment protocols used in some RCTs included in the reviews. It would be unreasonable to dismiss the use of TENS for labour pain until the discrepancy between clinical experience and clinical evidence is resolved (Johnson, 2000).

TENS and chronic pain

The widespread use of TENS for chronic pain is supported by a large number of clinical trials that suggest that TENS is useful for a wide range of chronic pain conditions. Conditions include chronic neuropathies (Thorsteinsson et al., 1977), postherpetic neuralgia (Nathan and Wall, 1974), trigeminal neuralgia (Bates and Nathan, 1980), phantom limb and stump pain (Finsen et al., 1988; Katz and Melzack, 1991; Thorsteinsson, 1987), musculoskeletal pains (Lundeberg, 1984) and arthritis (Mannheimer and Carlsson, 1979; Mannheimer, Lund and Carlsson, 1978). Myers, Woolf and Mitchell (1977) and Sloan et al. (1986) have shown that TENS relieves pain associated with fractured ribs.

Systematic reviews of TENS and chronic pain conclude that it is difficult to determine TENS effectiveness due to the lack of good quality trials (Flowerdew and Gadsby, 1997; Gadsby and Flowerdew, 1997; McQuay and Moore, 1998b; Reeve, Menon and Corabian, 1996). Reeve, Menon and Corabian (1996) reported that nine of 20 RCTs provided evidence that TENS was more effective than sham TENS ($n = 7$) or no treatment ($n = 2$) for a range of conditions (Table 17.4). Eight of 20 RCTs showed evidence that TENS was no more effective than sham TENS ($n = 6$) or acupuncture. It was not possible to classify the outcome of three RCTs. Reeve, Menon and Corabian (1996) concluded that the evidence was inconclusive and that the methodological quality of these trials was poor.

McQuay et al. (1997) also reported that there was limited evidence to assess the effectiveness of TENS in outpatient services for chronic pain. Ten of 24 RCTs provided evidence that TENS effects were better than sham TENS, placebo pills or control points such as inappropriate electrode placements (McQuay and Moore, 1998b). Fifteen RCTs compared TENS with an active treatment and only three reported that TENS provided benefit greater than the active treatment. However, over 80% of trials included in the review by McQuay and Moore (1998b) delivered TENS for less than 10 hours per week and 67% of trials delivered less than ten TENS treatment sessions. McQuay and Moore (1998b) concluded that TENS may provide some benefit in chronic pain patients if large enough (appropriate) doses are used.

Perhaps the most common use for TENS is in the management of low back pain. However,

contradictory findings are found in the literature. Marchand et al. (1993) concluded that conventional TENS was significantly more efficient than placebo TENS in reducing pain intensity but not pain unpleasantness in 42 patients with back pain. In contrast, a RCT by Deyo et al. (1990b) concluded that treatment with TENS was no more effective than treatment with a placebo in 145 patients with chronic low back pain. A systematic review by Flowerdew and Gadsby (Flowerdew and Gadsby, 1997; Gadsby and Flowerdew, 1997) included only six RCTs; 62 trials were excluded as they were either non-randomised or failed to compare active TENS with a credible placebo. The meta-analysis showed that more patients improved with AL-TENS (86.70%) than with conventional TENS (45.80%) or placebo (36.40%), with greater odds ratios for AL-TENS vs. placebo (7.22) than conventional TENS vs. placebo (1.62). However, the odds ratio for AL-TENS was based on the findings of only two studies, neither of which applied AL-TENS to produce muscle contractions (Gemignani et al., 1991; Melzack, Vetere and Finch, 1983, see Johnson (1998) for critical review). Flowerdew and Gadsby (1997) concluded that TENS reduces pain and improves the range of movement in patients suffering chronic low back pain although a definitive RCT is still necessary in the field. Thus, at present the evidence for TENS effectiveness for chronic pain as generated from systematic reviews is inconclusive.

There is an increasing use of TENS for angina, dysmenorrhoea, pain associated with cancer and pain in children. Conventional TENS is used for angina with electrodes placed directly over the painful area of the chest (Börjesson et al., 1997; Mannheimer et al., 1982; Fig. 17.14). Mannheimer et al. (1985); Mannheimer, Emanuelsson and Waagstein (1990) have shown that TENS increases work capacity, decreases ST segment depression, and reduces the frequency of anginal attacks and nitroglycerin consumption when compared with control groups. A variety of types of TENS have been reported to be successful in the management of dysmenorrhea (Dawood and Ramos, 1990; Kaplan et al., 1994; Lewers et al., 1989; Milsom, Hedner and

Mannheimer, 1994; Neighbors *et al.*, 1987). Most often electrodes are applied over the lower thoracic spine and sometimes on acupuncture points (Fig. 17.14, see Walsh (1997a, p. 86) for review). Success with TENS has also been reported in the palliative care setting with both adults (Avellanosa and West, 1982; Hoskin and Hanks, 1988) and children (Stevens *et al.*, 1994). TENS can be used for metastatic bone disease, for pains caused by secondary deposits and for pains due to nerve compression by a neoplasm (see Thompson and Filshie (1993) for review). In these circumstances electrodes should be placed on healthy skin near to the painful area or metastatic deposit providing sensory function is preserved or alternatively the affected dermatome. TENS has been shown to be useful in the management of a variety of pains in children including dental pain (Harvey and Elliott, 1995; Oztas, Olmez and Yel, 1997; teDuits *et al.*, 1993), minor procedures such as wound dressing (Merkel, Gutstein and Malviya, 1999) and venipuncture (Lander and Fowler-Kerry, 1993).

PRINCIPLES UNDERLYING APPLICATION

The basic principles of the practical application of electrical stimulation are described in Chapter 15.

Electrode positions

As conventional TENS is operating via a segmental mechanism TENS electrodes are placed to stimulate Aβ fibres which enter the same spinal segment as the nociceptive fibres associated with the origin of the pain. Thus, electrodes are applied so that currents permeate the site of pain and this is usually achieved by applying electrodes to straddle the injury or painful area (Fig. 17.14). Electrodes should always be applied to healthy innervated skin. If it is not possible to deliver currents within the site of pain, due to absence of a body part following amputation, a skin lesion or altered skin sensitivity, electrodes can be applied proximally over the main nerve trunk arising from the site of pain. Alternatively, electrodes can be applied over the spinal cord at the spinal segments related to origin of pain. Electrodes can also be applied at a site which is contralateral to the site of pain in conditions such as phantom limb pain and trigeminal neuralgia where the affected side of the face may be sensitive to touch.

Accurate placement of pads can be time consuming. Berlant (1984) has described a useful method of determining optimal electrode sites for TENS. The therapist applies one TENS electrode to the patient at a potential placement site. The second electrode is held in the hand of the therapist who uses the index finger to probe the skin of the patient to locate the best site to place the second electrode. When the TENS device is switched on and the amplitude slowly increased the patient or therapist, or both, will feel TENS paraesthesia when the circuit is made by touching the patient's skin. As the therapist probes the patient's skin with the index finger the intensity of TENS paraesthesia will increase whenever nerves on the patient's skin run superficial. This will help to target an effective electrode site.

Dual-channel devices using four electrodes or large-sized electrodes should be used for pains covering large areas. However, if the pain is generalised and widespread over a number of body parts it may be more appropriate to use AL-TENS at a relevant myotome as this may produce a more generalised analgesic effect (Johnson, 1998). Dual-channel stimulators are useful for patients with multiple pains such as low back pain and sciatica or for pains which change in their location and quality as during childbirth.

Electrical characteristics

The efficiency of different electrical characteristics of TENS to selectively activate different types of fibre was discussed earlier. For conventional TENS, selective activation of Aβ fibres is determined through the report of a strong but comfortable electrical paraesthesia without muscle contraction. Pulse frequencies anywhere between 1 and 250 p.p.s. can achieve this although clinical trials consistently report frequencies between 10 and 200 p.p.s. to be effective and popular with patients. In practice, each patient may have an individual preference for pulse frequencies and pulse patterns and will turn to these settings on subsequent treatment sessions (Johnson, Ashton and Thompson, 1991b). As no relationship between pulse frequency and pattern used by patients and the magnitude of analgesia or their medical diagnosis has yet been found it is likely that encouraging patients to experiment with TENS settings will produce the most effective outcome (Johnson, Ashton and Thompson, 1991a).

Timing and dosage

Clinical trials report that maximum pain relief occurs when the TENS device is switched on and that analgesic effect usually disappears quickly once the device is switched off. Thus, patients using conventional TENS patients should be encouraged to use TENS whenever the pain is present. For ongoing chronic pain this may mean that patients use TENS over the entire day. In a study of long-term users of TENS Johnson, Ashton and Thompson (1991a) reported that 75% used TENS on a daily basis and 30% reported using TENS for more than 49 hours a week. When TENS is used continuously in this way it is wise to instruct the patient to monitor skin condition under the electrodes on a regular basis and take regular (although short) breaks from stimulation. It is advisable to apply electrodes to new skin on a daily basis. If TENS is administered in an outpatients clinic a dosing regimen of 20 minutes at daily, weekly or monthly intervals is likely to be ineffective.

Some patients report poststimulation analgesia although the duration of this effect varies widely, lasting anywhere between 18 hours (Augustinsson, Carlsson and Pellettieri, 1976) and 2 hours (Johnson, Ashton and Thompson, 1991a). This may reflect natural fluctuations in symptoms and the patient's expectation of treatment duration rather than specific TENS-induced effects. It is believed that post-TENS analgesia is longer for AL-TENS than for conventional TENS and this is supported by initial findings in experimental studies (Johnson, Ashton and Thompson, 1992a). However, more work is needed to establish the time course of analgesic effects of different types of TENS.

Giving a patient a trial of TENS for the first time

All new TENS patients should be given a supervised trial of TENS prior to use (Table 17.5). The purpose of the trial is to ensure TENS does not aggravate pain and to give careful instruction on equipment use and expected therapeutic outcome. Patients should be allowed to familiarise themselves on the use of TENS and therapists should use the session to check that patients can apply TENS appropriately. The initial trial can help to determine whether a patient is likely to respond to TENS and it should also be seen as an opportunity to troubleshoot problems arising

Table 17.5 Suggested characteristics to use for a patient trying TENS for the first time

	Conventional TENS	AL-TENS	Intense TENS
Electrode placement	Straddling site of pain or over main nerve bundle proximal to pain	Over muscle or motor point myotomally related to the site of pain	Straddling site of pain or over main nerve bundle proximal to pain
Pulse pattern	Continuous	Burst	Continuous
Pulse frequency	80–100 p.p.s.	80–100 p.p.s.	200 p.p.s.
Pulse duration	100–200 μs	100–200 μs	1000 μs
Pulse amplitude (intensity)	Increase intensity to produce a strong but comfortable tingling	Increase intensity to produce a strong but comfortable muscle twitch	Increase intensity to produce an uncomfortable tingling which is just bearable
Duration of stimulation in first instance	At least 30 minutes	No more than 20 minutes	No more than 5 minutes

from poor response. Ideally, the trial should last a minimum of 30–60 minutes as it may take this length of time for a patient to respond.

When using TENS on a new patient for the first time it is advisable to deliver conventional TENS as most long-term users select this type of TENS (Table 17.5). A set of audio speakers (or headphones) can be plugged into the output sockets of some TENS devices to demonstrate the sound of pulses and improve patient understanding of output characteristics of the TENS device. Following the initial trial, patients should be instructed to administer TENS in 30 minute sessions for the first few times although once they have familiarised themselves with the equipment they should be encouraged to use TENS much as they like. Patients should also be encouraged to experiment with all stimulator settings so that they achieve the most comfortable pulse frequency, pattern and duration (Table 17.6).

An early review of progress, ideally within a few weeks, can serve to ensure correct application, provide further instruction and recall TENS devices which are no longer required. Most non-responders return borrowed devices at the next clinic visit (Johnson, Ashton and Thompson, 1992b). Assessing TENS effectiveness at regular intervals is vital for tracking the location and continued use of devices. Some clinics and manufacturers allow patients to borrow TENS devices for a limited period with a view to purchasing the device. A point of contact should always be made available for patients who encounter problems.

Declining response to TENS

Some TENS users claim that the effectiveness of TENS declines over time although the exact proportion of patients is not known (see Table 92-1 in Sjölund, Eriksson and Loeser (1990) for

Table 17.6 Suggested advice following the initial trial

	Conventional TENS	AL-TENS	Intense TENS
Electrode positions	Straddle site of pain but if not successful try main nerve bundle, across spinal cord or contralateral positions—dematomal	Over muscle belly at site of pain but if not successful try motor point at site of pain, contralateral positions—myotomal	Straddle site of pain but if not successful try over main nerve bundle
Pulse pattern	Patient preference	Burst but if not successful or uncomfortable try amplitude modulated	Continuous but if not successful or uncomfortable try frequency or duration modulated
Pulse frequency	Patient preference, usually 10–200 p.p.s.	Above fusion frequency of muscle 80–100 p.p.s. within the burst	High, e.g. 200 p.p.s.
Pulse duration	Patient preference, usually 100–250 µs	Patient preference, usually 100–250 µs	Highest possible but if uncomfortable gradually reduce duration
Pulse amplitude (intensity)	Strong but comfortable sensation without visible muscle contraction	Strong but comfortable sensation with visible muscle contraction	Highest tolerable sensation with limited muscle contraction
Dosage	As much and as often as is required—have a break every hour or so	About 30 minutes at a time as fatigue may develop with ongoing muscle contractions	15 minutes at a time as the stimulation may be uncomfortable
Analgesic effects	Occur when stimulator on	Occur when stimulator on and for a while once the stimulator has been switched off May exacerbate pain	Occur when stimulator on and for a while once the stimulator has been switched off May exacerbate pain
General advice	Experiment with settings to maintain strong comfortable sensation	Experiment with settings (except burst) to maintain a phasic twitch	Experiment with settings to maintain highest tolerable sensation

summary of studies). Eriksson, Sjölund and Nielzen (1979) found that effective pain relief was achieved by 55% of chronic pain patients at 2 months, 41% at 1 year and 30% at 2 years. Loeser, Black and Christman (1975) reported that only 12% of 200 chronic pain patients obtained long-term benefits with TENS despite 68% of patients achieving initial pain relief. Woolf and Thompson (1994) suggest that the magnitude of pain relief from TENS may decline by up to 40% for many patients over a period of a year.

There may be many reasons for the decline in TENS effects with time including dead batteries, perished leads or a worsening pain problem. However, there is evidence that some patients habituate to TENS currents owing to a progressive failure of the nervous system to respond to monotonous stimuli. Pomeranz and Niznick (1987) have shown that repetitive delivery of TENS pulses at 2 p.p.s. produces habituation of late peaks (>50 ms) of SEPs. This implies that for some people the nervous system filters out monotonous stimuli associated with TENS. However, they found that delivering currents randomly to six different points on the body using a TENS-like device called a Codetron markedly reduced the habituation response (Table 17.2). Fargas-Babjak and colleagues (Fargas-Babjak, Rooney and Gerecz, 1989; Fargas-Babjak, Pomeranz and Rooney, 1992) performed a 6 week double-blind randomised placebo controlled pilot trial of the effectiveness of Codetron on osteoarthritis of the hip/knee and reported beneficial effects. Some TENS manufacturers have tried to overcome the problem of habituation by including random pulse delivery or frequency-modulated pulse delivery settings to their standard TENS devices. However, these devices have met with varied success.

If patients report that they are responding less well to TENS over time it may be worth experimenting with the electrical characteristics of TENS or with electrode placements to try and improve analgesia. It may also be worth considering temporary withdrawal of TENS treatment so that an objective assessment of the contribution of TENS to pain relief can be made. When this is done patients may report that their pain worsens in the absence of TENS, demonstrating that TENS was in fact beneficial.

HAZARDS AND CONTRAINDICATIONS

Contraindications

Contraindications to TENS are few and mostly hypothetical (Box 17.2) with few reported cases of adverse events associated with TENS in the literature. Nevertheless, therapists should be cautious when giving TENS to certain groups of patients.

• Those suffering from epilepsy (Scherder, Van Someren and Swaab, 1999): if the patient were to experience a problem while using TENS, from a legal perspective it might be difficult to exclude TENS as a potential cause of the problem.

• Women in the first trimester of pregnancy: TENS effects on fetal development are as yet unknown (although there are no reports of it being detrimental). To reduce the risk of inducing labour, TENS should not be administered over a pregnant uterus although TENS is routinely administered on the back to relieve pain during labour.

• Patients with cardiac pacemakers: this is because the electrical field generated by TENS could interfere with implanted electrical devices.

Box 17.2 Contraindications

• Undiagnosed pain (unless recommended by a medical practitioner)
• Pacemakers (unless recommended by a cardiologist)
• Heart disease (unless recommended by a cardiologist)
• Epilepsy (unless recommended by a medical practitioner)
• Pregnancy:
 — first trimester (unless recommended by a medical practitioner)
 — over the uterus

Do not apply TENS:
• over the carotid sinus
• on broken skin
• on dysaesthetic skin
• Internally (mouth)

Rasmussen *et al.* (1988) reported that TENS did not interfere with pacemaker performance in 51 patients although TENS may induce artifacts in monitoring equipment (Hauptman and Raza, 1992; Sliwa and Marinko, 1996). Chen *et al.* (1990) reported two cases of a Holter monitor detecting interference of a cardiac pacemaker by TENS and in both instances the sensitivity of the pacemaker was reprogrammed to resolve the problem. These authors suggest that careful evaluation and extended cardiac monitoring should be performed when using TENS with pacemakers. Therapists wishing to administer TENS to a patient with a cardiac pacemaker or any cardiac problem should always discuss the situation with a cardiologist.

- TENS should not be applied internally (mouth), or over areas of broken or damaged skin.
- Therapists should ensure that a patient has normal skin sensation prior to using TENS as if TENS is applied to skin with diminished sensation the patient may be unaware that they are administering high-intensity currents and this may result in a minor electrical skin burn.
- TENS should not be delivered over the anterior part of the neck as currents may stimulate the carotid sinus leading to an acute hypotensive response via a vasovagal reflex. TENS currents may also stimulate laryngeal nerves, leading to a laryngeal spasm.

Hazards

- Patients may experience skin irritation with TENS such as reddening beneath or around the electrodes. This is commonly due to dermatitis at the site of contact with the electrodes resulting from the constituents of electrodes, electrode gel or adhesive tape (Corazza *et al.*, 1999; Fisher, 1978; Meuleman, Busschots and Dooms Goossens, 1996a, b). The development of hypoallergenic electrodes has markedly reduced the incidence of contact dermatitis. Patients should be encouraged to wash the skin (and electrodes when indicated by the manufacturer) after TENS and to apply electrodes to fresh skin on a daily basis.

- It is crucial that patients are educated on the appropriate administration of TENS. For example, patients (and therapists) should be encouraged to follow set safety procedures when applying and removing TENS (Box 17.3) to reduce the chance of an electric shock. If patients are to borrow a TENS device from a clinic they should be informed that they should not use TENS while operating vehicles or potentially hazardous equipment. In particular, drivers of motor vehicles should never use TENS while driving as a sudden surge of current may cause an accident. From a legal perspective it would be wise for TENS users to place their TENS device in a glove compartment whenever driving as the cause of an accident may be attributed to TENS if it were attached to a drivers belt (even if it was switched off). TENS can be used at bedtime providing the device has a timer so that it automatically switches off. Patients should be warned not to use TENS in

---

Box 17.3 Safety protocols for TENS

Protocol for the safe application of TENS
- Check contraindications with patient.
- Test skin for normal sensation using blunt/sharp test.
- TENS device should be switched off and electrode leads disconnected.
- Set electrical characteristics of TENS while device is switched off (see Tables 17.5 and 17.6).
- Connect electrodes to pins on lead wire and position electrodes on patient's skin.
- Ensure TENS device is still switched off and connect the electrode wire to the TENS device.
- Switch the TENS device ON.
- Gradually (slowly) increase the intensity until the patient experiences the first 'tingling' sensation from the stimulator.
- Gradually (slowly) increase the intensity further until the patient experiences a 'strong but comfortable' tingling sensation.
- This intensity should not be painful or cause muscle contraction (unless intense TENS or AL-TENS are being used).

Protocol for the safe termination of TENS
- Gradually (slowly) decrease the intensity until the patient experiences no tingling sensation.
- Switch the TENS device OFF.
- Disconnect the electrode wire from the TENS device.
- Disconnect electrodes from the pins on lead wire.
- Remove the electrodes from the patient's skin.

the shower or bath and keep TENS appliances out of the reach of children.

SUMMARY

TENS is used extensively in health care to manage painful conditions because it is cheap, safe and can be administered by patients themselves. Success with TENS depends on appropriate application and therefore patients and therapists need an understanding of the principles of application. When used in its conventional form TENS is delivered to selectively activate Aβ afferents leading to inhibition of nociceptive transmission in the spinal cord. It is claimed that the mechanism of action and analgesic profile of AL-TENS and intense TENS differ from conventional TENS and they may prove useful when conventional TENS is providing limited benefit. Systematic reviews of RCTs report that there is weak evidence to support the use of TENS in the management of postoperative and labour pain. However, these findings have been questioned as they contrast with clinical experience and it would be inappropriate to dismiss the use of TENS in acute pain until the reasons for the discrepancy between experience and published evidence is fully explored. Systematic reviews are more positive about the effectiveness of TENS in chronic pain. However, better-quality trials are required to determine differences in the effectiveness of different types of TENS and to compare the cost effectiveness of TENS with conventional analgesic interventions and other electrotherapies.

REFERENCES

Abram, SE, Reynolds, AC, Cusick, JF (1981) Failure of naloxone to reverse analgesia from transcutaneous electrical stimulation in patients with chronic pain. *Anesthesia and Analgesia* **60**: 81–84.

Ali, J, Yaffe, C, Serrette, C (1981) The effect of transcutaneous electric nerve stimulation on postoperative pain and pulmonary function. *Surgery* **89**: 507–512.

Augustinsson, L, Bohlin, P, Bundsen, P, *et al.* (1976a) Analgesia during delivery by transcutaneous electrical nerve stimulation. *Lakartidningen* **73**: 4205–4208.

Augustinsson, L, Carlsson, C, Pellettieri, L (1976b) Transcutaneous electrical stimulation for pain and itch control. *Acta Neurochirurgica* **33**: 342.

Augustinsson, L, Bohlin, P, Bundsen, P, *et al.* (1977) Pain relief during delivery by transcutaneous electrical nerve stimulation. *Pain* **4**: 59–65.

Avellanosa, AM, West, CR (1982) Experience with transcutaneous electrical nerve stimulation for relief of intractable pain in cancer patients. *Journal of Medicine* **13**: 203–213.

Bates, J, Nathan, P, (1980) Transcutaneous electrical nerve stimulation for chronic pain. *Anaesthesia* **35**: 817–822.

Bayindir, O, Paker, T, Akpinar, B, Erenturk, S, Askin, D, Aytac, A (1991) Use of transcutaneous electrical nerve stimulation in the control of postoperative chest pain after cardiac surgery. *Journal of Cardiothoracic and Vascular Anesthesia* **5**: 589–591.

Benedetti, F, Amanzio, M, Casadio, C *et al.* (1997) Control of postoperative pain by transcutaneous electrical nerve stimulation after thoracic operations. *Annals of Thoracic Surgery* **63**: 773–776.

Berlant, S (1984) Method of determining optimal stimulation sites for transcutaneous electrical nerve stimulation. *Physical Therapy* **64**: 924–928.

Bjordal, J, Greve, G (1998) What may alter the conclusions of systematic reviews? *Physical Therapy Reviews* **3**: 121–132.

Börjesson, M, Eriksson, P, Dellborg, M, Eliasson, T, Mannheimer, C (1997) Transcutaneous electrical nerve stimulation in unstable angina pectoris. *Coronary Artery Disease* **8**: 543–550.

Bundsen, P, Ericson, K (1982) Pain relief in labor by transcutaneous electrical nerve stimulation. Safety aspects. *Acta Obstetrica Gynecologica Scandanavia* **61**: 1–5.

Bundsen, P, Carlsson, C, Forssman, L, Tyreman, N (1978) Pain relief during delivery by transcutaneous electrical nerve stimulation. *Praktika Anaesthesia* **13**: 20–28.

Carroll, D, Tramer, M, McQuay, H, Nye, B, Moore, A (1996) Randomization is important in studies with pain outcomes: systematic review of transcutaneous electrical nerve stimulation in acute postoperative pain. *British Journal of Anaesthesia* **77**: 798–803.

Carroll, D, Moore, A, Tramer, M, McQuay, H (1997a) Transcutaneous electrical nerve stimulation does not relieve labour pain: updated systematic review. *Contemporary Reviews in Obstetrics and Gynecology* **9(3)**: 195–205.

Carroll, D, Tramer, M, McQuay, H, Nye, B, Moore, A (1997b) Transcutaneous electrical nerve stimulation in labour pain: a systematic review. *Bristish Journal of Obstetrics and Gynaecology* **104**: 169–75.

Chabal, C, Fishbain, DA, Weaver, M, Heine, LW (1998) Long-term transcutaneous electrical nerve stimulation (TENS) use: impact on medication utilization and physical therapy costs. *Clinical Journal of Pain* **14**: 66–73.

Champagne, C, Papiernik, E, Thierry, J, Nooviant, Y, (1984) Electrostimulation cerebrale transutanee par les courants de Limoge au cors de l'accouchement. *Annales Francaises d'Anesthesie et de Reanimation* **3**: 405–413.

Chen, D, Philip, M, Philip, PA, Monga, TN (1990) Cardiac pacemaker inhibition by transcutaneous electrical nerve stimulation. *Archives of Physical Medicine and Rehabilitation* **71**: 27–30.

Chia, Y, Arulkumaran, S, Chua, S, Ratnam, S (1990) Effectiveness of transcutaneous electric nerve stimulator for pain relief in labour. *Asia Oceania Journal of Obstetrics and Gynaecology* **16**: 145–151.

Chiu, JH, Chen, WS, Chen, CH et al. (1999) Effect of transcutaneous electrical nerve stimulation for pain relief on patients undergoing hemorrhoidectomy: prospective, randomized, controlled trial. *Diseases of the Colon and Rectum* **42**: 180–185.

Chung, JM, Fang, ZR, Hori, Y, Lee, KH, Willis, WD (1984a) Prolonged inhibition of primate spinothalamic tract cells by peripheral nerve stimulation. *Pain* **19**: 259–275.

Chung, JM, Lee, KH, Hori, Y, Endo, K, Willis, WD (1984b) Factors influencing peripheral nerve stimulation produced inhibition of primate spinothalamic tract cells. *Pain* **19**: 277–293.

Conn, I, Marshall, A, Yadav, S, Daly, J, Jaffer, M (1986) Transcutaneous electrical nerve stimulation following appendicectomy: the placebo effect. *Annals of the Royal College of Surgery of England* **68**: 191–192.

Corazza, M, Maranini, C, Bacilieri, S, Virgili, A (1999) Accelerated allergic contact dermatitis to a transcutaneous electrical nerve stimulation device. *Dermatology* **199**: 281.

Dawood, M, Ramos, J (1990) Transcutaneous electrical nerve stimulation (TENS) for the treatment of primary dysmenorrhea: a randomized crossover comparison with placebo TENS and ibuprofen. *Obstetrics and Gynecology* **75**: 656–660.

Deyo, R, Walsh, N, Schoenfeld, L, Ramamurthy, S (1990a) Can trials of physical treatments be blinded? The example of transcutaneous electrical nerve stimulation for chronic pain. *American Journal of Physical and Medical Rehabilitation* **69**: 6–10.

Deyo, R, Walsh, N, Martin, D, Schoenfeld, L, Ramamurthy, S (1990b) A controlled trial of transcutaneous electrical nerve stimulation (TENS) and exercise for chronic low back pain. *New England Journal of Medicine* **322**: 1627–1634.

Duggan, AW, Foong, FW (1985) Bicuculline and spinal inhibition produced by dorsal column stimulation in the cat. *Pain* **22**: 249–259.

Duranti, R, Pantaleo, T, Bellini, F (1988) Increase in muscular pain threshold following low frequency-high intensity peripheral conditioning stimulation in humans. *Brain Research* **452**: 66–72.

Eriksson, M, Sjölund, B (1976) Acupuncture-like electroanalgesia in TNS resistant chronic pain. In: Zotterman, Y (ed). *Sensory Functions of the Skin*. Oxford/New York; Pergamon Press, pp 575–581.

Eriksson, MB, Sjölund, BH, Nielzen, S (1979) Long term results of peripheral conditioning stimulation as an analgesic measure in chronic pain. *Pain* **6**: 335–347.

Facchinetti, F, Sforza, G, Amidei, M, et al. (1986) Central and peripheral β-endorphin response to transcutaneous electrical nerve stimulation. *NIDA Research Monographs* **75**: 555–558.

Fargas-Babjak, A, Rooney, P, Gerecz, E (1989) Randomised control trial of Codetron for pain control in osteoarthritis of the hip/knee. *Clinical Journal of Pain* **5**: 137–141.

Fargas-Babjak, A, Pomeranz, B, Rooney, P (1992) Acupuncture-like stimulation with Codetron for rehabilitation of patients with chronic pain syndrome and osteoarthritis. *Acupuncture and Electrotherapeutic Research* **17**: 95–105.

Finsen, V, Persen, L, Lovlien, M, et al. (1988) Transcutaneous electrical nerve stimulation after major amputation. *Journal of Bone and Joint Surgery* **70**: 109–112.

Fishbain, A, Chabal, C, Abbott, A, Wippermann-Heine, L, Cutler, R (1996) Transcutaneous electrical nerve stimulation treatment outcome in long-term users. In: *8th World Congress on Pain*, IASP Vancouver, Canada, p. 86.

Fisher, A (1978) Dermatitis associated with transcutaneous electrical nerve stimulation. *Cutis* **21**: 24, 33, 47.

Flowerdew, M, Gadsby, G (1997) A review of the treatment of chronic low back pain with acupuncture-like transcutaneous electrical nerve stimulation and transcutaneous electrical nerve stimulation. *Complementary Therapies in Medicine* **5**: 193–201.

Gadsby, G, Flowerdew, M (1997) The effectiveness of transcutaneous electrical nerve stimulation (TENS) and acupuncture-like transcutaneous electrical nerve stimulation (AL-TENS) in the treatment of patients with chronic low back pain. *Cochrane Library* **1**: 1–139.

Garrison, D, Foreman, R (1994) Decreased activity of spontaneous and noxiously evoked dorsal horn cells during transcutaneous electrical nerve stimulation (TENS). *Pain* **58**: 309–315.

Garrison, D, Foreman, R (1996) Effects of transcutaneous electrical nerve stimulation (TENS) on spontaneous and noxiously evoked dorsal horn cell activity in cats with transected spinal cords. *Neuroscience Letters* **216**: 125–128.

Gemignani, G, Olivieri, I, Ruju, G, Pasero, G, (1991) Transcutaneous electrical nerve stimulation in ankylosing spondylitis: a double-blind study. *Arthritis and Rheumatology* **34**: 788–789.

Grim, L, Morey, S (1985) Transcutaneous electrical nerve stimulation for relief of parturition pain. A clinical report. *Physical Therapy* **65**: 337–340.

Hansson, P, Ekblom, A, Thomsson, M, Fjellner, B (1986) Influence of naloxone on relief of acute oro-facial pain by transcutaneous electrical nerve stimulation (TENS) or vibration. *Pain* **24**: 323–329.

Harrison, R, Woods, T, Shore, M, Mathews, G, Unwin, A (1986) Pain relief in labour using transcutaneous electrical nerve stimulation (TENS). A TENS/TENS placebo controlled study in two parity groups. *British Journal of Obstetrics and Gynaecology* **93**: 739–746.

Harvey, M, Elliott, M (1995) Transcutaneous electrical nerve stimulation (TENS) for pain management during cavity preparations in pediatric patients. *ASDC Journal of Dentistry for Children* **62**: 49–51.

Hauptman, P, Raza, M (1992) Electrocardiographic artifact with a transcutaneous electrical nerve stimulation unit. *International Journal of Cardiology* **34**: 110–112.

Hoskin, PJ, Hanks, GW (1988) The management of symptoms in advanced cancer: experience in a hospital-based continuing care unit. *Journal of the Royal Society of Medicine* **81**: 341–344.

Howson, D (1978) Peripheral neural excitability. Implications for transcutaneous electrical nerve stimulation. *Physical Therapy* **58**: 1467–1473.

Hymes, A, Raab, D, Yonchiro, E, Nelson, G, Printy, A (1974) Electrical surface stimulation for control of post operative pain and prevention of ileus. *Surgical Forum* **65**: 1517–1520.

Ignelzi, RJ, Nyquist, JK (1976) Direct effect of electrical stimulation on peripheral nerve evoked activity: implications in pain relief. *Journal of Neurosurgery* **45**: 159–165.

Jeans, ME (1979) Relief of chronic pain by brief, intense transcutaneous electrical stimulation—a double blind study. In: Bonica, JJ, Liebeskind, JC, Albe-Fessard, DG (eds) *Advances in Pain Research and Therapy*, vol. 3, Raven Press, New York, pp 601–606.

Johannsen, F, Gam, A, Hauschild, B, Mathiesen, B, Jensen, L (1993) Rebox: an adjunct in physical medicine? *Archives in Physical and Medical Rehabilitation* **74**: 438–440.

Johnson, MI (1998) The analgesic effects and clinical use of acupuncture-like TENS (AL-TENS). *Physical Therapy Reviews* **3**: 73–93.

Johnson, MI (1997) Transcutaneous electrical nerve stimulation (TENS) in the management of labour pain: the experience of over ten thousand women. *British Journal of Midwifery* **5**: 400–405.

Johnson, MI (2000) The clinical effectiveness of TENS in pain management. *Critical Reviews in Physical Therapy and Rehabilitiation* **12**: 131–149.

Johnson, MI, Ashton, C, Bousfield, D, Thompson, J (1989) Analgesic effects of different frequencies of transcutaneous electrical nerve stimulation on cold-induced pain in normal subjects. *Pain* **39**: 231–236.

Johnson, MI, Ashton, CH, Bousfield, DR, Thompson, JW (1991) Analgesic effects of different pulse patterns of transcutaneous electrical nerve stimulation on cold-induced pain in normal subjects. *Journal of Psychosomatic Research* **35**: 313–321.

Johnson, MI, Ashton, CH, Thompson, JW (1991b) The consistency of pulse frequencies and pulse patterns of transcutaneous electrical nerve stimulation (TENS) used by chronic pain patients. *Pain* **44**: 231–234.

Johnson, MI, Ashton, CH, Thompson, JW (1991a) An in-depth study of long-term users of transcutaneous electrical nerve stimulation (TENS). Implications for clinical use of TENS. *Pain* **44**: 221–229.

Johnson, MI, Ashton, CH, Thompson, JW (1992a) Analgesic effects of acupuncture like TENS on cold pressor pain in normal subjects. *European Journal of Pain* **13**: 101–108.

Johnson, MI, Ashton, CH, Thompson, J (1992b) Long term use of transcutaneous electrical nerve stimulation at Newcastle Pain Relief Clinic. *Journal of the Royal Society of Medicine* **85**: 267–268.

Johnson, MI, Ashton, CH, Thompson, JW, Weddell, A, Wright Honari, S (1992) The effect of transcutaneous electrical nerve stimulation (TENS) and acupuncture on concentrations of β endorphin, met enkephalin and 5 hydroxytryptamine in the peripheral circulation. *European Journal of Pain* **13**: 44–51.

Johnson, MI, Penny, P, Sajawal, MA (1997) An examination of the analgesic effects of microcurrent stimulation (MES) on cold-induced pain in healthy subjects. *Physiotherapy Theory and Practice* **13**: 293–301.

Kane, K, Taub, A (1975) A history of local electrical analgesia. *Pain* **1**: 125–138.

Kantor, G, Alon, G, Ho, H (1994) The effects of selected stimulus waveforms on pulse and phase characteristics at sensory and motor thresholds. *Physical Therapy* **74**: 951–962.

Kaplan, B, Peled, Y, Pardo, J *et al.* (1994) Transcutaneous electrical nerve stimulation (TENS) as a relief for dysmenorrhea. *Clinical and Experimental Obstetrics and Gynecology* **21**: 87–90.

Katz, J Melzack, R (1991) Auricular transcutaneous electrical nerve stimulation (TENS) reduces phantom limb pain. *Journal of Pain and Symptom Management* **6**: 73–83.

Kubista, E, Kucera, H, Riss, P (1978) The effect of transcutaneous nerve stimulation on labour pain. *Geburtschilfe Frauenheilkunde* **38**: 1079–1084.

Lander, J, Fowler-Kerry, S (1993) TENS for children's procedural pain. *Pain* **52**: 209–216.

Lee, E, Chung, I, Lee, J, Lam, P, Chin, R (1990) The role of transcutaneous electrical nerve stimulation in management of labour in obstetric patients. *Asia Oceania Journal of Obstetrics and Gynaecology* **16**: 247–254.

Levin, M, Hui-Chan, C (1993) Conventional and acupuncture-like transcutaneous electrical nerve stimulation excite similar afferent fibers. *Archives of Physical and Medical Rehabilitation* **74**: 54–60.

Lewers, D, Clelland, J, Jackson, J, Varner, R, Bergman, J (1989) Transcutaneous electrical nerve stimulation in the relief of primary dysmenorrhea. *Physical Therapy* **69**: 3–9.

Lewis, SM, Clelland, JA, Knowles, CJ, Jackson, JR, Dimick, AR (1990) Effects of auricular acupuncture-like transcutaneous electric nerve stimulation on pain levels following wound care in patients with burns: a pilot study. *Journal of Burn Care and Rehabilitation* **11**: 322–329.

Loeser, J, Black, R, Christman, A (1975) Relief of pain by transcutaneous electrical nerve stimulation. *Journal of Neurosurgery* **42**: 308–314.

Long, DM (1973) Electrical stimulation for relief of pain from chronic nerve injury. *Journal of Neurosurgery* **39**: 718–722.

Long, DM (1974) External electrical stimulation as a treatment of chronic pain. *Minnesota Medicine* **57**: 195–198.

Longobardi, A, Clelland, J, Knowles, C, Jackson, J (1989) Effects of auricular transcutaneous electrical nerve stimulation on distal extremity pain: a pilot study. *Physical Therapy* **69**: 10–17.

Lundeberg, T (1984) A comparative study of the pain alleviating effect of vibratory stimulation, transcutaneous electrical nerve stimulation, electroacupuncture and placebo. *American Journal of Chinese Medicine* **12**: 72–79.

Macdonald, ARJ, Coates, TW (1995) The discovery of transcutaneous spinal electroanalgesia and its relief of chronic pain. *Physiotherapy* **81**: 653–660.

McDowell, BC, Lowe, AS, Walsh, DM, Baxter, GD, Allen, JM (1995) The lack of hypoalgesic efficacy of H-wave therapy on experimental ischaemic pain. *Pain* **61**: 27–32.

McDowell, BC, McCormack, K, Walsh, DM, Baxter, DG, Allen, JM (1999) Comparative analgesic effects of H-wave therapy and transcutaneous electrical nerve stimulation on pain threshold in humans. *Archives of Physical Medicine and Rehabilitation* **80**: 1001–1004.

McQuay, H, Moore, A (1998a) Judging the quality of trials. In: McQuay, H, Moore, A (eds) *An Evidence-based Resource for Pain Relief*, Oxford University Press, Oxford, pp 10–13.

McQuay, H, Moore, A (1998b) TENS in chronic pain. In: McQuay, H, Moore, A (eds) *An Evidence-Based Resource for Pain Relief*. Oxford University Press, Oxford, p 207.

McQuay, HJ, Moore, RA, Eccleston, C, Morley, S, Williams, AC (1997) Systematic review of outpatient services for chronic pain control. *Health Technology Assessment* **1**: 1–135.

Macefield, G, Burke, D (1991) Long-lasting depression of central synaptic transmission following prolonged high-frequency stimulation of cutaneous afferents: a mechanism for post-vibratory hypaesthesia. *Electroencephalography and Clinical Neurophysiology* **78**: 150–158.

Mannheimer, C, Carlsson, C (1979) The analgesic effect of transcutaneous electrical nerve stimulation (TNS) in patients with rheumatoid arthritis. A comparative study of different pulse patterns. *Pain* **6**: 329–334.

Mannheimer, C, Lund, S, Carlsson, C (1978) The effect of transcutaneous electrical nerve stimulation (TNS) on joint pain in patients with rheumatoid arthritis. *Scandinavian Journal of Rheumatology* **7**: 13–16.

Mannheimer, C, Carlsson, C, Ericson, K, Vedin, A, Wilhelmsson, C (1982) Transcutaneous electrical nerve stimulation in severe angina pectoris. *European Heart Journal* **3**: 297–302.

Mannheimer, C, Carlsson, C, Emanuelsson, H, Vedin, A, Waagstein, F, Wilhelmsson, C (1985) The effects of transcutaneous electrical nerve stimulation in patients with severe angina pectoris. *Circulation* **71**: 308–316.

Mannheimer, C, Emanuelsson, H, Waagstein, F (1990) The effect of transcutaneous electrical nerve stimulation (TENS) on catecholamine metabolism during pacing-induced angina pectoris and the influence of naloxone. *Pain* **41**: 27–34.

Marchand, S, Charest, J, Li, J, Chenard, J, Lavignolle, B, Laurencelle, L (1993) Is TENS purely a placebo effect? A controlled study on chronic low back pain. *Pain* **54**: 99–106.

Melzack, R, Wall, P (1965) Pain mechanisms: A new theory. *Science* **150**: 971–979.

Melzack, R, Vetere, P, Finch, L (1983) Transcutaneous electrical nerve stimulation for low back pain. A comparison of TENS and massage for pain and range of motion. *Physical Therapy* **63**: 489–493.

Merkel, SI, Gutstein, HB, Malviya, S (1999) Use of transcutaneous electrical nerve stimulation in a young child with pain from open perineal lesions. *Journal of Pain and Symptom Management* **18**: 376–381.

Meuleman, V, Busschots, AM, Dooms-Goossens, A (1996) Contact allergy to a device for transcutaneous electrical neural stimulation (TENS). *Contact Dermatitis* **35**: 53–54.

Meyerson, B (1983) Electrostimulation procedures: effects presumed rationale, and possible mechanisms. In: Bonica, J, Lindblom, U, Iggo, A (eds.) *Advances in Pain Research and Therapy*, vol 5. Raven, New York, pp 495–534.

Miller-Jones, C (1980) Transcutaneous nerve stimulation in labour. *Anaesthesia* **35**: 372–375.

Milsom, I, Hedner, N, Mannheimer, C (1994) A comparative study of the effect of high-intensity transcutaneous nerve stimulation and oral naproxen on intrauterine pressure and menstrual pain in patients with primary dysmenorrhea. *American Journal of Obstetrics and Gynecology* **170**: 123–129.

Myers, RA, Woolf, CJ, Mitchell, D (1977) Management of acute traumatic pain by peripheral transcutaneous electrical stimulation. *South African Medical Journal* **52**: 309–312.

Nardone, A, Schieppati, M (1989) Influences of transcutaneous electrical stimulation of cutaneous and mixed nerves on subcortical and cortical somatosensory evoked potentials. *Electroencephalography and Clinical Neurophysiology* **74**: 24–35.

Nash, T, Williams, J, Machin, D (1990) TENS: does the type of stimulus really matter? *Pain Clinic* **3**: 161–168.

Nathan, PW, Wall, PD (1974) Treatment of post-herpetic neuralgia by prolonged electric stimulation. *British Medical Journal* **3**: 645–647.

Neighbors, L, Clelland, J, Jackson, J, Bergman, J, Orr, J (1987) Transcutaneous electrical nerve stimulation for pain relief in primary dysmenorrhea. *Clinical Journal of Pain* **3**: 17–22.

Nesheim, B (1981) The use of transcutaneous electrical nerve stimulation for pain relief during labour. A controlled clinical study. *Acta Obstetrica Gynecologia* **60**: 13–16.

Odendaal, CL, Joubert, G (1999) APS therapy—a new way of treating chronic backache—a pilot study. *South African Journal of Anaesthesiology and Analgesia* **5**.

Oztas, N, Olmez, A, Yel, B (1997) Clinical evaluation of transcutaneous electronic nerve stimulation for pain control during tooth preparation. *Quintessence International* **28**: 603–608.

Pomeranz, B, Niznick, G (1987) Codetron, a new electrotherapy device overcomes the habituation problems of conventional TENS devices. *American Journal of Electromedicine* **first quarter**: 22–26.

Pope, G, Mockett, S, Wright, J (1995) A survey of electrotherapeutic modalities: Ownership and use in the NHS in England. *Physiotherapy* **81**: 82–91.

Rasmussen, M, Hayes, D, Vlietstra, R, Thorsteinsson, G (1988) Can transcutaneous electrical nerve stimulation be safely used in patients with permanent cardiac pacemakers? *Mayo Clinical Procedures* **63**: 443–445.

Reeve, J, Menon, D, Corabian, P (1996) Transcutaneous electrical nerve stimulation (TENS): a technology assessment. *International Journal of Technology Assessment Health Care* **12**: 299–324.

Reynolds, DV (1969) Surgery in the rat during electrical analgesia induced by focal brain stimulation. *Science* **164**: 444–445.

Rieb, L, Pomeranz, B (1992) Alterations in electrical pain thresholds by use of acupuncture-like transcutaneous electrical nerve stimulation in pain-free subjects. *Physical Therapy* **72**: 658–667.

Robertson, V, Spurritt, D (1998) Electrophysical agents: Implications of their availability and use in undergraduate clinical placements. *Physiotherapy* **84**: 335–344.

Sandkühler, J (2000) Long-lasting analgesia following TENS and acupuncture: Spinal mechanisms beyond gate control. In: Devor, M, Rowbotham, MC, Wiesenfeld-Mallin, Z (eds) *9th World Congress on Pain: Progress in Pain Research and Management*, vol. 16. IASP, Austria, pp 359–369.

Sandkühler, J, Chen, JG, Cheng, G, Randic, M (1997) Low-frequency stimulation of afferent Aδ-fibers induces long-term depression at primary afferent synapses with substantia gelatinosa neurons in the rat. *Journal of Neuroscience* **17**: 6483–6491.

Scherder, E, Van Someren, E, Swaab, D (1999) Epilepsy: a possible contraindication for transcutaneous electrical nerve stimulation. *Journal of Pain and Symptom Management* **17**: 152–153.

Schulz, KF, Chalmers, I, Hayes, RJ, Altman, DG (1995) Empirical evidence of bias. Dimensions of methodological quality associated with estimates of treatment effects in controlled trials. *Journal of the American Medical Association* **273**: 408–412.

Schuster, G, Infante, M (1980) Pain relief after low back surgery: the efficacy of transcutaneous electrical nerve stimulation. *Pain* **8**: 299–302.

Shealy, CN, Mortimer, JT, Reswick, JB (1967) Electrical inhibition of pain by stimulation of the dorsal columns: preliminary clinical report. *Anesthesia and Analgesia* **46**: 489–491.

Sjölund, B (1985) Peripheral nerve stimulation suppression of C-fiber-evoked flexion reflex in rats. Part 1: Parameters of continuous stimulation. *Journal of Neurosurgery* **63**: 612–616.

Sjölund, B (1988) Peripheral nerve stimulation suppression of C-fiber-evoked flexion reflex in rats. Part 2: Parameters of low-rate train stimulation of skin and muscle afferent nerves. *Journal of Neurosurgery* **68**: 279–283.

Sjölund, B, Terenius, L, Eriksson, M (1977) Increased cerebro-spinal fluid levels of endorphins after electro-acupuncture. *Acta Physiologica Scandinavica* **100**: 382–384.

Sjölund, BH, Eriksson, MB (1979) The influence of naloxone on analgesia produced by peripheral conditioning stimulation. *Brain Research* **173**: 295–301.

Sjölund, B, Eriksson, M, Loeser, J (1990) Transcutaneous and implanted electric stimulation of peripheral nerves. In: Bonica JJ (ed) *The Management of Pain*, Vol II, Lea & Febiger, Philadelphia, pp 1852–1861.

Sliwa, J, Marinko, M (1996) Transcutaneous electrical nerve stimulator-induced electrocardiogram artifact. A brief report. *American Journal of Physical and Medical Rehabilitation* **75**: 307–309.

Sloan, J, Muwanga, C, Waters, E, Dove, A, Dave, S (1986) Multiple rib fractures: transcutaneous nerve stimulation versus conventional analgesia. *Journal of Trauma* **26**: 1120–1122.

Stevens, M, Dalla Pozza, L, Cavalletto, B, Cooper, M, Kilham, H (1994) Pain and symptom control in paediatric palliative care. *Cancer Survey* **21**: 211–231.

Stewart, P (1979) Transcutaneous electrical nerve stimulation as a method of analgesia in labour. *Anaesthesia* **34**: 361–364.

Stillings, D (1975) A survey of the history of electrical stimulation for pain to 1900. *Medical Instrumentation* **9**: 255–259.

teDuits, E, Goepferd, S, Donly, K, Pinkham, J, Jakobsen, J (1993) The effectiveness of electronic dental anesthesia in children. *Pediatric Dentistry* **15**: 191–196.

Thomas, I, Tyle, V, Webster, J, Neilson, A (1988) An evaluation of transcutaneous electrical nerve stimulation for pain relief in labour. *Australia and New Zealand Journal Obstetric Gynaecology* **28**: 182–189.

Thompson, J (1989) The pharmacology of transcutaneous electrical nerve stimulation (TENS). *Intractable Pain Society Forum* **7**: 33–39.

Thompson, J, Filshie, J (1993) Transcutaneous electrical nerve stimulation (TENS) and acupuncture. In: Doyle, D, Hanks, G and MacDonald, N (eds) *Textbook of Palliative Medicine*, Oxford University Press, Oxford, pp 229–244.

Thorsteinsson, G (1987) Chronic pain: use of TENS in the elderly. *Geriatrics* **42**: 75–77, 81–82.

Thorsteinsson, G (1990) Can trials of physical treatments be blinded? The example of transcutaneous electrical nerve stimulation for chronic pain. *American Journal of Physical and Medical Rehabilitation* **69**: 219–220.

Thorsteinsson, G, Stonnington, HH, Stillwell, GK, Elveback, LR (1977) Transcutaneous electrical stimulation: a double-blind trial of its efficacy for pain. *Archives of Physical Medicine and Rehabilitation* **58**: 8–13.

Tulgar, M, McGlone, F, Bowsher, D, Miles, J (1991b) Comparative effectiveness of different stimulation modes

in relieving pain. Part II. A double-blind controlled long-term clinical trial. *Pain* **47**: 157–162.

Tulgar, M, McGlone, F, Bowsher, D, Miles, J (1991a) Comparative effectiveness of different stimulation modes in relieving pain. Part I. A pilot study. *Pain* **47**: 151–155.

van der Ploeg, J, Vervest, H, Liem, A, Schagen van Leeuwen, J (1996) Transcutaneous nerve stimulation (TENS) during the first stage of labour: a randomized clinical trial. *Pain* **68**: 75–78.

Vincenti, E, Cervellin, A, Mega, M (1982) Comparative study between patients treated with transcutaneous electric stimulation and controls during labour. *Clinical and Experimental Obstetrics and Gynaecology* **9**: 95–97.

Wall, PD, Sweet, WH (1967) Temporary abolition of pain in man. *Science* **155**: 108–109.

Walsh, D (1997a) Review of clinical studies on TENS. In: Walsh, D (ed) *TENS. Clinical Applications and Related Theory*. Churchill Livingstone, New York, pp 83–124.

Walsh, D (1997b) Non-analgesic effects of TENS. In: Walsh, D (ed) *TENS. Clinical Applications and Related Theory*. Churchill Livingstone, New York, pp 125–138.

Walsh, D (ed) (1997c) *TENS. Clinical Applications and Related Theory*. Churchill Livingstone, New York;

Walsh, D (1997d) TENS: physiological principles and stimulation parameters. In: Walsh, D (ed) *TENS. Clinical Applications and Related Theory*. Churchill Livingstone, New York; pp 25–40.

Walsh, D (1997e) Review of experimental studies on TENS. In: Walsh, D (ed) *TENS. Clinical Applications and Related Theory*. Churchill Livingstone, New York; pp. 63–81.

Walsh, DM, Lowe, AS, McCormack, K, Willer, JC, Baxter, GD, Allen, JM (1998) Transcutaneous electrical nerve stimulation: effect on peripheral nerve conduction, mechanical pain threshold, and tactile threshold in humans. *Archives of Physical Medicine and Rehabilitation* **79**: 1051–1058.

Warfield, C, Stein, J, Frank, H (1985) The effect of transcutaneous electrical nerve stimulation on pain after thoracotomy. *Annals of Thoracic Surgery* **39**: 462–465.

Wattrisse, G, Leroy, B, Dufossez, F, Tai, RBH (1993) Electrostimulation cerebrale transcutanee: etude comparative des effets de son association a l'anesthesie peridurale par bupivacaine-fentanyl au cours de l'analgesie obstetricale. *Cahiers d'Anesthesthesiologie* **41**: 489–495.

Woolf, C, Thompson, J (1994) Segmental afferent fibre-induced analgesia: transcutaneous electrical nerve stimulation (TENS) and vibration. In: Wall, P, Melzack, R (eds) *Textbook of Pain*, Churchill Livingstone, New York, pp 1191–1208.

Woolf, CJ, Mitchell, D, Myers, RA, Barrett, GD (1978) Failure of naloxone to reverse peripheral transcutaneous electroanalgesia in patients suffering from acute trauma. *South African Medical Journal* **53**: 179–180.

Woolf, CJ, Mitchell, D, Barrett, GD (1980) Antinociceptive effect of peripheral segmental electrical stimulation in the rat. *Pain* **8**: 237–252.

Woolf, C, Thompson, S, King, A (1988) Prolonged primary afferent induced alterations in dorsal horn neurones, an intracellular analysis in vivo and in vitro. *Journal of Physiology* **83**: 255–266.

18

Interferential current for pain control

Shea Palmer
Denis Martin

INTRODUCTION

Interferential current (IC) was developed in the 1950s by Dr Hans Nemec in Vienna, and became increasingly popular in the UK during the 1970s (Ganne, 1976). Although the actual definition of IC is not standardised in the literature, it may be described as the transcutaneous application of alternating medium-frequency electrical currents, amplitude modulated at low frequency for therapeutic purposes. From this definition it should be seen that IC is a form of transcutaneous electrical nerve stimulation (see Ch. 17).

IC has been reported to have the advantage of reducing the skin resistance, and thus the discomfort normally incurred by traditional low-frequency currents, whilst still producing low-frequency effects within the tissues (Low and Reed, 2000). IC has also been claimed to permit the treatment of deep tissues (Goats, 1990; Hansjuergens, 1986; Low and Reed, 2000; Nikolova, 1987; Willie, 1969). Both of the above claims, which are unique to IC, are largely unsubstantiated and have been challenged (Alon, 1987).

A survey carried out in England revealed that IC was available in 97.2% of physiotherapy clinical sites (Pope, Mockett and Wright, 1995). In Australia this figure has been reported to be between 77% (Robertson and Spurritt, 1998) and 85% (Lindsay *et al.*, 1990). In addition to this wide availability, 90% of physiotherapy clinicians with access to IC have been reported to use it at least once per day (Lindsay *et al.*, 1990). In terms of the conditions treated with IC, 91% of respondents to one survey had used IC to relieve pain (67% for acute pain, and 78% for chronic pain) (Johnson and Tabasam, unpublished study, 1998); 31% considered IC to be the 'most effective treatment' for pain relief, and 44% said that it was their 'personal preference' over other modalities used to relieve pain. In a follow-up study using a treatment-logging system (Tabasam and Johnson, unpublished study, 2000), 25.7% of treatments were found to be for acute pain, 50.1% for chronic pain, and 16.0% for reduction of swelling. In another survey 87.5% of clinicians reported using IC to treat non-specific low back pain, with 44.1% describing it as the first choice of treatment modality (Foster et al., 1999).

These studies illustrate both a high rate of access to IC stimulators, and also a high rate of usage. Importantly, it is interesting to note the prevalence of its usage for pain. It could be argued that this evidence indicates a perceived benefit to patients in terms of IC-mediated effects on pain. Clinical trials, however, still remain scarce and largely inconclusive. Most reports of the effectiveness of IC are anecdotal remarks in electrotherapy textbooks (Savage, 1984; Kahn, 1987; Nikolova, 1987) or in largely descriptive journal articles (Belcher, 1974; De Domenico, 1982; Ganne, 1976; Goats, 1990; Willie, 1969). This chapter will attempt to summarise the literature surrounding pain relief with IC.

A fundamental issue in the chapter is whether IC is a singular, distinctive form of treatment, or simply another type of TENS.

PHYSICAL PRINCIPLES OF INTERFERENTIAL CURRENT

IC is essentially a medium-frequency current (normally approximately 4000 Hz) that rhythmically increases and decreases in amplitude at low frequency (adjustable between 0 and 200–250 Hz). IC is produced by mixing two medium-frequency currents that are slightly out of phase, either by applying them so that they 'interfere' within the tissues, or alternatively by mixing them within the stimulator prior to application ('premodulated' current). One current is normally of fixed frequency, for example at 4000 Hz, and the other current is adjustable, for example between 4000 and 4200 Hz. Theoretically, the two currents summate or cancel each other out in a predictable manner, producing the resultant amplitude-modulated 'interferential current'. The frequency of the resultant current will be equal to the mean of the two original currents, and will vary in amplitude at a frequency equal to the difference between these two currents. This latter frequency is known as the 'amplitude-modulated frequency' (AMF) or 'beat frequency'. Figure 18.1 illustrates the production of IC, where two

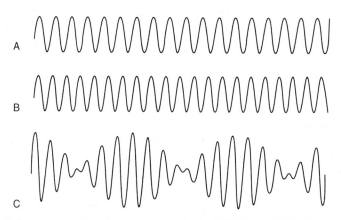

Figure 18.1 Interference between two medium-frequency currents, A: 4000 Hz and B: 4100 Hz produces a resultant 'interferential current' C: 4050 Hz and an amplitude modulated frequency of 100 Hz.

currents of 4000 and 4100 Hz are mixed, resulting in a medium-frequency current of 4050 Hz that is amplitude modulated at a frequency of 100 Hz.

TREATMENT PARAMETERS

Amplitude-modulated frequency

The amplitude-modulated frequency (AMF) or 'beat frequency' is traditionally considered to be the effective component of IC, mimicking low-frequency currents and creating differential stimulation of nerve and tissue types (De Domenico, 1982; Ganne, 1976; Goats, 1990; Hansjuergens, 1986; Low and Reed, 2000; Nikolova, 1987; Szehi and David, 1980; Willie, 1969). The theory of IC is that the medium-frequency components simply act as 'carrier' currents, bringing the low frequency AMF into the tissues (De Domenico, 1982), where the body must be able to demodulate it. The mechanisms of this demodulation have not been established (Johnson, 1999).

Claims of the AMF as the effective component of IC have been challenged (Johnson, 1999; Martin, 1996; Martin and Palmer, unpublished study, 1995; Palmer et al., 1999). It has been demonstrated that alteration of the AMF has little effect on the threshold activation of sensory, motor and pain responses (Martin and Palmer, unpublished study, 1995; Palmer et al., 1999). IC certainly did not follow the very clear frequency-dependent effects displayed by TENS in these studies. These observations suggested that the AMF does not, in fact, mimic low-frequency stimulation. In addition, a 0 Hz AMF (pure 4000 Hz current) displayed similar effects to when an AMF was used. It was concluded from this latter observation that it was the medium-frequency component of IC, and not the AMF, that was the dominant stimulating parameter. The mean sensory thresholds (the point at which the current was first reported as being perceived) from Palmer et al. (1999) are presented in Figure 18.2.

These results may be explained by consideration of Table 18.1, which illustrates the effect of altering the AMF on the other components of IC.

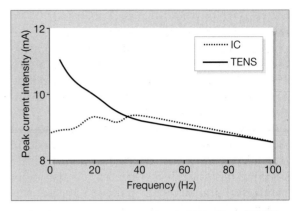

Figure 18.2 Mean sensory thresholds for IC and TENS.

Table 18.1 Interferential current characteristics with a range of amplitude-modulated frequencies (4000 Hz carrier frequency)

Amplitude-modulated frequency (AMF)	Resultant medium frequency (Hz)	Resultant medium-frequency phase duration (μs)
100	4050	123.5
40	4020	124.4
30	4015	124.5
20	4010	124.7
15	4007.5	124.8
10	4005	124.9
5	4002.5	124.9
0	4000	125

This highlights the fact that the resultant current frequency, and thus the phase duration, change little. If the medium frequency *is* the main stimulating parameter then it is perhaps not surprising that the effect of the AMF might prove not to be as important as traditionally thought, and the available evidence supports this. Anecdotally, however, it is obvious that the sensation induced by IC stimulation changes with different AMF settings. Low AMFs, for example, elicit a 'beating' or 'tapping' sensation, whilst higher AMFs elicit a 'buzzing' or 'tingling' sensation. This proposes some ability of sensory nerves to differentiate between different AMF settings. It has been found that that individuals experienced a 5 Hz AMF setting as being significantly more uncomfortable than either 50 or 100 Hz, though with no significant difference between the level of discomfort at 50 and 100 Hz (Martin and Palmer, 1996).

The AMF, therefore, may have a role in altering perceived comfort (Martin and Palmer, 1996), but the main component of stimulation seems to be the medium frequency (Martin and Palmer, unpublished study, 1995; Palmer *et al.*, 1999). The AMF may be a synergistic partner in stimulation with IC, along with the medium frequency, but its role may be minor. As AMF selection has traditionally been a major component of clinical decision making with IC, this observation has important significance.

AMF settings across a wide range of settings between 1 and 130 Hz have been recommended in the literature for the treatment of pain, with little consensus. Clinically, however, it was found that in the south-west of Scotland the most popular AMF used for pain relief was 130 Hz (38% of replies) (Scott and Purves, 1991), although a 'great range' of AMF settings were used. In another study, when IC was applied at a fixed frequency, it was reported that the mean was 85 Hz in a range of 1–150 Hz (Tabasam and Johnson, unpublished study, 2000). This included treatment for all conditions, however, and was not specific to pain relief.

In conclusion, recent evidence has questioned the importance of the AMF. Most subjects appear to prefer higher (50–100 Hz) to lower AMF settings (5 Hz) and the most commonly used frequencies clinically are also in this higher band. It is therefore difficult, and perhaps unnecessary, to recommended specific AMF settings. Initially it may prove beneficial to use one that is most comfortable for the patient and carefully evaluate the effects of treatment.

Frequency sweep

A frequency sweep is available on most IC stimulators, where the AMF is altered over time. A sweep may be set between two prefixed AMFs, for example between 50 and 10 Hz. The pattern of change in frequency can also be adjusted on most machines. For example, it may be set to increase and decrease slowly over a period of 6 seconds (normally depicted by $6 \wedge 6$),

or to give a 1 second stimulation at one frequency and then to automatically switch to the other frequency ($1 \int 1$).

A frequency sweep has been claimed to reduce adaptation (Low and Reed, 2000; Nikolova, 1987; Savage, 1984). It has been suggested, however, that evidence for the importance of a frequency sweep with IC treatment is, at best, only weak (Johnson, 1999). One unpublished study by Martin and Palmer (1995), albeit small, has offered evidence to challenge the role of sweep in adaptation. These authors demonstrated that the inclusion of a frequency sweep had no effect on the amount of adaptation experienced by subjects. This study requires replication, but empirical evidence for a frequency sweep reducing adaptation is certainly lacking.

A frequency sweep has also been claimed to allow stimulation of a greater range of excitable tissues (Low and Reed, 2000; Savage, 1984) extending the scope of potential treatment effects. In an investigation of the effect of frequency sweep pattern, it was found that cold-pain threshold increased with a $6 \wedge 6$ sweep pattern when compared with a $1 \int 1$ pattern or sham stimulation (Johnson and Wilson, 1997). Although the results of this study were not subjected to statistical analysis, it suggested a possible effect of frequency sweep. A later, larger unpublished study by Tabasam and Johnson (1999) contradicted these results, finding no effect of frequency sweep on cold-induced pain. It has been reported (Tabasam and Johnson, unpublished study, 2000) that 95.7% of treatments by physiotherapists which employed a frequency sweep used a $6 \wedge 6$ pattern.

Due to a lack of experimental evidence, and the argument in the previous section that the AMF may be of limited importance, it is again difficult, and perhaps unnecessary, to recommend the inclusion or selection of specific frequency sweeps. If used clinically, the effectiveness of frequency sweep may be monitored by careful assessment.

Quadripolar/bipolar application

IC may be produced either by applying the two medium frequency currents via four electrodes (quadripolar method) so that they intersect in the tissues, or alternatively by mixing the two currents in the stimulator prior to application via two electrodes (premodulated or bipolar method). It is claimed that a quadripolar application of IC produces modulated current in a 'clover-leaf' pattern, as depicted in Figure 18.3, with the 'leaves' set up at right angles to the two medium-frequency currents (Kahn, 1987; Low and Reed, 2000; Savage, 1984).

Treffene (1983) found that there was a good correlation between the expected and actual pattern of IC fields in a homogeneous water medium. The amplitude-modulated current was set up not only in the central area between electrodes, however, but also beneath the electrodes. To ascertain what happens within a non-homogeneous environment Demmink (unpublished study, 1995) measured the distribution of quadripolar IC fields within pork tissue, discovering the pattern to be uneven and unpredictable, and the degree of modulation to be unreliable and haphazard. Additionally, the current did not follow a straight line between electrodes in each circuit. From this evidence, it was concluded that the pattern of IC depicted in textbooks could not be held as a true, reliable and predictable representation of that produced in biological tissue.

It has been claimed that bipolar IC displays a different distribution within tissues compared with quadripolar application (Hansjuergens, 1986; Savage, 1984). Whereas quadripolar IC is claimed to be created deep within the tissues, bipolar IC will be distributed similarly to conventional electrical stimulation (Savage, 1984), with maximal current intensities underneath the electrodes, progressively decreasing with distance (Hansjuergens, 1986). It has also been suggested that the wide dispersal of the area of interference with bipolar IC might also reduce the effectiveness of treatment (Goats, 1990). A haphazard distribution of modulated current, with modulation also occurring beneath the electrodes, seems to invalidate claims of the supremacy of quadripolar application, however. A bipolar application ensures that modulation is always 100% (Low and Reed, 2000), although, as discussed previously, the AMF may not prove to be critical in any case. Kloth (1991) pointed out that there were no controlled clinical studies to support claims of the superiority of either application method. A bipolar application has been found to be most commonly used by physiotherapists (79% of treatments) (Tabasam and Johnson, unpublished study, 2000).

Recommendation of the choice of either bipolar or quadripolar application probably centres on practical considerations. The use of two electrodes has been argued to provide the easier alternative (Martin, 1996).

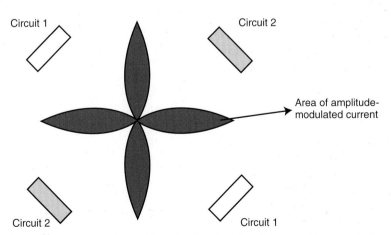

Figure 18.3 'Clover-leaf' pattern with quadripolar IC application. 'Interferential current' is theoretically created at right angles to the two medium-frequency currents.

Suction versus plate electrodes

IC is often applied via electrodes that are held in place using an intermittent suction unit. Alternatively, flat carbon rubber electrodes may be used. Tabasam and Johnson (unpublished study, 2000) revealed that 90% of IC treatments in their survey used carbon rubber electrodes, but no literature has investigated the relative merits of either technique. Suction electrodes have been reported to have the advantage of allowing application to large flat areas or to patients who are relatively immobile (Savage, 1984). The suction has also been claimed to stimulate cutaneous nerves and cause vasodilation (Low and Reed, 2000). Such claims remain to be validated and there is also no indication of whether suction provides any additional effect to the putative effects of IC.

In recommendations for selection, ease of application should probably guide the choice of method. Flat carbon rubber electrodes may be easier to apply to peripheral limbs, when they may be held in position by bandages or elasticated Velcro® straps. On the other hand there may be anatomical areas that are less accessible and in these cases the suction option may be advantageous.

Current intensity

Most authors advocate a current intensity that produces a 'strong but comfortable' sensation (Goats, 1990; Nikolova, 1987; Savage, 1984; Wadsworth and Chanmugam, 1980). In an unpublished study from our lab, however, it was observed that the peak current intensity producing 'strong but comfortable' sensation in the forearm varied significantly between individuals and over time. Factors such as the area treated and the size and placement of electrodes will also determine the sensation induced by specific current intensities.

By definition, 'strong but comfortable' stimulation should be determined by subject report rather than peak current intensity settings. Intensity should be slowly turned up until the patient signals that the required sensation has been reached. Periodic adjustment of the

intensity is recommended to compensate for any adaptation (Goats, 1990; Robinson and Snyder-Mackler, 1995; Savage, 1984).

Treatment duration

Ten to fifteen minutes treatment with IC, with no longer than 20 minutes to one area, has been suggested (Savage, 1984). Other authors have recommended 10 minutes for most painful conditions (Wadsworth and Chanmugam, 1980). Treatment time has been reported by clinicians to be between 11 and 15 minutes in the majority (60.5%) of cases (Tabasam and Johnson, unpublished study, 2000). The development of these recommended and clinically used treatment durations has an unclear theoretical basis, however, and may be the result of practical constraints as opposed to scientific rationale (Johnson, 1999). There is some evidence that IC has short-lived effects, with increased experimentally induced cold-pain threshold returning to baseline levels within 10 to 20 minutes (Johnson and Tabasam, 1999; Johnson and Wilson, 1997; Tabasam, Johnson and Turja, unpublished study, 1998). The applicability of these observations to the clinical situation continues to stimulate debate. If the reader accepts a fair degree of validity, then it may temper any expectancy of lasting pain relief following such short treatment sessions. This has yet to be specifically investigated clinically, however. The advent of small, portable IC stimulators, as opposed to the traditional application via large, expensive and bulky stimulators in outpatient departments, is to be welcomed. These smaller stimulators will allow IC to be used for longer periods, as recommended for TENS (McQuay et al., 1997).

On existing knowledge, recommendation of specific treatment durations is potentially misleading. Time constraints in the clinical setting often limit the use of IC to 10–20 minutes.

Conclusions

It is clear from this overview that there is a wide array of possible application methods of IC, with little rationale or evidence for many of them. In some cases, such as for the claimed importance of the AMF, the available evidence actually contradicts traditional theory. The wide choice of parameters with IC makes the investigation of its efficacy all the more difficult and makes their selection for clinical use confusing. On the other hand, if the reader accepts their limited importance, then comparison of different applications is eased and clinical choice is simplified.

THEORETICAL PAIN RELIEF MECHANISMS WITH IC

Chapter 5 of this text describes in general terms the physiological mechanisms associated with pain. The following highlights the five main theoretical mechanisms quoted in the literature to support the analgesic effects of IC. These include the following.

• **The 'pain gate' theory.** Developed by Melzack and Wall in 1965, this theory suggests that impulses in large diameter sensory nerves (Aβ fibres) inhibit dorsal horn neurons normally responsive to nociceptive afferent nerves (C and Aδ fibres). This effectively 'closes the gate' to nociceptive impulses (Wall, 1999). IC has been proposed to initiate pain relief via stimulation of these sensory nerves (De Domenico, 1982; Goats, 1990; Rennie, 1988; Shafshak, El-Sheshai and Soltan, 1991).

• **Increased circulation.** IC has been claimed to improve the circulation of blood and swelling, which may wash away the chemicals that stimulate nociceptive nerve endings (De Domenico, 1982; Goats, 1990; Rennie, 1988; Shafshak, El-Sheshai and Soltan, 1991). Reduced swelling may concomitantly reduce tissue pressure. These phenomena are reported to occur because of mild muscle contraction or action on the autonomic nervous system, decreasing the tone of blood vessels (Low and Reed; Shafshak, El-Sheshai and Soltan, 1991).

• **Descending pain suppression.** This mechanism may be mediated through stimulation of afferent Aδ and C fibres (De Domenico, 1982; Goats, 1990; Low and Reed, 2000; Rennie, 1988).

This increases activity in descending fibres from the raphe nuclei, releasing inhibitory neurotransmitters at the spinal level (Goats, 1990; Rennie, 1988). Resulting analgesia may be long lasting, but pain may initially increase owing to stimulation of nociceptive Aδ and C fibres (Goats, 1990).

• **Physiological block of nerve conduction.** Stimulation of peripheral nociceptive fibres at rates above their maximum conduction frequency may cause cessation of action potential propagation (De Domenico, 1982; Goats, 1990; Low and Reed, 2000; Rennie, 1988; Shafshak, El-Sheshai and Soltan, 1991), caused by increased stimulation threshold and synaptic fatigue (Goats, 1990).

• **Placebo.** Placebo responses have been identified in the literature as a potential factor with IC stimulation (De Domenico, 1982; Goats, 1990; Low and Reed, 2000; Rennie, 1988; Taylor et al., 1987).

Evidence for theoretical analgesic mechanisms with IC

Conclusive evidence for the specific theoretical analgesic mechanisms outlined above is elusive. Much of the literature equates IC with TENS (Johnson, 1999; Kloth, 1991) carrying with it an assumption that the stimulus characteristics of the two modalities are comparable. This has been demonstrated not to be the case (Palmer et al., 1999). The use of literature on claimed frequency-specific effects of TENS to explain the mechanisms of action of IC may not, therefore, be appropriate. The evidence for each of the theoretical analgesic mechanisms with IC outlined in the last section will now be addressed in turn.

• **The 'pain gate' theory.** IC is capable of stimulating large diameter peripheral nerve fibres, evidenced by the sensation produced. It is logical, therefore, to suggest that this mechanism may be activated.

• **Increased circulation.** Two experimental studies have found no evidence of increased tissue perfusion with IC stimulation (Indergand and Morgan, 1995; Nussbaum, Rush and

Disenhaus, 1990). Another found that IC significantly increased blood flow, but that this effect was no greater than placebo or TENS stimulation (Olson *et al.*, 1999). One study, which observed increased arterial circulation and skin perfusion during and after IC (Lamb and Mani, 1994), was unable to determine whether these effects were caused by muscle stimulation or by effects on the sympathetic nervous system. IC at 10–20 Hz has been found to increase cutaneous blood flow significantly (after 12 minutes) compared with other IC settings (10–100 Hz and 80–100 Hz), control and placebo stimulation (Noble *et al.*, 2000). At 21 minutes, however, the 10–20 Hz group was not significantly different from controls. The evidence to date, therefore, is contradictory as to the effect of IC on circulation. Conclusive published evidence for the influence of IC in reducing swelling is also elusive. Only one experimental study specifically examined the influence of IC stimulation on swelling (Christie and Willoughby, 1990), finding no significant effect after open reduction and internal fixation of the ankle.

• **Descending pain suppression.** No evidence for the effectiveness of IC in eliciting these claimed mechanisms has been found in the literature.

• **Physiological block of nerve conduction.** Authors have been careful to point out that physiological block of nerve fibres has not been demonstrated with IC stimulation (De Domenico, 1982; Ganne, 1986). An interesting review of the literature by Ganne (1986) on conduction block with electrical stimulation concluded that there was no evidence for this phenomenon. Howson (1978) also stated that the published evidence suggested insufficient blockage of small fibre activity to account for substantial pain reduction with electrical stimulation. Both these authors concluded, therefore, that pain relief with electrical stimulation most probably depended upon maximising normal responses of nerve fibres rather than blocking them. It has been observed that IC did not significantly alter conduction velocity in the ulnar and median nerves (Belcher, 1974), or did it affect RIII nociceptive or H reflexes in the sural nerve (Cramp *et al.*, 2000).

These results question the claims of conduction block with IC stimulation.

• **Placebo.** As in the majority of medical interventions, a placebo effect with the application of IC is to be expected. Taylor *et al.* (1987) concluded that IC treatment involved a large placebo component owing to the observation that some 65% of subjects in their placebo group gave a subjective report of an improvement in pain. Other authors (Shafshak, El-Sheshai and Soltan, 1991; Stephenson and Johnson, 1995) have suggested, however, that, in the context of their specific experimental conditions, placebo was unlikely to be a major factor. Like the other claimed mechanisms, therefore, the extent of placebo responses with IC stimulation remains unclear.

A summary of the theoretical analgesic mechanisms and suggested AMFs for eliciting these effects is given in Table 18.2. This clearly demonstrates that there is little agreement on optimal treatment parameters. In a combination of claims, a frequency of 100 Hz, for example, might be expected to activate the pain gate, increase circulation and block nociceptive fibre transmission. Johnson (1999) has similarly observed the multiplicity of claims of the actions of specific AMFs.

There is currently scant evidence to support specific mechanisms by which IC is claimed to operate owing to a lack of appropriate investigation. Although a mechanism involving the stimulation of peripheral nerves in line with the gate theory is likely to be related to IC, the more radical explanation of blocking of nerve conduction is unlikely to contribute to pain relief with this modality. Other mechanisms such as descending pain suppression, increased circulation and placebo cannot be easily discounted, although they do require verification.

EVIDENCE FOR ANALGESIC EFFECTS OF IC

Evidence for the analgesic effects of IC can be gleaned from both laboratory and clinical investigations.

Table 18.2 Claimed analgesic mechanisms and suggested AMFs

Theoretical analgesic mechanism	Suggested AMF (author)
'Pain gate'/ sensory fibre stimulation	1–100 Hz (Wadsworth and Chanmugam, 1980) 80–100 Hz (De Domenico, 1982) 90–100 Hz (Savage, 1984) 100 Hz (Goats, 1990)
Increased circulation/ sympathetic fibre stimulation	0–100 Hz (Willie, 1969) 100 Hz (Ganne, 1976, Nikolova, 1987) 100 Hz, 90–100 Hz, 1–10 Hz (Wadsworth and Chanmugam, 1980) > 80 Hz (De Domenico, 1982) 0–5 Hz (Savage, 1984)
Descending pain suppression/ nociceptive fibre stimulation	10–25 Hz (De Domenico, 1982) 130 Hz (Savage, 1984) 15 Hz (Goats, 1990)
Physiological block of nociceptive fibres	C fibres > 50 Hz; Aδ fibres > 40 Hz (De Domenico, 1982) 40 Hz large diameter/< 40 Hz small diameter (Goats, 1990)
Placebo response	None specifically implicated

Laboratory investigations

A number of studies of the effects of IC on experimental pain have been undertaken. The value of these studies is that they can indicate the presence of effects in a controlled environment, which if also found in the clinical environment could be associated with a benefit to people with pain.

Ischaemic pain

There is some unpublished evidence (Johnson and Tabasam, unpublished studies, 1999) that IC is more effective than either control or placebo stimulation in reducing experimental ischaemic pain intensity and affect. This finding is not consistent within the literature however (Scott and Purves, 1991).

Cold-induced pain

A cold-pressor test model of experimental pain has been used frequently to investigate the effects of IC. Cold pain is interesting because it is mediated by both C and Aδ fibre nerve pathways (Verduga and Ochoa, 1992; Yarnitsky and Ochoa, 1990). Any change in the experience of cold pain may, therefore, indicate more global effects on the perception of activity within peripheral nociceptive pathways.

A number of studies have demonstrated the ability of IC to decrease reported perception of pain using the cold-pressor test (Johnson and Tabasam, 1999 also unpublished study, 1999; Johnson and Wilson, 1997; Stephenson and Johnson, 1995; Tabasam and Johnson, unpublished study, 1999), although the results are often dependent on the outcome measure used. Together these studies suggest that modulation of specific elements of the experience of cold-induced pain may be possible with IC treatment.

Quantitative sensory testing

Quantitative sensory testing (QST) allows the assessment of, and differentiation between, the perception of activity within C and Aδ fibre nerve pathways (Palmer et al., 2000; Price, 1996; Verdugo and Ochoa, 1992). Assessment of specific thermal thresholds (the very first perception of a thermal sensation) gives information on the perception of activity within these neural pathways. Warm sensation (WS), for example, is mediated by C fibres (Morin and Bushnell, 1998; Verdugo and Ochoa, 1992; Yarnitsky and Ochoa, 1990, 1991), cold sensation (CS) by Aδ fibres (Verdugo and Ochoa, 1992; Yarnitsky and Ochoa, 1991), heat pain (HP) by C fibres (Morin and Bushnell, 1998; Verdugo and Ochoa, 1992; Yarnitsky and Ochoa, 1991), and cold pain (CP) by a mixture of C and Aδ fibres

(Verdugo and Ochoa, 1992; Yarnitsky and Ochoa, 1990). Effects of modalities on specific sensations may, therefore, indicate effects on specific nerve fibre types. QST has previously been shown to be sensitive to TENS (Eriksson, Rosén and Sjölund, 1985; Marchand, Bushnell and Duncan, 1991) and vibration (Yarnitsky et al., 1997).

Despite initial reports of an effect of 100 Hz IC on the perception of CP and CS (Palmer et al., unpublished study, 1999), a larger follow-up study found no significant effect of a range of IC AMFs (0, 5 and 100 Hz) in altering the perception of activity in these peripheral pathways compared with controls, 5 Hz and 100 Hz TENS, or placebo stimulation (Palmer et al., unpublished study, 2000). The use of these assessment techniques on patients, however, will advance the systematic investigation of IC and other interventions for the reduction of pain.

IC compared with TENS

At the beginning of the chapter we proposed that a key issue is whether IC is superior or even different to TENS, a question which has been highlighted by other authors in the field (Alon, 1987; Johnson, 1999). The controlled environment of a laboratory is a suitable arena for comparing IC and TENS on fundamental effects. A number of studies on experimental pain have been conducted to investigate this topic.

It has been observed that IC and TENS had different effects on cold-induced pain, with TENS increasing threshold but not altering pain intensity ratings, whereas IC decreased intensity ratings but had no effect on threshold (Salisbury and Johnson, 1995). Another study, however, discovered no significant differences between the effects of IC and TENS on cold-induced pain (Johnson and Tabasam, 1999). Tabasam and Johnson (unpublished study, 1999) found that both IC and TENS reduced the intensity of ischaemic pain compared with placebo, but again that there was no significant difference between the two modalities. Using quantitative sensory testing methods, it has been observed that IC and TENS were equally ineffective compared with control and placebo stimulation in

altering the perception of activity within peripheral nerve pathways (Palmer et al., unpublished study, 2000). Effects of IC and TENS on RIII and H reflexes have also been shown to be similar (Cramp et al., 2000).

This evidence suggests, therefore, that conclusive differences between IC and TENS on mechanisms related to the experience of pain remain to be demonstrated.

This overview proposes some evidence that IC stimulation may alter some but not all elements of the pain experience associated with ischaemic and cold induced pain, which is consistent with IC having a clinical use. IC's effects on experimental pain may not, however, be different to those of TENS.

Clinical investigations

The evidence for the effects of IC on pain in clinical populations will be investigated in this section.

Osteoarthritis

IC stimulation coupled with an exercise programme has been compared with short-wave diathermy (SWD) coupled with an exercise programme, and with an exercise programme alone (Quirk, Newman and Newman, 1985). All experimental groups exhibited significant improvement in pain scores over the course of treatment, but there were no significant differences between groups. Due to methodological issues, there are questions about the degree of scientific merit of the evidence in this study. However, perhaps the best interpretation is that it does not suggest an additive effect of IC over exercise alone.

IC has also been compared with placebo stimulation for patients with osteoarthritis (OA) of the knee (Young et al., 1991). The authors observed that, although there were significant decreases in measured indices of pain, active IC stimulation was no more effective than placebo. Again issues related to the methodology make it difficult to comment conclusively on the merits of the results but they do not support IC effects as being other than placebo.

Another approach investigated the effect that personality has on the response to IC treatment of OA knee pain (Shafshak, El-Sheshai and Soltan, 1991). There was no significant difference in personality types associated with 'responders' to treatment (50% or more relief for at least 5 days after treatment) and 'non-responders' (25% or less relief for at least 5 days after treatment). The authors concluded that personality did not affect the response to IC treatment, and that placebo responses may be a minor factor in IC treatment. This supposition, however, relies on an as-yet unfounded premise that personality characteristics are major factors in the placebo response.

The effects of bipolar and quadripolar IC have been assessed in eight patients with bilateral OA of the knee (Ní Chiosoig, Hendricks and Malone, 1994). The authors reported statistically significant improvements in pain after six treatments and at the end of the treatment period, but no statistically significant differences between the bipolar and quadripolar groups. It was suggested that bipolar IC, however, produced faster improvements, displaying a 73.14% reduction in pain, as opposed to 37% with quadripolar IC after six treatments. At 12 treatments, however, the figures were very similar, with 83.0% and 81.8% reduction for bipolar and quadripolar respectively. A combination of methodological issues such as small sample size and lack of a control group limits definitive conclusions, but an optimistic interpretation of the results may suggest a potential difference in the effectiveness of IC applied by these two methods. Interestingly the authors reported that six out of eight individuals preferred bipolar IC.

In conclusion, with regard to pain associated with OA, claims of any benefit from IC must be judged against a background of scientific evidence of poor quantity and quality.

Jaw pain

The effects of IC and placebo stimulation in patients with jaw pain have been investigated (Taylor et al., 1987). Both groups reported improvements in pain over the three treatments administered, but the difference between groups was not significant. The authors concluded that treatment of chronic jaw pain with IC displayed a high placebo component, with IC being no better than placebo.

Fracture pain

In a study of the effectiveness of IC on pain and range of movement following fracture of the proximal humerus (Martin, Palmer and Heath, 2000), three treatment groups were used: (1) active IC with exercise and mobilisation, (2) placebo IC with exercise and mobilisation, and (3) exercise and mobilisation alone. No significant differences between treatment groups were observed but there were statistically significant improvements in all outcome measures over time. It was concluded that IC, when used in conjunction with exercise and mobilisation, did not provide any additional benefit over and above that achieved by placebo IC, or exercise and mobilisation alone. However, incomplete randomisation and the small subject numbers in this study again prevent definitive answers. The results do have interesting parallels with those of Quirk, Newman and Newman (1985), who found that IC had no additional effect over exercise alone on pain associated with knee joint OA.

Low back pain

Werners, Pynsent and Bulstrode (1999) compared IC with mechanical traction and massage on patients with low back pain. Significant improvements were observed at 3 months, but there were no significant differences between the groups. The lack of control or placebo groups in this study makes it impossible to gauge the clinical significance of the results, which may be due to natural progression, equal effectiveness (or ineffectiveness) of the two modalities, equivalent placebo responses, or a combination of these situations.

Hurley et al. (2000) also studied the effects of IC on low back pain. Subjects were randomly assigned to one of three groups: (1) IC to the 'painful area' and use of *The Back Book* (1997) ($n = 18$), (2) IC to the 'spinal nerve root' plus *The Back Book* ($n = 22$), and (3). *The Back Book* in isolation ($n = 20$). (*The Back Book*, produced by The Stationery Office, is an evidence-based information booklet which has been shown by Burton *et al.* (1999) to reduce disability in people with acute back pain.) From their results the authors suggested that the use of IC applied over the painful area should be challenged, and that the combined use of *The Back Book* with IC applied over the spinal nerve root be recommended for maximum effectiveness. The results are interesting, but do not justify claims that *'the clinical efficacy of'* [IC] *'for patients with LBP has been established'*. As was reported previously (Martin, Palmer and Heath, 2000; Quirk, Newman and Newman, 1985), there was no strong evidence in this study for the role of IC when used as an addition to a treatment programme.

In summary, there seems to be scant clinical evidence for the effectiveness of IC in the management of pain. The studies reviewed are not of a high standard, and are few in number. The perceived clinical effectiveness of this modality demonstrated by its high availability and usage has not, to date, been subject to rigorous scientific scrutiny.

METHODS OF APPLICATION

The principles of application are outlined in Chapter 15. Dosages are based on the information provided above, both in the section describing treatment parameters and under that discussing efficacy.

HAZARDS

Adverse effects

A number of adverse effects have been reported with IC treatment; these include (Kitchen, 2000a, b; Partridge and Kitchen, 1999):

- burns
- increased pain
- general malaise
- nausea
- vomiting
- dizziness/faintness
- migraine/headache
- neurological effects.

Theoretically, IC should be incapable of producing a burn as it is an evenly alternating current, but clearly there is a reaction in some patients, the mechanisms of which have yet to be established. Stimulation of the autonomic nervous system may account for some of the more general effects reported. At present there are no adequate screening tools to identify patients who may experience undesirable reactions to IC.

Contraindications

These include:

- patients where disturbance of a thrombus, spread of infection or cancerous cells, or haemorrhage might result
- pacemakers
- the abdomen during pregnancy
- the chest wall in patients with cardiac problems.

These recommendations are based on prudence as opposed to scientific evidence, however.

CONCLUSIONS

This chapter has introduced the characteristics of interferential current, the theoretical mechanisms involved in producing pain relief with this method of electrical stimulation and the evidence for these mechanisms. A review has also been made of the laboratory and clinical investigations of the efficacy of IC in producing analgesia.

Many fundamental questions remain to be clarified. It is still not clear whether IC is, indeed, efficacious in treating pain, or which aspects of the pain experience are affected. The experimental evidence, especially for cold pain, suggests some modulatory influence, but this has not been demonstrated convincingly in the clinical situation. There is also the key question of whether IC is any more effective than TENS for contributing to the management of pain. Initial work would suggest that it may not be, but this requires further clarification.

When considering the literature for TENS, the best evidence from systematic reviews suggests that it is not effective for the relief of acute pain; in the management of chronic pain, McQuay *et al.* (1997) report that much larger trials are needed and that TENS needs to be applied for long periods of time, rather than in short-duration treatment packages. This latter view is shared by Johnson (1999), who stated that analgesic effects have been demonstrated to occur only whilst TENS is active. Taking the lead from the TENS evidence, therefore, there is little to suggest that the traditional application of IC in short treatment sessions provides optimal conditions for efficacy. All of these questions represent hurdles in the way of gaining a truer understanding of interferential current as a singular, distinctive treatment modality deserving of its own niche in the field of electrotherapy.

REFERENCES

Alon, G (1987) Interferential current news. *Physical Therapy* **67**(2): 280–281.

Belcher, JF (1974) Interferential therapy. *New Zealand Journal of Physiotherapy* **6**: 29–34.

Burton, AK, Waddell, G, Tillotson, KM *et al.* (1999) Information and advice to patients with back pain can have a positive effect. A randomised controlled trial of a novel educational booklet in primary care. *Spine* **24**(23): 2484–2491.

Christie, AD, Willoughby, GL (1990) The effect of interferential therapy on swelling following open reduction and internal fixation of ankle fractures. *Physiotherapy Theory and Practice* **6**: 3–7.

Cramp, FL, Noble, G, Lowe, AS *et al.* (2000) A controlled study of the effects of transcutaneous electrical nerve stimulation and interferential therapy upon the RIII nociceptive and H-reflexes in humans. *Archives of Physical Medicine and Rehabilitation* **81**: 324–333.

De Domenico, G (1982) Pain relief with interferential therapy. *Australian Journal of Physiotherapy* **28**(3): 14–18.

Eriksson, MBE, Rosén, I, Sjölund, B (1985) Thermal sensitivity in healthy subjects is decreased by a central mechanism after TENS. *Pain* **22**: 235–242.

Foster, NE, Thompson, KA, Baxter, GD *et al.* (1999) Management of non-specific low back pain by physiotherapists in Great Britain and Ireland. A descriptive questionnaire of current clinical practice. *Spine* **24**(13): 1332–1342.

Ganne, JM (1976) Interferential therapy. *Australian Journal of Physiotherapy* **22**(3): 101–110.

Ganne, JM (1986) Interferential therapy. *Australian Journal of Physiotherapy* **32**(1): 63–65.

Goats, GC (1990) Interferential current therapy. *British Journal of Sports Medicine* **24**(2): 87–92.

Hansjuergens, A (1986) Interferential current clarification. *Physical Therapy* **66**(6): 1002.

Howson, DC (1978) Peripheral neural excitability—implications for transcutaneous electrical nerve stimulation. *Physical Therapy* **58**(12): 1467–1473.

Hurley, DA, Minder, P, McDonough, SM *et al.* (2000) Evidence for interferential therapy for acute low back pain. *Physiotherapy* **86**(1): 36.

Indergand, HJ, Morgan, BJ (1995) Effect of interference current on forearm vascular resistance in asymptomatic humans. *Physical Therapy* **75**(4): 306–312.

Johnson, M, Wilson, H (1997) The analgesic effects of different swing patterns of interferential currents on cold-induced pain. *Physiotherapy* **83**(9): 461–467.

Johnson, MI (1999) The mystique of interferential currents when used to manage pain. *Physiotherapy* **85**(6): 294–297.

Johnson, MI, Tabasam, G (1999) A double blind placebo controlled investigation into the analgesic effects of interferential currents (IFC) and transcutaneous electrical nerve stimulation (TENS) on cold-induced pain in healthy subjects. *Physiotherapy Theory and Practice* **15**: 217–233.

Kahn, J (1987) *Principles and Practice of Electrotherapy.* Churchill Livingstone, New York.

Kitchen, S (2000a) Audit of the unexpected effects of electrophysical agents. Interim report: responses to December 1999. *Physiotherapy* **86**(3): 152–155.

Kitchen, S (2000b) Audit of the unexpected effects of electrophysical agents. Interim report: responses January to June, 2000. *Physiotherapy* **86**(10): 509–511.

Kloth, LC (1991) Interference current. In: Nelson, RM, Currier, DP (eds) *Clinical Electrotherapy.* Appleton & Lange, Connecticut, pp 221–260.

Lamb, S, Mani, R (1994) Does interferential therapy affect blood flow? *Clinical Rehabilitation* **8**: 213–218.

Lindsay, D, Dearness, J, Richardson, C *et al.* (1990) A survey of electromodality usage in private physiotherapy practices. *Australian Journal of Physiotherapy* **36**(4): 249–256.

Low, J, Reed, A (2000). *Electrotherapy Explained. Principles and Practice*, 3rd edn. Butterworth Heinemann, Oxford.

McQuay, HJ, Moore, RA, Ecclestone, C, Morley, S, de C Williams, AC (1997) Systematic review of outpatient services for chronic pain control. *Health Technology Assessment* **1**(6): i–iv, 1–135.

Marchand, S, Bushnell, MC, Duncan, GH (1991) Modulation of heat pain perception by high frequency TENS. *Clinical Journal of Pain* **7**: 122–129.

Martin, D (1996) Interferential current. In: Kitchen, S, Bazin, S (eds) *Clayton's Electrotherapy*, 10th edn. WB Saunders, New York, pp 306–315.

Martin, D, Palmer, S (1996) The effect of beat frequency on perceived comfort during stimulation of healthy subjects with interferential current. *Physiotherapy* 82(11): 639.

Martin, D, Palmer, S, Heath, C (2000) Interferential current as an adjunct to exercise and mobilisation in the treatment of proximal humerus fracture pain: lack of evidence of an additional effect. *Physiotherapy* 86(3): 147.

Melzack, R, Wall, P (1965) Pain mechanisms: a new theory. *Science* 150(3699): 971–979.

Morin, C, Bushnell, MC (1998) Temporal and qualitative properties of cold pain and heat pain: a psychophysical study. *Pain* 74: 67–73.

Ní Chiosoig, F, Hendriks, O, Malone, J (1994) A pilot study of the therapeutic effects of bipolar and quadripolar interferential therapy, using bilateral osteoarthritis as a model. *Physiotherapy Ireland* 15(1): 3–7.

Nikolova, L (1987) Treatment with interferential current. Churchill Livingstone, Singapore.

Noble, JG, Henderson, G, Cramp, AF *et al.* (2000) The effect of interferential therapy upon cutaneous blood flow in humans. *Clinical Physiology* 20(1): 2–7.

Nussbaum, E, Rush, P, Disenhaus, L (1990) The effects of interferential therapy on peripheral blood flow. *Physiotherapy* 76(12): 803–807.

Olson, SL, Perez, JV, Stacks, LN *et al.* (1999) The effects of TENS and interferential current on cutaneous blood flow in healthy subjects. *Physiotherapy Canada* **Winter**: 27–31.

Palmer, S, Martin, D, Steedman, W *et al.* (1999) Interferential current and transcutaneous electrical nerve stimulation frequency: effects on nerve excitation. *Archives of Physical Medicine and Rehabilitation* 80: 1065–1071.

Palmer, S, Martin, D, Steedman, W *et al.* (2000) C and Aδ-fibre mediated thermal perception: response to the rate of temperature change using method of limits. *Somatosensory and Motor Research* 17(4): 325–333.

Partridge, CJ, Kitchen, SS (1999) Adverse effects of electrotherapy used by physiotherapists. *Physiotherapy* **85**(6): 298–303.

Pope, GD, Mockett, SP, Wright, JP (1995) A survey of electrotherapeutic modalities: ownership and use in the NHS in England. *Physiotherapy* 81(2): 82–91.

Price, DD (1996) Selective activation of A-delta and C nociceptive afferents by different parameters of nociceptive heat stimulation: a tool for analysis of central mechanisms of pain. *Pain* 68: 1–3.

Quirk, A, Newman, RJ, Newman, KJ (1985) An evaluation of interferential therapy, shortwave diathermy and exercise in the treatment of osteoarthrosis of the knee. *Physiotherapy* 71(2): 55–57.

Rennie, S (1988) Interferential current therapy. In: Peat, M (ed) *Current Physical Therapy*. BC Decker, Philadelphia, pp 196–206.

Robertson, VJ, Spurritt, D (1998) Electrophysical agents: implications of their availability and use in undergraduate clinical placements. *Physiotherapy* 84(7): 335–344.

Robinson, AJ, Snyder-Mackler, L (1995) Clinical electrophysiology: electrotherapy and electrophysiologic testing, 2nd edn. Williams & Wilkins, Baltimore.

Salisbury, L, Johnson, M (1995) The analgesic effects of interferential therapy compared with TENS on experimental cold induced pain in normal subjects. *Physiotherapy* 81: 741.

Savage, B (1984) *Interferential Therapy*. Faber & Faber, London.

Scott, S, Purves, C (1991) The effect of interferential therapy in the relief of experimentally induced pain: a pilot study. In: *Proceedings of the 11th International Congress of the World Confederation for Physical Therapy, Book II*; pp 743–745.

Shafshak, T, El-Sheshai, AM, Soltan, HE (1991) Personality traits in the mechanisms of interferential therapy for osteoarthritic knee pain. *Archives of Physical Medicine and Rehabilitation* 72: 579–581.

Stationery Office (1997) *The Back Book*. The Stationery Office, Norwich.

Stephenson, R, Johnson, M (1995) The analgesic effects of interferential therapy on cold-induced pain in healthy subjects: a preliminary report. *Physiotherapy Theory and Practice* 11: 89–95.

Szehi, E, David, E (1980) The stereodynamic interferential current—a new electrotherapeutic technique. *Electromedica* 38: 13–17.

Taylor, K, Newton, R, Personius, W *et al.* (1987) Effects of interferential current stimulation for treatment of subjects with recurrent jaw pain. *Physical Therapy* 67(3): 346–350.

Treffene, RJ (1983) Interferential fields in a fluid medium. *Australian Journal of Physiotherapy* 29(6): 209–216.

Verdugo, R, Ochoa, JL (1992) Quantitative somatosensory thermotest: a key method for functional evaluation of small calibre afferent channels. *Brain* 115: 893–913.

Wadsworth, H, Chanmugam, APP (1980) *Electrophysical Agents in Physiotherapy. Therapeutic and Diagnostic Use*. Science Press, Marrickville, NSW.

Wall, P (1999) *Pain: The Science of Suffering*. Weidenfield & Nicolson, London.

Werners, R, Pynsent, PB, Bulstrode, CJK (1999) Randomised trial comparing interferential therapy with motorised lumbar traction and massage in the management of low back pain in a primary care setting. *Spine* 24(15): 1579–1584.

Willie, CD (1969). Interferential therapy. *Physiotherapy* **55**(12): 503–505.

Yarnitsky, D, Ochoa, JL (1990) Release of cold-induced burning pain by block of cold-specific afferent input. *Brain* 113: 893–902.

Yarnitsky, D, Ochoa, JL (1991) Warm and cold specific somatosensory systems: psychophysical thresholds, reaction times and peripheral conduction velocities. *Brain* 114: 1819–1826.

Yarnitsky, D, Kunin, M, Brik, R *et al.* (1997) Vibration reduces thermal pain in adjacent dermatomes. *Pain* 69(1–2): 75–77.

Young, SL, Woodbury, MG, Fryday-Field, K *et al.* (1991) Efficacy of interferential current stimulation alone for pain reduction in patients with osteoarthritis of the knee: a randomized placebo control clinical trial. *Physical Therapy* 71(6): S52.

19

Diagnostic and assessment applications

Oona Scott
(Part 1 Electrophysiological testing)
Steve Young
Kate Ballard
(Part 2 Wound assessment)

INTRODUCTION

A number of modalities considered in this text may be used as assessment or diagnostic tools by the therapist, either to test the integrity of structures or to assess progress, or both. Part 1 addresses ways in which neuromuscular structures may be tested for their integrity using electrical stimulation; Part 2 addresses methods of assessing tissue repair and evaluating circulatory efficiency using ultrasound.

PART 1
ELECTROPHYSIOLOGICAL
TESTING

INTRODUCTION

This section provides an overview of a number of electrophysiological tests used in the clinical setting to assist both diagnosis and evaluation of responses to therapeutic intervention in peripheral nerve and muscle disorders. The past 30 years have seen major advances both in our understanding of the basic and applied physiological properties of peripheral nerves and skeletal muscles and in developing tools to use for investigating these properties. (The references at the end of this chapter provide a list of key texts used as source material.)

HUMAN MUSCLE FUNCTION STUDIES

Assessment of muscle strength

Muscle strength is usually measured as the ability of a subject to generate maximum tension for a short duration, such as 5–10 seconds (see Ch. 8 Introduction). Muscle strength is a physiological concept and is a function of the number and size of motor units that constitute the muscle. The simplest definition of strength is the ability to develop force against an unyielding resistance in a single contraction of unrestricted duration. Essentially the magnitude of a maximum voluntary contraction (MVC) is determined by a combination of neural, mechanical and muscular factors.

Voluntary muscle activation

The ability to activate all of the motor units of a muscle can be tested using twitch interpolation (Enoka, 1993; Rutherford et al., 1986). Electrically elicited twitch contractions are superimposed as the individual attempts to perform an MVC (Fig. 19.1). If there is a detectable increase in force, the interpretation is that the muscle was not maximally activated. Maximum activation may be brought about through greater motor unit recruitment or a higher rate of motor unit firing. In healthy subjects, early gains of muscle strength have been attributed to altered neural drive, sometimes known as the learning effect (Jones et al., 1989; Komi, 1986). In untrained subjects, increases in muscle strength on repeated assessment and in the first few weeks of training may be due to this learning effect.

Determination of contractile properties of whole muscle

Figure 19.2 shows the response of the tibialis anterior muscle to electrical fatigue testing. At the same time, rapid developments in molecular biochemistry and immunocytochemical techniques have made it possible not only to identify the histochemistry of different types of fibre but also to relate changes in muscle mass and contractile characteristics of skeletal muscle to overall function and metabolism.

Techniques developed to measure the isometric tensions developed in both voluntary and electrically elicited contractions were first described by Merton (1954) and Desmedt et al. (1968) and then by Edwards et al. (1977). Using standardised equipment and a simple strain gauge arrangement, it is possible to measure:

- MVC with and without superimposed twitches
- response to short trains of stimulation at 1, 10, 20 and 40 Hz
- response to fatigue testing by stimulation at 40 Hz for 250 ms, every second for 5 minutes
- the time course of muscle contraction
- loss of force and changes in integrated electromyogram (EMG) activity during a 60 s voluntary fatigue test.

The indications are that these isometric measurements of muscle strength, fatigue resistance and contractile properties can provide valuable information reflecting muscle composition and function.

ELECTROMYOGRAPHY STUDIES

Electromyography refers to methods of studying the electrical activity of muscles. Recordings are made of muscle unit action potentials (MUAPs) as they pass from neuromuscular junctions along muscle to activate individual muscle fibres within motor units. The output is recorded as an EMG.

Clinically, it has been useful to be able to demonstrate when a particular muscle was contracting. The normal pattern of electrical activity could be recognised, and it also became possible to recognise departures from normal, and to associate these with nerve–muscle disorders. Needle electrodes, by recording activity from a much smaller area than surface electrodes, made it possible to study the activity of single motor units. Because all of the muscle fibres for a given motor unit discharge almost simultaneously, one aggregate spike is picked up, usually the output of the greater density of

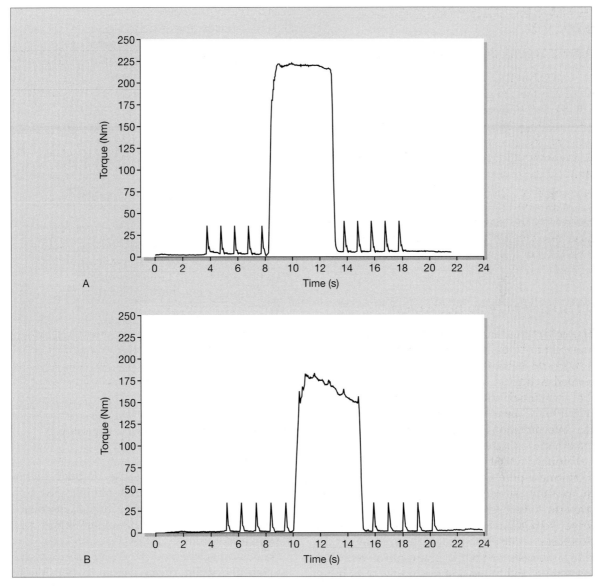

Figure 19.1 Maximum voluntary contraction (MVC) of the quadriceps femoris with superimposed twitches. A: Full activation. B: Detectable force—less than full activation.

fibres from the same motor unit nearest to the tip of the needle electrode. The waveform may be complex as additional spikes will have different amplitudes and sizes depending on the distance of the active fibres from the electrode.

Surface electrodes (discs, usually silver–silver chloride) are attached to the skin overlying the muscle or nerve from which activity is to be recorded. More recently, malleable, self-adhesive electrodes have been developed commercially. These have the advantage of being both very light and easy to apply. The potential difference between two electrodes is recorded through a differential amplifier, a third electrode being used to connect the patient to earth. The recorded signal represents the sum of the individual

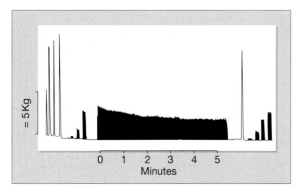

Figure 19.2 A typical trace of force measurements of the human tibialis muscle showing maximum voluntary contraction and the response to stimulation at 1, 10, 20 and 40 Hz, before and after fatigue testing, and the response to fatigue testing by stimulation at 40 Hz for 250 ms, every second for 5 minutes. (See p. 302.)

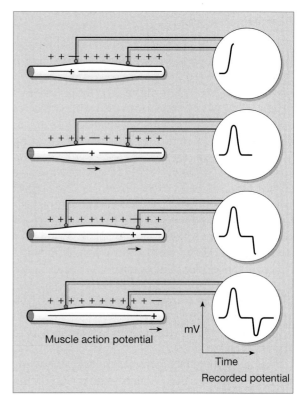

Figure 19.3 Representation of changes in potential difference of muscle action potentials being recorded by external electrodes.

potentials produced by all of the nerve or muscle fibres that are activated. The MUAPs or potential differences are very small, usually only a few microvolts (Fig. 19.3).

The surface EMG signal can be analysed in terms of two fundamental variables: amplitude and frequency. The first step in determining amplitude involves full-wave rectification. *Rectification* means that the EMG signal is converted into a signal that contains only positive voltages and the rectified signal is then filtered with a low-pass filter (Winter, 1990). This provides a linear envelope or 'moving average' because it follows the trend of the EMG. The area of the linear envelope can be computed providing an assessment of the amplitude of the signal. Sometimes known as the *time domain*, the amplitude of the signal is documented as being positively correlated to the force production. However, care has to be taken in interpreting the relationship between tension generated by the muscle and this signal. A known standard such as the amplitude of the signal in a maximum contraction can be used for purposes of comparison.

The frequency content of the recorded signal is related to the numbers of active motor units as well as to their constituent firing rates. Recruitment of an individual motor unit results in the generation of a MUAP of specific size,

shape and frequency. Because of their higher conduction velocities, MUAPs travelling on fast-twitch fibres have inherently higher frequency content than those on slow-twitch fibres (see Kamen and Caldwell, 1996).

To determine the power density spectrum, the frequency domain of the EMG, a fast fourier transform function is used. This function determines the power of frequencies in any set period of time. Three parameters provide useful measures of the spectrum: the median frequency, which is the frequency that divides the power density spectrum into two regions of equal power, the mean power frequency, which is the average frequency, and the bandwidth of the spectrum or width of the frequency window of the band pass filter; this puts limits on the range of frequencies to be recorded and analysed (for further information see Basmajian and Luca, 1985).

The tendon jerk

The tendon jerk, or monosynaptic stretch reflex, is a spinal reflex and is used clinically to observe the response of a muscle to percussion (a tap) on its tendon and to determine neuronal status at a spinal level. Conventionally, two types of neurons were thought to be involved. A tap to the tendon initiates a burst of impulses passing along the group Ia afferent nerve fibres from the primary sensory endings in the muscle spindle (see section Afferent input to the central nervous system in Ch. 4). These are the fastest-conducting afferent neurons. Among the spinal connections of the afferent nerves are excitatory synapses on motoneurons supplying the same muscle. These motoneurons are the second type of neuron involved in the reflex; they complete the reflex arc by forming the efferent pathway via the α motoneurons, neuromuscular junctions and resulting contraction of the skeletal muscle fibres.

The afferent axons project directly on to the motoneurons without necessarily involving inter-neurons. The motoneurons so activated innervate the extrafusal or skeletal fibres of the muscle that was originally stretched and the action potentials relayed down the motor nerves cause the muscle to contract.

The afferent neurons branch within the dorsal horn of the spinal cord. A side branch (collateral) projects to an inhibitory interneuron in the spinal chord. This inhibits motoneurons innervating the antagonist muscles. The time delay between the dorsal root and the excitatory post-synaptic potential in the excited motoneuron is about 1 ms. A further 1 ms elapses before the inhibitory postsynaptic potential is recorded in the motoneurons supplying fibres in the antagonist muscle.

The H reflex

The H reflex is a monosynaptic reflex response to electrical stimulation of spindle afferent (Ia) fibres and was first described by Hoffman in 1918. Hoffman stimulated the tibial nerve with a low-intensity stimulus which mediated a monosynaptic response in the soleus muscle. This low-intensity stimulus selectively activates the Ia afferent fibres. Figure 19.4 shows the typical M and H waves elicited in human soleus muscle by stimulating the tibial nerve.

It was originally thought that the H reflex was analogous to the stretch reflex. Essentially, the H reflex stimulates the Ia afferent fibres, bypassing the muscle spindles, which are directly stimulated by the tendon tap. It is thought that the H reflex provides an indication of the excitability of the α motoneuron pool.

The stimulus used to evoke the H reflex should be of lower intensity than is required to elicit a maximal M response (see next section), otherwise the H reflex will be blocked. Blocking occurs because antidromic (opposite-direction) impulses evoked in motoneurons by direct stimulation collide with orthodromic (same-direction) impulses evoked reflexively in these axons in response to stimulation of the spindle afferent fibres. Latency depends on the site of stimulation; it is approximately 30 ms for the soleus and 16 ms for the flexor carpi radialis.

A means of standardising the intensity of stimulation is to present the results in terms of an H/M ratio. Use of the direct motor response (M wave) is well documented in studies investigating human H reflexes. If the position and intensity of the stimulating electrode are not altered, the size of the M wave has been found to be consistent.

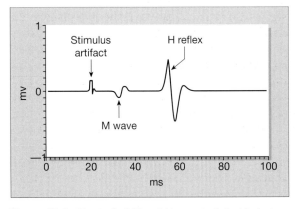

Figure 19.4 The typical M and H waves elicited in human soleus muscle by stimulating the tibial nerve.

The M wave

If motor fibres of a peripheral nerve are stimulated electrically, a response is evoked in the muscles that they supply. This potential is called the M wave. The interval (latency) from the time of application of the signal to muscle contraction represents the conduction time—that is, the time that the impulse takes to travel along the nerve fibres, across the neuromuscular junction and along the muscle fibres to the recording electrodes.

The latency of a submaximal response may be longer than a maximal response. The stimulus must evoke a maximal motor response because, with an inadequate signal, an H reflex may be elicited and mistaken for an M response of prolonged latency. A maximal M response is accomplished by increasing the intensity gradually until the response is maximal, and then increasing the intensity by an additional 30%.

The F wave

This is evoked in muscle by electrical stimulation of the peripheral nerve by which it is supplied. It occurs as a result of a motoneuron discharge elicited by antidromic (opposite-direction) activation rather than by any reflex phenomenon. It has a latency similar to that of the H reflex (see above), but it requires a more intense stimulus and is not blocked if the stimulus evokes a maximal M response in the muscle. It is smaller than the M response and may not be elicited by every stimulus that is applied, even if they are of the same intensity. It can be elicited in deafferented muscles and its latency decreases as the electrode is moved proximally.

SENSORY AND MOTOR NERVE CONDUCTION STUDIES

Both sensory and motor nerve conduction velocities can be recorded and this measurement is routinely performed in patients where peripheral nerve problems are suspected. The passage of an action potential along a nerve fibre generates a change in potential in the surrounding extracellular field. This potential is smaller than the action potential recorded across the membrane of the nerve and is initially negative because sodium ions are leaving the extracellular fluid to enter the axoplasm.

Sensory nerve conduction studies

To account for the neural events involved in the perception of touch, we can start by recording signals from a neuron that terminates in the skin. Brief electrical pulses of 0.1 V amplitude, lasting for 0.001 second (1 millisecond) move up the nerve at a speed up to 80 metres per second (m/s). Although the impulses in a cell responsive to touch are virtually identical to those in other nerve cells, the significance and meaning are specific for that cell. They convey to the brain that a particular part of the skin has been pressed.

Adrian (1946) showed that the frequency of impulse firing in a nerve cell is a measure of the intensity of the stimulus. The stronger the pressure applied to the skin, the higher is the frequency and the better maintained the firing of the cell. Information is provided about the modality of the stimulus (by the particular type of sensory neuron it influences), its location (by the position and the connections of the sensory cell), and its intensity (by the frequency of firing).

Techniques have been developed for stimulating the sensory digital nerves using ring electrodes while recording the impulses, either as they pass under a pair of electrodes placed more proximally from the nerve trunk or with reference to a single electrode placed over the nerve and another placed at a distance from the nerve. The position of the nerve trunk is located by using a stimulating electrode and then finding the point at which the muscle potential is minimal.

The detection of the nerve action potential is facilitated by use of an electronic averaging technique. The waveform is typically triphasic with a small positive onset, which coincides with the arrival of the impulse at the more distal of the two electrodes. However, latency is often more satisfactorily measured to the peak of the negative deflection, which is best used directly as a measure of latency rather than being converted into conduction velocity (Buchtal and Rosenfalck, 1966). Peak-to-peak amplitude of the potential should also be measured. The amplitude relates to the number of sensory nerve fibres activated, the distribution of their conduction velocities and the distance of the nerve from the recording electrodes.

Motor nerve conduction studies

These involve the use of electrical stimulation and either surface or needle electrodes. Nerves are stimulated where they are relatively superficial with surface electrodes. Deeply situated nerves such as the sciatic nerve at the gluteal fold need to be stimulated with needle electrodes. If bipolar stimulation is used, two small stimulating electrodes, the anode (positive) and cathode (negative), are placed 2–3 cm apart over the nerve with the cathode distal to the anode. For monopolar stimulation, the cathode is positioned over the nerve and a large anode is placed more distally and at a significant distance from it.

Pulse duration can be varied from 0.05 to 2 ms; the frequency of stimulation is also variable, but either 1 or 2 Hz would be common. The two recording electrodes are placed on the muscle innervated by the nerve that is being stimulated, with one being as close to the motor point of the muscle as possible (see section Basis for the therapeutic use of electrical stimulation in Ch. 8). The motor point, the position on the skin where maximum contraction can be achieved, is often found at the junction of the proximal third with the distal two-thirds of the muscle belly.

The response is typically biphasic, with a negative onset. Conventionally, the negative phase is recorded as an upward deflection. The amplitude of the negative component is usually slightly reduced when the nerve is stimulated proximally rather than distally. This is attributable to variation in time of the action potentials, because of their differing conduction velocities. The amplitude is recorded as a compound action potential since it is compounded of contributions from the many action potentials of individual nerve fibres.

The velocity at which the impulse is propagated along the fastest-conducting motor fibres can be determined by stimulating the nerve at two separate points and recording the evoked responses of the muscle it supplies. The stimulus is given at two points and the distance between the two points is measured. To determine the conduction velocity, the distance between the two points is measured and divided by the time difference.

Magnetic stimulation

Magnetic stimulation is one of the most recent developments in the field of electrodiagnosis. Originally designed (Merton et al., 1982) for the stimulation of peripheral nerves, magnetic stimulation has been applied widely for painless stimulation of the brain, spinal cord and nerve roots. Magnetic stimulators use a magnetic field that varies over time and passes unchanged through skin and bone to induce currents in excitable tissue. When such activation is applied to the brain, neurons in the cortex can be activated and a motor response elicited in the targeted muscle. Magnetic stimulation has been used to examine central motor pathway conductivity and to assess excitatory and inhibitory influences of descending nerve pathways.

Strength–duration curves

The strength–duration relationship can be determined by applying rectangular pulses of differing pulse widths to a peripheral nerve. The current required to produce a muscle twitch is recorded along with the relationship between the intensity of the current required to produce a muscle contraction and the time for which it is applied. This test has clinical applications and can be used to determine the state of innervation and to monitor reinnervation of skeletal muscle following trauma to peripheral nerves (see section Motoneuron to muscle activation in Ch. 4).

REFERENCES

Adrian, ED (1946) *The Physical Background of Perception.* Clarendon Press, Oxford.

Basmajian, JV, Luca, CJ (1985) *Muscles Alive. Their Functions Revealed by Electromyography*, 5th edn. Williams & Wilkins, Baltimore, MD.

Buchtal, F, Rosenfalck, A (1966) Spontaneous electrical activity of human muscle. *Electroencephalography and Clinical Neurophysiology* **20**: 321.

Desmedt, JE (1968) The isometric twitch of human muscle in the normal and dystrophic states. In: Milherat, AT (ed), *Exploratory Concepts in Muscular Dystrophy and Related Disorders.* Excerpta Medica Foundation, Amsterdam, pp 224–231.

Dubowitz, V (1985) *Muscle Biopsy. A Practical Approach*, 2nd edn. Baillière Tindall, London.

Dubowitz, V, Brooke, MH (1973) *Muscle Biopsy. A Modern Approach.* WB Saunders, Philadelphia.

Edwards, RHT, Young, A, Hoskings, GP, Jones, DA (1977) Human skeletal muscle function: description of tests and normal values. *Science in Molecular Medicine* **52**: 283–290.

Enoka, RM, Fuglevand, AJ (1993) Neuromuscular basis of the maximum force capacity of a muscle. In: Grabiner, MD (ed) *Current Issues in Biomechanics.* Human Kinetics, Champaign, IL, pp 215–235.

Jones, DA, Rutherford, OM, Parker, DF (1989) Physiological changes in skeletal muscle as a result of strength training. *Quarterly Journal of Experimental Physiology* **74**: 233–256.

Kamen, G, Caldwell, GE (1996) Physiology and interpretation of the electromyogram. *Journal of Clinical Neurophysiology* **13**(5): 366–384.

Komi, PV (1986) Training of muscle strength and power: interaction of neuromotoric, hypertrophic and mechanical factors. *International Journal of Sports Medicine* **7**: 10–15.

Merton, PA (1954) Voluntary strength and fatigue. *Journal of Physiology.* WB Saunders, Philadelphia.

Merton, PA, Morton, HB, Hill, DK, Marsden, CD (1982) Scope of a technique for electrical stimulation of human brain, spinal cord and muscle. *Lancet* **II**: 597–600.

Rothwell, J (1994) *Control of Human Voluntary Movement*, 2nd edn. Chapman & Hall, London.

Rutherford, OM, Jones, DA, Newham, DJ (1986) Clinical and experimental application of the percutaneous twitch superimposition technique for the study of human muscle activation. *Journal of Neurology, Neurosurgery and Psychiatry* **49**: 1288–1291.

Scott, OM, Hyde, SA, Vrbova, G, Dubowitz, V (1990) Therapeutic possibilities of chronic low frequency electrical stimulation in children with Duchenne muscular dystrophy. *Journal of Neurological Sciences* **95**: 171–182.

Winter, DA (1990) *Biomechanics and Motor Control of Human Movement*, 2nd edn. John Wiley & Sons, New York.

PART 2
WOUND ASSESSMENT

INTRODUCTION

Although this section will mainly address the use of ultrasound to scan wounds and assess blood flow, it will initially consider other ways of monitoring wound repair. There are a number of techniques available to the clinician for the assessment of wounds. These techniques tend to fall into one of two categories: invasive or non-invasive.

INVASIVE AND NON-INVASIVE METHODS OF ASSESSMENT

Invasive techniques

These techniques provide quantitative information regarding the wound and its stage in healing. These methods include:

- histological evaluation of excised tissue to identify and measure the number of cell types present during the healing process (Young, 1988)

- biochemical analysis of wound tissue biopsies and fluid to measure the various components involved in wound repair, for example collagen synthesis and deposition, messenger RNA synthesis, extracellular factors (Saperia, Glassberg and Lyons, 1986)

- tensile strength may be analysed by tissue breaking point or 'wound rupture stress' (Charles *et al.*, 1992)

- angiogenesis may be monitored by angiography (Young and Dyson, 1990).

Although these methods are able to yield quantitative data regarding wound healing they are invasive, involving biopsy, which results in the destruction of the tissue under investigation, thereby delaying wound healing. In addition, many patients find this procedure, at best, uncomfortable.

Non-invasive methods

These techniques tend to be less quantitative than the invasive methods; however, they are more acceptable to patients. Non-invasive methods include the following.

- **Transparency tracings.** A double layer of sterile acetate or polythene film is placed over the wound, and the outline is traced using a permanent marker pen. By using a double-layer film, the side which has been in contact with the wound can be discarded to prevent contact infection. The surface area of the wound can then be measured by either placing the acetate tracing on to the graph paper and counting the squares, or evaluated using a computer which scans and digitises the traced outline and calculates the surface area automatically. The disadvantage of using the tracing method is that it is very hard to define the edges of the wound and so the error can be high.

- **Photographic recording.** Wounds can be photographed instead of traced. The operator must place a ruler or some other object of known size next to the wound to provide a scale against which measurements can be made. The wound surface area can then be calculated from photographs using computerised image analysis. Although accuracy is increased using photographic rather than tracing methods, errors can still occur because, for example, of varying ambient light conditions leading to variations in exposure from film to film, or of distortions of the vertical and horizontal axes, which arise if the wound is on a curved surface.

- **Depth gauges.** A device known as the Kundin gauge (Kundin, 1989) has been developed that is able to measure the length, width and depth of a wound; from these the area and volume are calculated. This method is more accurate when used to measure circular and elliptical wounds. When used for irregular wounds, in which there is tracking and underlying cavities, the method often underestimates area and volume; this is the main disadvantage of this method. However, the method is easy to use, disposable, objective and inexpensive.

- **Volume.** The volume of wounds can be measured by making moulds of the wound. A variety of substances can be used, including hydrocolloid gel, silicone rubber, silastic foam and alginates (Convington *et al.*, 1989). The mould is then placed in water, and the volume displaced is the volume of the wound. The use of this method is restricted; it cannot be used over shallow wounds, or those which are circumferential around a limb, or for wounds with undermining and sinus formation. The orifice of the wound has to be sufficiently large to remove the material. Another method to measure volume is the use of saline (Berg *et al.*, 1990). The wound is covered by a film, and saline is injected into the wound. This is a simple and reproducible technique, but is not satisfactory for superficial sores.

- **Stereoscopic photography.** This is used to overcome projection errors from the curved skin surface to a flat screen. This method uses two cameras, so that a photograph is produced from which depth measurements can be recorded (Bulstrode, Goode and Scott, 1986). The area and volume of the wound can be calculated by a computer. The method is accurate and reproducible, and measurements of irregular defects in the wound, in three dimensions, can be made. However, the amount of specialised equipment and time involved restricts this method's application in clinical practice.

- **Thermal imaging.** This method detects infrared radiation emitted from the skin. The emission of the wound will, however, vary depending upon whether the wound has been exposed without a dressing, and if so for how long, and whether it is infected. It can be used to record temperature at the edges of a wound, to monitor blood perfusion, and could also be useful for monitoring the effect of antibiotic therapy in an infected wound.

- **Video image analysis.** Video cameras can be used to record lesions from different angles to provide optimum information, and to reduce the measurement problems caused by skin curvature (Smith, Bhat and Bulgrin, 1992). This method uses a video camera with a macrolens, linked to an image-processing computer which produces high-precision measurements of area, colour density and volume.

HIGH-FREQUENCY DIAGNOSTIC ULTRASOUND

One major drawback exists with most of the non-invasive techniques discussed up to this point: they produce data which describes the outer surface of the wound and surrounding uninjured skin only—none of the techniques give any indication as to the quality of the underlying reparative tissue. However, there now exists a non-invasive method that allows the clinician to look deep into the skin and wound bed, with a high degree of resolution, to assess the quality of the reparative tissue (Calvin *et al.*, 1997; Karim *et al.*, 1994; Whiston, Melhuish and Harding, 1993; Whiston *et al.*, 1993; Young and Koffman, 1997; Young, Erian and Dyson, 1996; Young *et al.*, 1993). This technique involves the use of a high-frequency ultrasound scanner (Fig. 19.5).

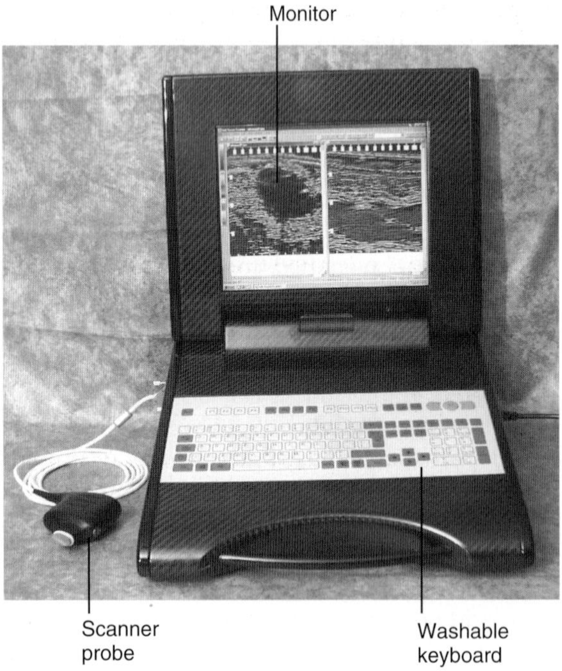

This is a simple procedure that is able to produce a high-resolution image of the dermis (Fig. 19.6) and wound bed (Fig. 19.7). The scan can be carried out through certain wound dressings such as semiocclusive or gel dressings (Fig. 19.8) when a coupling gel is applied,

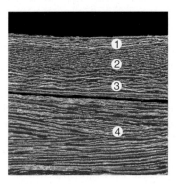

Figure 19.6 High-resolution image of the dermis. 1: Epidermis. 2: Dermis (papillary layer). 3: Dermis (reticular layer). 4: Tendon.

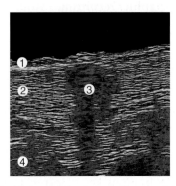

Figure 19.7 High-resolution image of a wound. 1: Epidermis. 2: Dermis. 3: Wound bed. 4: Subcutaneous fat.

Monitor

Scanner probe

Washable keyboard

Figure 19.5 High-frequency untrasound scanner (Longport Inc. USA)

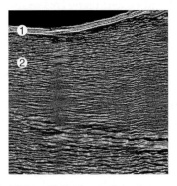

Figure 19.8 High-resolution image through a wound dressing. 1: Wound dressing. 2: New tissue.

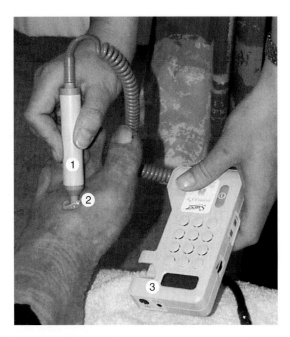

Figure 19.9 Doppler ultrasonography equipment. 1: Probe. 2: Ultrasound gel. 3: Doppler display.

thereby avoiding risks of infection and also offering protection to the delicate wound surface during the scanning procedure. An axial resolution of 65 μm and a lateral resolution of approximately 200 μm can be obtained. The images produced can be analysed using software built into the scanner. Using image analysis it is possible to monitor even small changes in a wound, even before they become clinically evident, and to recognise whether the wound is deteriorating or improving. This early detection can lead to large savings in treatment times. Wound depth can also be calculated using this technique (e.g. in burn injuries). This is a rapid, sensitive and repeatable method of quantifying wound healing.

DOPPLER ULTRASONOGRAPHY

This technique is used as a method of measuring blood flow in the peripheral arteries, and is used routinely in the assessment of leg ulcers. In combination with a full physical examination and clinical history the Doppler assessment gives an indication of arterial blood flow to the lower limb. It comprises an important part of the decision-making process of whether to apply compression therapy to a limb in order to reduce oedema, reverse venous hypertension and aid venous return. Doppler ultrasonography can play a critical part in the assessment process; if compression in the form of bandaging or intermittent compression pumps is applied to a limb with reduced arterial supply then the compression could further compromise the blood flow leading to tissue necrosis and possible amputation.

The device (Fig. 19.9) consists of a hand-held Doppler probe which emits ultrasound at a frequency within the range 2–10 MHz. The transmitted ultrasound beam is directed towards the blood vessel of interest. Ultrasound waves are reflected back and detected by the probe; the ultrasound waves reflect from the moving red blood cells. These reflections amplify the frequency shift and this is filtered by the Doppler to give a sound or graphic output.

The technique of performing a Doppler ultrasound assessment (Moffat and Harper, 1997; Vowden and Vowden, 1996) involves recording systolic pressure with a hand-held ultrasound Doppler at the foot or ankle. This reading (A) is taken at the dorsalis pedis, posterial tibial artery, anterior tibial artery and peroneal artery and the highest pressure recorded is then divided by the highest brachial artery reading (B) measured from testing both arms. The ratio is referred to as the ankle brachial pressure index (ABPI).

Generally a rate of 0.8 (= 80% flow to the lower limb) or higher indicates that it is safe to apply compression. A normal reading will be around one (Collier, 1999). Basic hand-held Doppler ultrasound machines retail at around £250.

REFERENCES

Berg, W, Traneroth, C, Gunnarsson, A, Lossing, C (1990) A method for measuring pressure sores. *Lancet* **335**: 1445–1446.

Bulstrode, CJK, Goode, JW, Scott, PJ (1986) Stereo-photogrammetry for measuring rates of cutaneous healing: a conventional technique. *Clinical Science* **71**: 4–443.

Calvin, M, Young, SR, Koffman, J, Dyson, M (1997) Pilot study using high frequency diagnostic ultrasound to assess surgical wounds in renal transplant patients. *Skin Research and Technology* **3**: 60–65.

Charles, D, Williams, K III, Perry, LC, Fisher, J, Rees, RS (1992) An improved method of *in vivo* wound disruption and measurement. *Journal of Surgical Research* **52**: 214–218.

Collier M (1999) Venous leg ulceration. In: Miller, M, Glover, D (eds) *Wound Management*. Nursing Times Books, London.

Covington, JS, Griffin, JW, Mendius, RK, Tooms, RE, Clifft, JK (1989) Measurement of pressure ulcer volume using dental impression materials. *Physical Therapy* **69**: 68–72.

Karim, A, Young, SR, Lynch, JA, Dyson, M (1994) A novel method of assessing skin ultrasound scans. *Wounds* **6**: 9–15.

Kundin, JI (1989) A new way to size up a wound. *American Journal of Nursing* **89**: 206–207.

Moffat, C, Harper, P (1997) Leg ulcers (ACE Series). Churchill Livingstone, New York.

Saperia, D, Glassberg, E, Lyons, RF (1986) Demonstration of elevated type I and II procollagen mRNA levels in cutaneous wounds treated with helium-neon laser. *Biochemical and Biophysical Research Communications* **136**: 1123–1128.

Smith, DJ, Bhat, S, Bulgrin, JP (1992) Video image analysis of wound repair. *Wounds* **4**: 6–15.

Vowden, K, Vowden, P (1996) Hand-held Doppler assessment for peripheral arterial disease. *Journal of Wound Care* **5**(3): 125–128

Whiston, RJ, Melhuish, J, Harding, KG (1993) High resolution ultrasound imaging in wound healing. *Wounds* **5**: 116–121.

Whiston, RJ, Young, SR, Lynch, JA, Harding, KG, Dyson, M (1993) Application of high frequency ultrasound to the objective assessment of healing wounds. In: *The 6th Annual Symposium on Advanced Wound Care*. Health Management Publications, pp 26–29.

Williams C (1995) HNE diagnostic Doppler ultrasound machines. *British Journal of Nursing* **4**(22): 1340–1344.

Young, SR (1988) *The Effect of Therapeutic Ultrasound on the Biological Mechanisms Involved in Dermal Repair.* PhD Thesis, University of London, pp 169–174.

Young, SR, Dyson, M (1990) The effect of therapeutic ultrasound on angiogenesis. *Ultrasound in Medicine and Biology* **16**: 261–269.

Young, SR, Koffman, J (1997) Sound reasons to prevent kidney rejection. *The Economist* **343**(8023): 134.

Young, SR, Lynch, JA, Leipins, PJ, Dyson, M (1993) Non-invasive method of wound assessment using high-frequency ultrasound imaging. In: *The 6th Annual Symposium on Advanced Wound Care*, Health Management Publications, pp 29–31.

Young, SR, Erian, A, Dyson, M (1996) High frequency diagnostic ultrasound: a noninvasive, quantitative aid for testing the efficacy of moisturizers. *International Journal of Aesthetic and Restorative Surgery* **4**: 1–5.

20

Electrical stimulation for wound healing: a review of current knowledge

Tim Watson

INTRODUCTION

Chronic wounds are a continuing problem within the health-care sector, and the costs of care are high. Effective care is therefore of great importance. Such wounds are treated in a wide variety of ways, one of which is based on the observed differences in electrical potential resulting from wounding and persisting through the stages of healing. This chapter will look at the current evidence for the efficacy of treatment using electrical stimulation.

The use of electrical stimulation as a means of enhancing wound healing is not a new approach. Reports dating back to the seventeenth century record the use of gold-leaf applications to cutaneous lesions associated with smallpox. Other workers have added to knowledge over the years, and it is the most recent view of this body of knowledge that is considered here.

Problems associated with chronic wounds

A relatively small proportion of wounds present with healing problems and most will heal spontaneously without major therapeutic intervention, including electrotherapy. However, some wound types are notoriously slow to heal, for example chronic venous ulcers and pressure sores. These tend to be lesions of long duration and are often resistant to many forms of treatment. They can result in significant medical, social and economical problems for patients, their relatives and the medical professionals involved.

The factors responsible for poor wound healing are legion and clearly beyond the scope of this chapter, but they remain central to the philosophy of the use of electrical stimulation as a modality to enhance healing. Interference with one or more levels of the cascade of events associated with any healing process can lead to inadequate healing and repair responses. Frank and Szeto (1983) summarised the possible general factors as follows:

- inability to form a blood clot or mount an adequate inflammatory reaction
- inability to produce new cells or scar components in adequate quantity or quality
- inability to organise the scar into an appropriate functional or cosmetic unit.

These factors can be considered on both a local and a systemic level. The local factors include infection, inadequate blood flow and nutrition, resulting in low oxygen levels and poor inflammatory response. Repeated wound stresses can also make a significant contribution. The systemic effects that may be detrimental include age-related changes, concurrent disease states and hormonal problems. Clearly, one could add to these lists with ever more detailed categories, but in principle there are a large number of factors which might be responsible for the interruption of a component of the healing process, and in doing so achieve a major healing dysfunction owing to the cascade nature of the normal healing events and the complex interactions between components of the processes.

Risk groups

The main groups of patients with superficial (i.e. skin) wounds likely to suffer from this delayed or prolonged healing can be divided into three major categories (Vodovnik and Karba, 1992):

1 spinal cord injury (with problems related to decreased movement, decreased sensation and disturbances in peripheral blood flow)
2 peripheral vascular disease (with ischaemia, tissue congestion and altered tissue viability)

3 the elderly (with decreased movement, altered blood flow and possibly additional multipathology).

Other groups have been identified using different criteria (e.g. Biedebach, 1989), but the high-risk patients are recognised as those presenting with concurrent problems which in some way inhibit or reduce the efficiency of the normal healing responses.

Variety of approaches

One of the main problems in reviewing the literature in this field is the wide variety of approaches adopted by the various research groups involved in both laboratory and clinical research. For the purposes of this chapter, the use of electrical stimulation to enhance or stimulate wound healing has been divided into three main (though somewhat arbitrary) approaches. Each approach described has reported beneficial clinical effects, and the available evidence at present does not appear to identify an optimal approach.

This chapter sets out to consider the effects of electrical stimulation on chronic skin wounds, particularly chronic venous ulcers, pressure sores and allied lesions. Additional work is available concerning electrical stimulation for promoting bone healing, though this aspect is not discussed in any detail (for additional reviews see Albert and Wong, 1991; Black, 1987; Gardner, Frantz and Schmidt, 1999; and Rubinacci *et al.*, 1988).

ELECTRICAL ACTIVITY IN THE SKIN RELATED TO WOUNDS AND HEALING

Skin batteries

There is good reason to believe that the human epidermis contains a skin battery capable of driving substantial currents into wounds. If wound healing is mediated at least in part by electrical signals, then the artificial exposure of wounds to electrical stimulation could be expected to alter the healing process (Weiss, Kirsner and Eaglstein, 1990).

Living tissues possess direct current electro-potentials that appear to regulate, at least in part, the healing process. Following tissue damage, a current of injury is generated that is thought to trigger biological repair. Exogenous electrical stimuli have been shown to enhance the healing of wounds both in humans and in animal models (e.g. Carley and Wainapel, 1985; Griffin *et al.*, 1991; and Weiss, Kirsner and Eaglstein, 1990).

The mammalian skin battery is quite powerful (at least in humans and guinea pigs) and it can maintain transcutaneous potential voltages of up to 80 mV (internally positive), and has a current-driving capacity of the order of 1 μA per millimetre of wound length (Jaffe and Vanable, 1984).

The work on skin batteries in mammals achieved a major forward step after the publication of the paper by Barker, Jaffe and Vanable, (1982) describing the skin battery of the guinea pig. They demonstrated a transcutaneous skin potential of 40–80 mV, the external surface being electrically negative compared with the sub-dermal tissues. The behaviour of the skin potential was then investigated following skin incision and it was established that the greater part of the skin resistance occurs across the stratum corneum, but that the potential is generated across the living epidermal layers (the stratum granulosum and basement membranes).

The transcutaneous potential at a wound that cuts right through the epidermis is zero, whilst a few millimetres away there is a normal voltage of 40–80 mV. There is a lateral voltage gradient, therefore, between the wound and the adjacent epidermis. This voltage gradient is steep, with an average value of 140 ± 20 mV/mm. Close to the wound, the outer surface of the living layer is electrically positive with respect to the outer surface of the living layer further from the wound (Jaffe and Vanable, 1984). These points are illustrated in Figure 20.1.

This work was extended by Foulds and Barker (1983) when they measured the transcutaneous potentials in 17 non-injured human volunteers. The surface potential was measured at 121 predetermined points in each subject, and referred to a common reference point which was subepidermal. The average potential for all sites on all subjects was 23 ± 9 mV, the surface always being negative with respect to the reference point. A consistent anatomical variation was demonstrated with the greatest potentials measured at the hands and the feet. No significant correlation was found between skin potential, and age or sex.

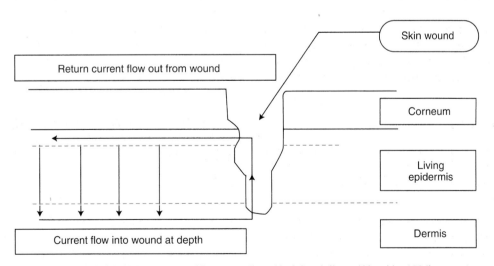

Figure 20.1 Current path with full-thickness wound in mammalian skin (after Jaffe and Vanable, 1984); current represents the movement of positive ions.

The skin potentials measured by Foulds and Barker (1983) were similar in magnitude and orientation to those measured in the guinea pig and some amphibian species. This skin potential appears to be capable of driving substantial currents into wounds and it is expected that lateral voltage gradients demonstrated in the guinea pig would also exist in human skin. It is suggested (Foulds and Barker, 1983; Jaffe and Vanable, 1984) that the lateral voltage gradients may be responsible for the epidermal cell migration across a healing wound.

Mammalian wounds heal more slowly when they are dry compared with when conditions are moist (Eaglstein and Mertz, 1978). Jaffe and Vanable (1984) noted that when wounds were allowed to become dry, the current was 'switched off' and the lateral voltage gradient was eliminated. Drying of the wound causes the resistance at the wound to increase and eliminates the potential drop at the wound margin (Barker, Jaffe and Vanable, 1982).

It is against this background that the electrical enhancement of wound healing is framed. The essential tenet is that normally healing wounds demonstrate electrical characteristics which can be superimposed in a variety of ways on those wounds that are not healing at the normal rate in an attempt to trigger the healing and repair process.

It has been suggested (Gentzkow and Miller, 1991) that the cascade of events which occur during and after the inflammatory/proliferative phases of healing may have been arrested in cases of chronic wounds. It was further suggested that the external electrical stimulation of these wounds produces effects that can 'restart' or 'jump-start' the healing phase.

The lateral voltage gradients associated with skin injury are within the limits of field strengths found to influence a variety of cells in several in vitro experiments. In addition to skin batteries, the piezoelectric potentials (stress-generated potentials), pyroelectric potentials (thermal-related potentials) and streaming potentials (interaction of charged fluids) can also be considered to exert an influence on the healing tissue (Charman, 1990a–e, 1991; Dayton and Palladino, 1989).

Skin battery changes on injury/healing

Bioelectric changes following injury have been demonstrated in several tissue types (predominantly bone, skin and nerve). The recorded potentials are different from those normally present in these tissues, though there does not appear to be any widely accepted explanation for the generation of such potentials (Watson, 1995). Their existence is generally accepted as being significant rather than just an epiphenomenon (Borgens, 1984) and it is considered by most authors that these potentials and subsequent current flow have a major role to play in initiating, controlling and terminating the repair process (Becker et al., 1962a,b, 1967, 1974a,b, 1977; Borgens, 1982; Burr, Harvey and Taffel, 1938; Foulds and Barker, 1983; Hinkle, McCaig and Robinson, 1981; Illingworth and Barker, 1980; Patel and Poo, 1982).

The bioelectric disturbances that occur on injury persist for various lengths of time depending on the tissue involved and the extent of the injury. Friedenberg and Brighton (1966), Wilber (1978), Illingworth and Barker (1980), Chang and Snellen (1982) and Chakkalakal, Wilson and Connolly (1988a,b) are amongst those who have monitored the electrical activity of damaged tissues as it progresses through its proliferative and healing processes. Each of these groups have reported progressive changes associated with the healing process and have obtained results from mammalian tissue.

The surface of a recent skin wound is electrically positive in relation to surrounding skin (Barnes, 1945; Illingworth and Barker, 1980) and, generally, it has been shown that this potential magnitude diminishes as healing progresses.

Many workers have considered the bioelectric correlates of injury/repair/regeneration in amphibians and other lower vertebrates. Borgens (1982, 1984) has established clear patterns of electrical behaviour in amphibians following limb amputation and subsequent regeneration.

Becker (1961) has demonstrated a difference in electrical behaviour between regenerating and non-regenerating species (Fig. 20.2). In regenerating systems (i.e. where the lost tissue is actually replaced with similar tissue), the initial injured positive polarity reverses to a high negative polarity and progressively returns to normal when the regeneration process is complete. In non-regenerating systems, the initial positive polarity slowly returns to normal with no phase of negative polarity (Becker, 1967). Whether this electrical activity is a consequence of local metabolic and physiological processes, or whether it acts as an initiator/control mechanism for the reparative process, has yet to receive unequivocal confirmation. Barker, Jaffe and Vanable (1982), Becker (1974a,b, 1982), Borgens and McCaig (1989), Kloth and McCulloch (1996), Vanable (1989), and Weiss, Kirsner and Eaglstein (1990), are amongst a growing body of researchers who present evidence for the latter view.

Further evidence to support the initiator/control theory is derived from studies (in animal models) where the natural electrical activity associated with tissue repair is inhibited or subjected to polarity reversal. The effect of this type of manipulation is either to slow down significantly, or more usually to inhibit completely, the normal repair process (Borgens, 1981).

The use of exogenous electrical potentials, fields and currents in order to facilitate tissue healing (in bone, nerve and skin) is becoming a clinically accepted technique. More than 80 papers have been identified which report research in this area. The results vary with tissue type, subjects and type of applied stimulus, but a high proportion claim significant enhancement of tissue healing.

One is led to the conclusions that tissues are electrically active, and that:

- following injury the behaviour of this electrical activity is modified
- as the repair process proceeds, there is a progressive return to a normal pattern of bioelectric behaviour.

Without necessarily considering the wider implications of the initiator/control concept, the physiological evidence is strong and gaining widespread acceptance.

BECKER'S GLOBAL DC THEORY

In addition to the evidence for local bioelectric phenomena, a more global bioelectric view is taken by some researchers in the field. Becker has produced a significant volume of literature expounding this aspect of bioelectric activity, highlighting the body-wide electric fields and current flow. Becker suggests that there are a series of equipotential lines that can be mapped from the body surface which reflect the organisation of a complex field with a spatial configuration which has a close relationship to the gross distribution of the central and peripheral nervous systems. In several species, including humans, the cranial, brachial and lumbar neuraxes were found to be electropositive, with an increasingly negative potential along the peripheral outflow (Becker, 1962). A complex pattern of axodendritic polarisation is proposed, with the steady DC potentials being transmitted by the Schwann cells in the periphery and the glial cells in the central nervous system. The nerves

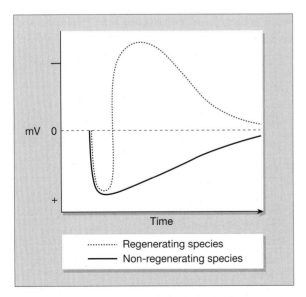

Figure 20.2 Difference between injury from regenerating and non-regenerating species (after Becker, 1974b, with permission of Elsevier Science).

are thought to be capable of carrying both action potentials (equated to digital signals) and slow DC potentials (equated to analogue signals). Local injury, trauma or disease is thought to lead to a disturbance of this body-wide potential pattern, acting as a stimulus for the healing, regenerative or reparative process appropriate to the tissue concerned (Figs 20.3 and 20.4).

Becker and colleagues (Becker and Spadaro, 1972; Becker, Spadaro and Marino, 1977) proposed a theoretical framework to model these events. First, an injury to a living system initiates a series of complex electrical currents at the site of injury, which are directly responsible for changes in both cell type and number. Secondly, the local electrical effect (the *current of injury*), is the primary response that is responsible for the appearance of new cells. The combination of these first two effects constitutes phase I of the model. Phase II involves the transmission of data to these new cells facilitating their ability to achieve the required repair and organisation into a self-regulating system. This theory does not deny the role of hormones and the numerous mediators involved in healing; instead, it suggests that there is a central monitoring and controlling role, which is electrical in nature, responsible for the initiation and management of the process (see Frank and Szeto, 1983 for a review).

The concept can be considered as a demand control model, with the injured tissue giving rise to an 'abnormal' potential, which initiates the tissue response. As healing and repair occur, the stimulus (the injury potential) diminishes, thus reducing the intensity of the stimulus for repair. This principle is illustrated below as a simple control diagram (after Black, 1987) (Fig. 20.5).

Becker's research remains controversial, but to many involved with electrical stimulation as a method of promoting tissue repair it is an attractive concept. The idea that the normal electrical activity of the tissues forms part of a global electrical network, which on disturbance provides a stimulus for repair and a simple feedback by which the reparative processes can be controlled, is attractive. Disturbance of this normal situation could be involved in delayed wound healing, thereby offering the opportunity to facilitate or enhance the process by external electrical intervention. Several studies have provided indirect evidence to support this theory including Chakkalakal, Wilson and Connolly (1988a, b); Chang and Snellen, (1982); and Weiss, Kirsner and Eaglstein (1990).

EVIDENCE OF EFFICACY

Studies have been conducted using cellular and animal models, as well as clinical trials.

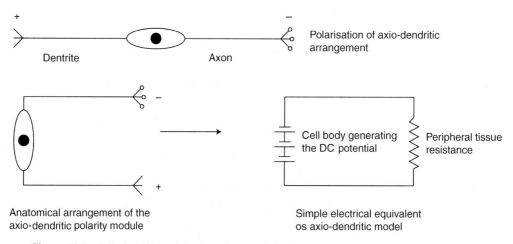

Dentrite

Axon

Polarisation of axio-dendritic arrangement

Cell body generating the DC potential

Peripheral tissue resistance

Anatomical arrangement of the axio-dendritic polarity module

Simple electrical equivalent os axio-dendritic model

Figure 20.3 Axio-dendritic polarisation of nerves (after Becker, Bachman and Friedman, 1962).

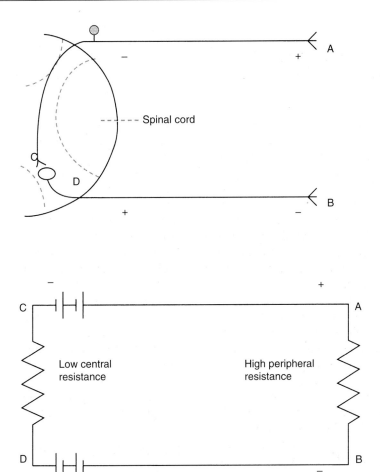

Figure 20.4 Physiological and electrical model of a neuron pair forming an elementary circuit (after Becker, Bachman and Friedman, 1962).

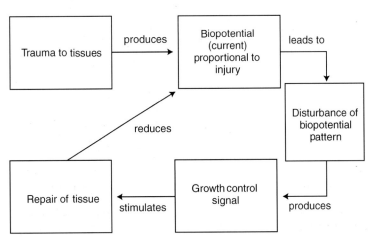

Figure 20.5 Control diagram for tissue repair stimulus/response (after Becker; Black, 1987).

Cellular studies

There is a substantial volume of published work concerning the effects of electrical stimulation on cell cultures and in vivo animal experiments. Numerous studies have demonstrated cellular responses to direct current, often at magnitudes comparable to those found physiologically.

Fibroblasts have been investigated by several groups, though not all studies have used human cultures. Dunn (1988) used DC stimulation when investigating fibroblast invasion of a collagen matrix placed in a skin wound in the guinea pig. It was found that fibroblast ingrowth and collagen fibre alignment were increased with DC stimulation compared with controls. The currents used were between 20 and 100 μA. Maximal fibroblast response was observed near the cathode.

Goldman and Pollack (1996) studied the effect of electrical stimulation (ES) on human fibroblasts in vitro. Various current intensities and frequencies were evaluated. A field strength of between 31 and 50 mV/mm was found to be effective at 10 Hz, but not at 100 Hz. The concept of frequency and amplitude windows appears to be supported by this work, and the effective parameters match those identified in the endogenous bioelectric state (Watson, 2000).

Erickson and Nuccitelli (1984) also used fibroblasts (from the quail embryo) and demonstrated cell migration towards the cathode when the cells were exposed to a DC field. The threshold field strength was found to be between 1 and 10 mV/mm. In addition to cell migration, they demonstrated changes in cell orientation, the fibroblasts realigning with their long axis perpendicular to the field direction. Field strengths of up to ten times greater than those necessary to induce fibroblast responses have been measured in vivo.

Ross, Ferrier and Aubin (1989) used human (adult) fibroblasts which were exposed to an electric field. Cellular alignment was noted with field strengths of 0.1 to 1.5 V/mm (100–1500 mV/mm), though they were unable to demonstrate mobility changes.

Gentzkow and Miller (1991) have reviewed several further studies involving fibroblasts.

These include the work of Bassett, Land and Hermann (1968) who showed that increases in DNA synthesis of 20% and of collagen synthesis (of up to 100%) occurred when fibroblasts were exposed to DC electric fields.

It has been suggested (Vodovnik, Miklavcic and Sersa, 1992) that cellular proliferation is modified by DC stimulation. If the proliferative rate is too low, it can be increased and, conversely, if the rate is too high then downregulation occurs with a reduced proliferative rate.

Cooper and Schliwa (1985) used epidermal cells (from fish) exposed to DC electric fields. The epidermal cells were observed to orientate in relation to the field and then to migrate towards the cathode. Chemotactic gradients were eliminated as a causal mechanism. The threshold for these effects was in the region of 0.5 V/cm (50 mV/mm), which represents some 1–4 mV per cell diameter. The demonstration by Winter (1964) that epithelial cells migrating from the periphery of an ulcer move in response to the voltage gradient is also pertinent to the discussion on the effects of electrical stimulation for wound healing.

In addition to fibroblasts and epidermal cells, several other cell types have been shown to respond to electrical stimuli. Cultured cartilage cells have shown an increase in cellular metabolism in response to a 1 μA DC stimulation (Okihana, Uchida and Shimorura, 1985) and mast cell numbers in healing wounds have been shown to be modified with DC stimulation (Reich et al., 1991). It was noted that a decrease in mast cell numbers followed pulsed electrical stimulation. No evidence was presented to show that the electrical stimulation had induced mast cell degranulation. The galvanotactic effect on neutrophils has been investigated by several groups (see Gentzkow and Miller, 1991). One interesting finding was that when tissues were inflamed, neutrophils were attracted to the cathode, suggesting a link between chemically mediated events and electrical responsiveness.

Cho et al. (2000) have demonstrated some fascinating effects of electrical stimulation (1 Hz, 2 V/cm) on the migration of human macrophages. The stimulation appears to change the migratory behaviour of the cells. The cells do not migrate any more rapidly, but their movement is less random.

Experimental results (predominantly from in vitro work) with neurons have demonstrated strong effects with DC electrical fields. Although not necessarily directly concerned with wound healing per se, it is important in the context of tissue repair, rather than simply skin lesion repair. Borgens (1988a, b) discussed at some length, the relationship between nerve injury potentials and degenerative and regenerative events. Long-term persistent injury potentials are thought to play a role in neuronal development and regeneration and, in addition, may have a modulating effect on the response of neurons to injury.

Patel (1986) demonstrated that neurites are attracted towards the cathode (−ve) pole in a DC field, and are repelled from the anode (+ve pole). Patel also discusses and develops a theoretical model that considers these effects in relation to the endogenous currents that could be present in damaged tissue. Pomeranz (1986) suggests that DC fields may enhance nerve growth in adult mammals. Significant results were achieved with cathodal (−ve) stimulation, whereas control and anodal stimulation experiments showed no effect. The effect was stronger for sensory than for motor nerves.

Other recent neuronal studies of interest include a well-cited paper by Hinkle, McCaig and Robinson (1981) describing neurite growth patterns in response to DC stimulation. Neurites were found to grow preferentially towards the cathode with field strengths of 7–190 mV/mm. The lower value appeared to be a threshold for their experiments (using frog neurites in vitro). In addition to the galvanotactic response, it was shown that greater numbers of neurons sprouted in the DC stimulation experiments and that fibroblasts were also stimulated, resulting in increased differentiation. Myoblasts were found to be responsive to greater field strengths (36–170 mV/mm) resulting in elongation and the development of a growth axis perpendicular to the field direction.

Finally, Patel and Poo (1982) demonstrated similar effects with cathodal galvanotaxis and preferential growth with neurons. The effects were reversible and did not appear to be related to electrode contaminants. This adds weight to the evidence for the effects of DC stimulation of neuronal cells.

Some results are conflicting, and not all publications report the exact stimulation parameters. However, there are common features including cellular orientation in relation to the field and cellular movement (galvanotaxis), usually towards the cathode.

Animal studies

Before considering the effects of electrical stimulation for wound healing in the clinical environment, it is pertinent to review some of the evidence generated from numerous animal experiments. It is difficult to extrapolate directly from this animal work as the wound-healing process is not identical, and although there are similarities between species there are no directly equivalent animal-healing models. The experimentation does, nevertheless, provide useful background material for the principles supporting clinical intervention.

A substantial number of studies have considered the electrical correlates of healing and regeneration in amphibian and vertebrate species. It is beyond the scope of this chapter to consider them in any depth, but the interested reader can read excellent recent reviews by Borgens and colleagues (Borgens, 1981, 1982; Borgens and McCaig, 1989; Borgens, Vanable and Jaffe, 1977; Borgens et al., 1989); and Sisken, (1983).

Chang and Snellen (1982) investigated the regenerative capacity in rabbit ears, noting that the naturally occurring potentials presented a similar pattern to the amphibian species in which true regenerative limb capacity had been retained. This pattern consists essentially of an initial wound-positive phase that lasts for approximately 1 week in the rabbit, which is followed by a wound-negative phase during the period of proliferative repair. The magnitude of the negative wound potential varied, and this variation appears to correlate with the regenerative ability, in that those animals which exhibited the largest negative wound potentials also demonstrated the most complete regeneration. The animals with negative potentials of smaller magnitude had less complete regeneration. Chang and Snellen (1982) observe that negative bioelectric activity accompanies growth and that whilst growth continues, the negative bioelectric potentials persist.

In an earlier series of experiments with rabbits (Wu *et al.*, 1967) the effects of electrical stimulation through a metallic suture in abdominal muscle lesions were investigated. Two suture materials were compared for effects: stainless steel and platinum. DC stimulation at 40–400 µA was used, and it was found that the rabbits with steel sutures gained greater wound strength than those with platinum sutures. The increases in wound strength did not appear to be related to stimulation polarity or intensity, and it was suggested therefore that the benefits of stimulation might be due to electrode products (Fe^{2+}) rather than the stimulation itself.

Skin incision work in rabbits is reported by Konikoff (1976) who used bilateral, full-thickness paravertebral incisions, with one side receiving DC stimulation whilst a sham treatment was delivered to the contralateral wound. A DC current of 20 µA was used and the wounds were tested at 1 week for tensile strength. The treated lesions required an average 53% increase in loading compared with the sham-treated wounds before separation. The polarity of the electrical stimulation was for the wound electrode to be made negative relative to the subcutaneous positive distal electrode.

Experiments with rats also feature in the animal-model research. Politis, Zanakis and Miller (1989) developed a full-thickness skin excision and replacement model. A necrotic area of skin resulted under control conditions following this procedure. After 1 week, the size of the necrotic area was compared in a control group and two treatment groups who had received DC stimulation with opposite-polarity currents. The group with the anode to the skin surface and the cathode implanted deep to the wound showed least necrosis (50%), whereas the reverse polarity stimulation group and the sham treatment group both had 80–90% necrosis after the same time period. The electrical stimulation was at 4.5 µA for 4 days following the operation.

Bach *et al.* (1991) also used a rat-skin wound model, comparing the effects of DC, AC and sham treatments on wound strength. The DC stimulation group used 1 V, 20 µA stimulation for 1 hour a day on days 4–8. The AC stimulation group used a sinusoidal current at 1 V peak, 100 µA, 300 Hz for 15 minutes/day on days 2–4. Neither type of electrical stimulation had a significant effect on wound strength when compared with controls, but both electrical stimulation groups showed significant increases in collagen content in and around the wound compared with the sham group. Some doubt has been raised as to the validity of measuring wound healing in terms of tensile strength alone (Forrest, 1983), although it has been used in numerous studies as a useful indicator.

Taskan *et al.* (1997) compared the effect of ultrasound and electrical stimulation in a rat wound model. Four groups were compared: real and sham ES, and real and sham ultrasound. Both real ES and US have beneficial effects, but the ES results were found to be superior to those attributed to the US.

Wound healing in pig skin has been extensively studied as it provides an animal model which more closely resembles human skin. Amongst the more recent studies, Im, Lee and Hoopes (1990) raised bilateral bipedicle skin flaps in pigs, the central portion of which is known to become ischaemic without intervention. This central zone was treated with electrical stimulation (pulsed DC) at 35 mA, 128 Hz, for 30 minutes twice a day over 9 days. The treatment protocol involved negative stimulation on days 1–3, positive stimulation on days 4–6 and negative stimulation again for days 7–9. The necrotic area in the treated animals was significantly less (13.2%) compared with that for the control group (28%).

The experimental work of Alvarez *et al.* (1983) also used a pig model, and compared the effects of DC stimulation, sham stimulation and no treatment on skin wounds that were evaluated for re-epithelialisation and collagen synthesis. They found that collagen content increased in the DC stimulation group and the epithelial covering was more rapid in the treatment group compared with the sham and no-treatment groups. In these experiments, the wound electrode was positive, with a dispersive (negative) electrode plate some distance from the lesion.

Stromberg (1988) reported the results of different electrical stimulation protocols on 13 skin wounds in pigs. They measured wound contraction and the open wound area. The stimulation groups received either DC stimulation with 35 mA unipolar square-wave stimulation for 30 minutes twice a day with the negative electrode at the wound, or an identical electrical stimulation but with the wound electrode polarity reversed every 3 days. The first group, with the consistently negative wound electrode, appeared to gain no benefit from the treatment, with a trend towards a retarded healing process. In contrast, in the second group the stimulated wound receiving an alternating wound electrode polarity demonstrated wound size decreases to 18% of the original size in 2 weeks, which was down to 5% of the original size by the end of 3 weeks of treatment.

Reger *et al.* (1999) compared the efficacy of DC and AC stimulation with a control condition on experimental skin ulcers in a pig model. Interestingly, both the AC and DC stimulation resulted in reduced healing time compared with the control condition, but the DC group showed the most rapid reduction in the wound area, and the AC stimulation showed the most rapid reduction in wound volume.

One animal study, which is not concerned directly with tissue healing, is of interest in that it demonstrates a fundamental physiological change associated with electrical stimulation. Reed (1988) investigated the effects of electrical stimulation on microvascular permeability changes in the hamster; the cheek pouch of the hamster offers a suitable model for microvascular changes which are observed relatively easily. Animals were given a dose of histamine in order to produce vasodilation and increased vascular permeability. The animals were divided into two groups, and one group received electrical stimulation in addition to the histamine. The stimulation consisted of a twin-pulse direct current given at 120 double pulses per second at peak voltages of 10, 30 and 50 V (giving currents of 10, 20 and 50 mA with average current densities of 0.02, 0.04 and 0.11 mA/mm^2). The pulses were of short duration and are illustrated in Figure 20.6. The effect of the electrical stimulation was to reduce the 'leakiness' from the vessels when compared with the histamine-only animals.

It is suggested that electrical stimulation of this type may be capable of retarding oedema formation. Chu *et al.* (1996) are amongst several groups who have reported the effects of electrical stimulation in relation to oedema formation following burn injury. Continuous DC stimulation was found to reduce oedema formation by up to 48% when applied up to 48 hours post burn injury.

There are many more animal studies reporting a wide variety of effects of electrical stimulation, and a more complete review is beyond the scope of this chapter.

Clinical trials

One of the problems with reviewing the literature concerning ES for wound healing is that there are multiple approaches, several variations with each area and a lack of controlled trials with large sample sizes. The mechanisms by which

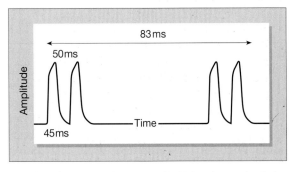

Figure 20.6 Current waveform for high-voltage stimulation (pulse rate = 120 double pulses per second).

ES achieves its results are still poorly understood and, although there are clearly links that can be established between the hypothetical effects of the treatment and the outcome of the intervention, the theoretical basis for the treatment remains tenuous in places. Nevertheless, the general trend of the clinical research reports is for beneficial effects to dominate, with only a minority of trials reporting zero or negative effects.

In clinical studies, there are three main approaches to the use of ES, though the differences within each group make direct comparison of the studies all but impossible. The main approaches are:

- the use of low-intensity direct current (LIDC)
- the use of pulsed LIDC
- the use of high-voltage pulsed galvanic stimulation (HVPGS) (also known as high-voltage pulsed current—HVPC).

The evidence for efficacy will be reviewed under these sections.

The polarity of stimulation may affect the outcome in clinical trials. Carey and Lepley (1962) have demonstrated that positive polarity stimulation attracts inflammatory cells to a wound site with an increase in the inflammatory reaction. Alvarez *et al.* (1983) have shown beneficial effects of ES on wound epithelialisation and collagen synthesis, encouraging cellular migration and stimulating collagen synthesis.

Decreased bacterial counts in wounds with negative-pole stimulation has been demonstrated by several groups working with patients in the clinical setting, often followed by stimulation of the healing response itself with the use of positive-pole stimulation (Carley and Wainapel, 1985; Dayton and Palladino, 1989; Gault and Gatens, 1976; Wolcott *et al.*, 1969). This approach has become popular, with several groups using combinations of negative-pole stimulation initially to reduce or eliminate bacterial infection, followed by positive-pole stimulation in order to enhance the proliferative process. This is sometimes further modified with alternating positive- and negative-pole stimulation when a healing plateau is reached.

LIDC

The measurement of small DC potentials associated with injury and the repair processes following musculoskeletal lesions (Barnes, 1945; Illingworth and Barker, 1980; Jaffe and Vanable, 1984) has resulted in a number of research groups using LIDC as a therapeutic tool in the management of non-healing or delayed-healing wounds.

DC stimulation was one of the first forms of ES to be used clinically, with reports as early as the seventeenth century concerning the application of charged gold leaf to smallpox lesions (see Dayton and Palladino, 1989). Many of the animal studies outlined above have used DC stimulation with encouraging results. The philosophy for the use of DC exogenous stimulation is that it can supplement or enhance the naturally occurring DC potentials associated with repair, and thereby stimulate the healing process, particularly in cases where the process is slow or appears to have stopped, as is the case with chronic venous ulcers and chronic pressure sores.

One of the first of the more recent research reports that involved the use of LIDC was by Assimacopoulos (1968) who treated chronic leg ulcers which had been resistant to all previous forms of therapy with DC stimulation. The ulcers were treated with negative polarity stimulation at currents up to 0.1 mA intensity. Complete healing was reported in 6 weeks. The main problem with this study was the very small sample ($n = 3$) and lack of any control group, thus limiting the strength of the results.

Soon after this, Wolcott *et al.* (1969) published the results of a more extensive study, in which 83 ischaemic ulcers were investigated. The DC stimulation involved three sessions a day, each of which lasted for 2 hours using current intensities of between 0.2 and 0.8 mA. One electrode (copper mesh) was placed in the wound, and the other on the skin surface proximally. The intensity of the stimulation was determined empirically as it was found that stimulation with too great an intensity resulted in a bloody exudate from the ulcer and stimulation with too low an intensity resulted in a serous exudate.

The intensity used fell between these two limits, being determined for each patient individually. The wound electrode was made negative initially, and maintained so for at least 3 days. If the ulcer was not infected at this stage, the electrode polarity was then reversed such that the wound electrode was made positive. Infected ulcers were stimulated with a negative wound electrode until the infection had cleared, and then for 3 further days; only then was the wound electrode made positive. All patients had the polarity of the wound electrode reversed each time a plateau was reached in the healing process.

The results from the 75 patients with a single ulcer were encouraging: 34 (45%) achieved 100% healing over 9.6 weeks with an average healing rate of 18.4% per week; of the remaining 41 ulcers, the mean healing rate was 9.3% per week and these patients achieved an average 64.7% healing over 7.2 weeks. Additional data were derived from a group of patients who presented with bilateral ulcers of comparable size and aetiology; these patients received ES to only one of the ulcers, the other acting as a control lesion. The results from these patients showed that six of the eight treated ulcers healed completely and the remaining two achieved 70% healing. The control ulcers from the same patients healed less well, with three of the eight showing no healing, a further three healing less than 50% and the remaining two healing by 75%. The average healing rate for the treated ulcers was 27% per week and for the control ulcers was 5% per week. Although these trial results are more convincing because of the increased sample size and the fact that there was a control group for part of the work, there are nevertheless pertinent issues which need to be highlighted. First, the control ulcers did also show signs of healing and this may either be due to the natural process at work, or be due to the effects of the ES to one ulcer causing the release of a systemic mediator substance which in turn stimulated the contralateral ulcer. It is not possible with this experimental design to differentiate between the possibilities. Secondly, a placebo effect cannot be discounted.

In addition to encouraging healing effects, the authors noted that there appeared also to be a strong antimicrobial effect associated with the initial wound-negative current application. Work on the bacteriostatic effects of LIDC by Rowley, McKenna and Wolcott (1974) demonstrated that the application of low-level direct electrical current to infected soft tissues retards the growth of bacteria which, coupled with normal defence mechanisms, enhances the destruction of infecting microorganisms. Further studies (Rowley, 1985) showed that LIDC enhances the destruction of infecting bacteria by retarding the growth of the bacteria and opening the capillary beds, therefore allowing the normal biological defences to act. In both of these reports, negative polarity stimulation was responsible for the bacteriostatic effects.

The work of Wolcott et al. (1969) is one of the most frequently cited in the field of ES for wound healing, and although there have been criticisms of the design and protocol (e.g. by Vodovnik and Karba, 1992) it remains an important paper. It is of interest that, although in principle the treatment was based on supplementing or enhancing the naturally occurring currents associated with healing, the polarity reversal on reaching a growth plateau does not appear to be based on a recognised physiological phenomenon. The published works which have measured rather than manipulated the potentials occurring with repair do not report multiple polarity reversals during the healing process (in non-regenerating species), and although in this study the effects were beneficial, the rationale for the approach is questioned.

A similar trial to that of Wolcott et al. was conducted by Gault and Gatens (1976) involving 76 patients with a total of 106 ischaemic ulcers of differing aetiology and location. Six patients presented with bilateral ulcers, providing a small control group. The treatment protocol was the same as the above study in that the wound electrode was negative initially and then changed to positive stimulation either after 3 days in the case of non-infected wounds or 3 days after the infection had been cleared in the case of infected wounds. The difference in this protocol was that once the positive stimulation had begun there was no reversal to the negative stimulation if a healing plateau was reached. For patients with a single ulcer, the mean healing rate was 28.4% per week (an improvement over the unilateral ulcer result from Wolcott's study). For the patients with bilateral ulcers, where one was treated with ES and one acted as a control, the mean healing rate of the control ulcers was 14.7% per week, and that of the treated ulcers was 30% per week. Wound asepsis was achieved typically in 3–7 days.

The third significant trial involving LIDC was a more rigorously controlled study by Carley and Wainapel (1985), using a similar but not identical protocol to Wolcott *et al.* (1969) and Gault and Gatens (1976). Thirty hospital inpatients were involved in the study, divided equally into a treatment and a control group by random selection. In addition to the equal size of groups, the patients were matched (paired) on the basis of age, diagnosis and wound aetiology, location and size.

The patients in the control group received conventional conservative therapy. The LIDC group received 2 hours of ES twice a day, 5 days a week in addition to the conventional therapy. The two stimulation sessions were separated by a 2–4 hour rest period when the machine gave no output but remained in situ. One electrode was placed at the wound site, and an indifferent or dispersive electrode was placed on the skin 15–25 cm proximally. The wound electrode had negative polarity for the first 3 days of the trial, after which time the polarities were reversed. The wound-positive arrangement was maintained until the wound healed or until there was a healing plateau, in which case the wound electrode was made negative again for a further 3 days and then reverted to positive. The current intensity was between 300 and 700 µA, determined empirically in the same manner as Wolcott *et al.* (1969). Wounds were measured and photographed on a weekly basis, and the programme continued for 5 weeks or until the ulcer had healed.

The results of the study showed that the patients in the LIDC group showed healing rates that were 1.5–2.5 times faster than those of their paired controls. The overall healing rate was two times greater. There was no significant difference between the wounds in the two groups at the commencement of the study and, in fact, the difference did not become apparent until week 3 of the study, after which it became progressively more significant.

In addition to the increased rate of healing, the scar tissue from the treatment group appeared to be stronger and there were fewer problems with wound infection. In the control group the healed tissue appeared thin and fragile and reopened in some patients. No patients in the treatment group required wound debridement during the trial period, whereas in the control group patients typically required repeated debridement. Patients in the LIDC group also reported decreased pain and discomfort compared with those in the control group.

The rationale for alternating the wound electrode polarity appears to be derived from the report by Rowley, McKenna and Wolcott (1974) concerning the effects of opposite polarities on rabbit wound healing. It was suggested that a negative-polarity wound electrode appears to encourage the resolution of infection, but does not stimulate healing, whereas the wound-positive electrode stimulates both infection and healing. Therefore, the suggestion that the wound electrode should be made negative until the infection cleared, then positive to promote the repair, has a rational basis. The alternating wound electrode polarity on reaching a healing plateau cannot be traced to the published literature, however.

Pulsed LIDC

Two recent publications have reported the use of pulsed LIDC for the treatment of chronic wounds. Mulder (1991) and Feedar, Kloth and Gentzkow (1991) both report the results from a randomised, double-blind, multicentre study with results presented from 47 patients with a total of 50 wounds. These wounds were of several different pathologies, covering nine different sites and at stages II–IV. Of the 50 wounds, 24 were allocated (randomly) to the control group and 26 to the treatment group. Patients in both groups were treated twice daily (with real or sham stimulation) using a small battery-powered device. Each session was for 30 minutes with a rest period of 4–8 hours between sessions. Treatment was thus applied 7 days a week for the first 4 weeks. The stimulation protocol was varied according to wound state (infected or non-infected) and wound stage (II–IV). The two pulse frequencies applied to the lesions are shown in Figure 20.7.

Infected wounds were treated at 128 pulses per second (p.p.s.) at a nominal current of 35 mA (measured at 29.2 mA through a 1 kΩ load) with a negative wound electrode. This stimulation was continued until the wound was infection free, and then continued for a further 3 days. Following this initial phase, the polarity of the wound electrode was alternated every 3 days until the wound reached stage II. After this time,

the pulse repetition rate was reduced to 64 p.p.s. and the wound electrode polarity was reversed daily. The initial part of the trial was conducted on a double-blind basis with neither the patient nor the investigator knowing whether real or sham treatment had been applied. After completion of this element, patients from the sham treatment (control) group were allowed to join the full-treatment programme along with any patient from the treatment group who had not achieved full healing.

The results were presented for the initial 4 week period and, additionally, for the follow-up study, with wound size reported as a percentage of the original size. Following the 4 week blind element, the treatment group wounds were 44% of their original size on average, whilst the control wounds averaged 67% of their initial size. The mean healing rate of the treated lesions was 14% per week compared with the control group healing rate of 8.25% per week. No wounds in

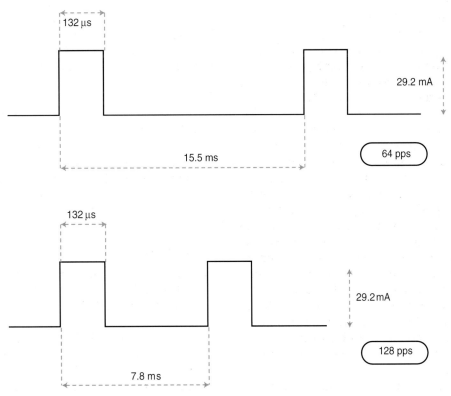

Figure 20.7 Pulse characteristics of monophasic pulsed currents used by Feedar, Kloth and Gentzkow, 1991.

the treatment group increased in size, compared with five wounds in the control group.

In the second phase, 14 wounds were crossed over to the stimulation protocol. The mean reduction in wound size during the sham treatment had been 11.3% at an average rate of 2.9% per week. After 4 weeks of active ES these wounds had reduced to 49% of their size at cross-over and had demonstrated a mean healing rate of 12.8% per week. With the exception of the ES parameters, all wounds in both groups were treated identically. The authors concluded that the results support the use of pulsed LIDC in the management of chronic dermal wounds at stages II, III and IV. The strength of the results is enhanced by the improvements in the cross-over group.

Weiss, Eaglstein and Falanga (1989) compared scar thickness and hypertrophic scar formation at the skin graft donor site in a small study of four patients. Each patient had bilateral split skin grafts taken from the anterior thigh. One site was given ES whilst the other acted as a control. The ES started on the day of surgery, and consisted of two sessions daily, each of 30 minutes' duration, which were continued for 7 days. The stimulation was delivered by a small unit as a pulsed DC stimulation at 128 p.p.s., the pulses being of 150 μs duration, at a peak current of 35 mA. The wound electrode was maintained at a positive polarity throughout the study. A combination of evaluation by three independent physicians and donor site punch biopsies at 2–3 months postsurgery provided data for the analysis.

The subjective findings strongly suggested that the scar at the donor sites which had been subjected to ES were softer, flatter and more cosmetically acceptable than the untreated scars. These differences were apparent by 1 month postsurgery and were persistent, but less marked at 6 months.

The biopsy data support the subjective (blinded) findings, the treated scars being on average 46% of the thickness of the untreated scars. Biopsies also showed fewer mast cells in the stimulated scars. The effect of ES under these conditions suggests that it can decrease fibrosis, possibly by reducing the number of mast cells.

HVPGS or HVPC

A more recent development in the use of ES for wound healing utilises a pulsed DC current applied at a high voltage—known as high-voltage pulsed galvanic stimulation (HVPGS) or high-voltage pulsed current (HVPC). The pulses are commonly 'twin pulses' of short duration and high intensity (100–500 V).

A study by Akers and Gabrielson (1984) reports the results of a comparative trial involving three treatment protocols with pressure ulcers in 14 patients. It is unfortunate that much of the critical information needed to replicate this study is omitted from the published report. The three treatment groups were whirlpool therapy once daily, whirlpool therapy plus ES twice daily, and ES alone twice daily. However, there was no control group and the initial condition of the patients in the three groups was not comparable in that the patients in the group receiving ES alone had sensory loss whilst those in the other groups still had some sensation. Also, the treatment parameters were not reported (i.e. electrode placement or polarity, stimulation intensity, characteristics, duration and patient numbers in each group). The results did not achieve statistical significance, but the underlying trend appeared to be that the group receiving ES alone achieved the best results, followed by the combined ES and whirlpool therapy group, and the least effective of the three treatments appears to have been the whirlpool therapy alone. The lack of significance was attributed to the wide variability in the results (and, one assumes, to the relatively small sample size).

A far more rigorous trial concerning the effects of HVPGS was reported by Kloth and Feedar (1988). A group of 16 patients with stage IV decubitus ulcers were recruited for the trial. All had lesions that had been unresponsive to previous treatment. Patients were allocated randomly to a treatment group ($n = 9$) or control (sham treatment) group ($n = 7$). The ES consisted of monophasic twin-pulse stimulation at 105 p.p.s. delivered at a voltage just below that required to achieve visible muscle contraction

(100–175 V). These stimulation parameters are reported as being arbitrarily set. ES was given for one 45 minute session a day for 5 days a week. Control group patients had electrodes placed in the same way, but the machine output was set to zero. Electrode polarity was set initially for the wound electrode to be positive, with the negative electrode placed on the skin surface proximally. If a healing plateau was reached during the trial, the wound electrode was made negative and the treatment continued. If a second plateau was reached, the electrode polarity was reversed daily thereafter. Whichever electrode was placed at the wound site, the relative arrangement was maintained in that the positive electrode was always placed cephalad in relation to the negative electrode.

All patients in the treatment group achieved complete healing of their ulcers (on average over 7.3 weeks at a mean healing rate of 44.8% per week). The control group patients did less well, with an increase in mean wound size of almost 29% between the first and last treatments. A subgroup of patients who were in the control group went on to complete a course of ES following the main trial; the three patients achieved full healing of their ulcers over 8.3 weeks with an average healing rate of 38% per week.

Griffin *et al.* (1991) assessed the effects of HVPC on pressure ulcer healing in a group of patients with spinal cord injury. Seventeen patients were assigned randomly to either a treatment or a control (sham treatment) group. ES treatments were carried out for 1 hour a day for 20 consecutive days with repeated wound assessments during this period. HVPC was delivered by means of a negative wound electrode with the stimulator delivering 100 p.p.s. at an intensity of 200 volts using similar twin pulses to the previous studies. The percentage change (decrease) in ulcer size for the treatment group was significantly greater at days 5, 15 and 20. The average change for all ulcers in the treatment group was an 80% size reduction compared with a 52% decrease for the control group.

Interestingly, Kincaid (1989) published a series of results highlighting the effects of HVPC on cultured bacterial species in a series of in vitro experiments. Three commonly isolated bacterial strains were exposed to positive and negative HVPC. All three strains were affected equally by 2 hours of HVPC above 250 volts. Cathodal (−ve) exposure resulted in bacterial death, whilst at the anode (+ve) toxic electrochemical end products appeared to be responsible for the bacterial demise. The authors suggested that HVPC could have significant antibacterial effects in the clinical environment.

Comparative studies

Stefanovska *et al.* (1993) conducted a comparative study involving three patient groups (DC stimulation, AC stimulation and a control group) with 250 patients, 170 of whom were spine-injured patients with 'pressure wounds'. The ES groups received conventional therapy in addition to the stimulation. DC stimulation utilised a 600 µA current for 2 hours daily, whilst the AC group patients were treated with low-frequency pulsed currents for 2 hours daily. (Further details of parameters are provided in the report.) The results suggested that the AC stimulation group achieved better results than the DC and control groups.

A recent study reported by Baker *et al.* (1997) compared the effect of asymmetric biphasic and symmetric biphasic square-wave pulsed stimulation with a control group. Eighty patients with open ulcers were involved in the study, the results of which demonstrated a significant increase in the healing rate, almost 60% in the group given the asymmetric stimulation. Symmetric pulse stimulation, in contrast, showed no significant advantage over the control condition.

Brief review of electrical stimulation for other tissue

Although the main emphasis of this chapter has been related to the effects of ES on wound healing for skin lesions, two further pieces or work deserve mention as they concern collagen repair—a tissue also involved in wound repair.

Both studies concern patellar tendon repair, both in animal models.

Stanish *et al.* (1985) considered the effects of ES as a method of stimulating tendon healing in the dog. Using a controlled surgical lesion of the patellar tendon in nine dogs, this comparative study evaluated the effects of: immobilisation alone, early mobilisation alone, and early mobilisation with ES using a constant current at $20\,\mu A$. The control and treated tendons were tested for breaking strength 8 weeks postoperatively and the results were reported as the percentage strength of the operated tendon, compared with the control tendon from the opposite limb of the same animal. The results clearly favoured the group receiving the early mobilisation combined with ES (92% of normal strength at 8 weeks), the immobilisation group and the early mobilisation group both having a much reduced strength (47% and 49% of normal respectively). The groups were small ($n = 3$), but the results appear to suggest a strong combined effect of ES together with early movement.

Akai *et al.* (1988) also conducted a study involving deliberate surgical insult to the patellar tendon, but this time in the rabbit. The study aimed to evaluate the effects of a constant direct current on healing from both a biomechanical and a biochemical aspect. Forty-five rabbits were used for the two types of test and, in addition, samples from a further 16 rabbits who underwent no surgery were used as baseline controls. A controlled lesion was produced bilaterally in the experimental animals. A treatment unit was implanted at the time of surgery with electrodes attached to both operated tendons, though only one was connected to the stimulator. The active stimulation consisted a cathodal ($-$ve) stainless steel electrode sutured at the tendon defect. The second electrode was implanted to the lateral aspect of the joint. A direct current of $10\,\mu A$ was passed through the electrodes to one knee only. Animals were sacrificed at various times following the surgery, and the results show that the tensile stiffness of the treated tendons was significantly higher than that for the control (sham-treated) tendons at week 5 after surgery.

Differences in the collagen production showed a trend for different peaks, but these were not statistically significant. By week 7, both the treated and the control tendons had achieved the same collagen mass as the intact (non-operated) tendons. However, there were marked differences between the group in terms of the ratio of type III collagen (which contributes to tissue elasticity) to type I collagen (which contributes to tissue strength). The non-operated tendons showed a negligible amount of type III collagen, whereas both operated groups (treated and sham treated) showed an increased percentage of type III. There was also a difference between the two operated groups, in that the tendons which had been exposed to ES had significantly less type III collagen at 3, 5 and 7 weeks. In conclusion, the dominant effect of ES under the conditions described appeared to be to promotion of early remodelling of the repair, producing a more mature collagen type at an earlier stage.

CONCLUSIONS AND CLINICAL IMPLICATIONS

The exact mechanism by which ES appears to enhance wound healing has not been established. Many components of the physiological response have been identified however, and are supported by the research to a greater or lesser extent. The clinical results support the use of ES in a variety of forms as a method which contributes to the management of chronic skin ulceration. Nevertheless it would be inappropriate to suggest that ES alone would produce significant changes in chronic wound healing. In addition to ES, other wound management factors may contribute to healing. Given the limited number of controlled trials, it is difficult to quantify the strength of the ES effect.

The effects and possible mechanisms of ES have been discussed in many of the publications cited in this chapter. Some of these effects are directly supported by the research, whilst some remain speculative.

Frank and Szeto (1983) suggest that electrical stimulation can affect soft tissue healing by inhibiting negative healing factors, by speeding normal healing processes, or by creating new and improved healing pathways, thus improving both the rate and the endpoint of scar formation of tissue regeneration.

Dayton and Palladino (1989) suggest that the possible effects of ES on wounds include reduction of bacteria (due to local pH changes, bactericidal ion release from the electrode, or phagocytic stimulation), increased rate of wound healing, increased wound strength, improved scar quality and pain relief.

Biedebach (1989) suggests both a local tissue response and a general vasodilatory response, which may be neuronal or chemically mediated. Animal studies support the idea of a local tissue response, together with DNA, ATP and protein (collagen) synthesis increases, following the passage of current through the tissue. There is also some evidence for this being a CNS-mediated mechanism, for instance the demonstration that in spinal injury patients the response to ES is less marked than in other patients (Wolcott et al., 1969). Additionally, there is evidence for a chemically mediated mechanism. Bourguignon and Bourguignon (1987) in one study demonstrated activation of fibroblasts by ES and in a separate study showed the effects of ES on T lymphocytes, with increased Ca^{2+} levels, and kinase activity, receptor clustering and increased DNA synthesis. It is suggested that calcium ions may act as the mediator for many of the changes in cell activation which have been observed, with this ion acting as a second messenger. It is possible that increased cellular Ca^{2+} uptake not only results in increased cellular motility (via the actin and myosin in cytoskeleton) but is also linked to cellular energy production (ATP) via mitochondrial mechanisms (see Ch. 2).

Dunn (1988) has suggested that the effects of ES in accelerating wound healing may be a consequence of:

- modification of endogenous bioelectricity
- activation or attraction of inflammatory cells
- presence of electrode-breakdown products
- attraction of connective tissue cells
- enhanced cell replication

- enhanced cell biosynthesis
- inhibition of infectious microorganisms.

Lundberg, Kiartansson and Samuelsson (1988) demonstrated significant changes in capillary-filling mechanisms in tissue with venous stasis, with subsequent reduction of oedema and stasis, whilst Griffin et al. (1991), in acknowledging the lack of a confirmed mode of action of ES in relation to wound healing, suggest that there are several attractive hypotheses. These include the attraction of connective tissue and inflammatory cells, modification of endogenous electrical potentials of tissue, stimulation of cellular biosynthesis and replication, bactericidal effects, enhanced circulation and the generation of a cellular electrophysiological effect. Some changes at electrode sites (e.g. pH changes, ion release from electrodes) may be making a contribution during LIDC, but it is suggested from the available evidence that these reactions have not been demonstrated in a series of in vitro experiments with HVPC.

A wide range of ES applications have apparently been responsible for enhanced soft tissue (particularly skin) healing. Scepticism has often been voiced (quite reasonably) as many of these trials have lacked controls, have failed to report important stimulation parameters and often involve relatively small numbers of subjects. In a recent critical review, Sheffet, Cytryn and Louria (2000) have suggested that a power analysis shows that a sample of at least 164 patients would be required to make a comparison and allow attention to be paid to critical variables. Confounding variables such as electrode contamination and the strength of the placebo effect could be responsible for a proportion of the results, but the accumulating evidence for the beneficial effects of electrical stimulation under a variety of applications suggests that a 'real' effect is likely. When the internal (endogenous) electrical activity of the body is considered, the electrical links between physiological processes and electrical activity are unlikely to be epiphenomenal. This being the case, externally applied electrical and electromagnetic stimulation in its numerous guises could reasonably be responsible for an alteration in healing responses. The exact mechanisms remain unexplained, but the clinical results support the tenet that external energy intervention can have significant effects. Important questions remain, however, and much further work is needed to identify the most important parameters. For instance, the stimulation could be used as a trigger to stimulate the process using amplitude or frequency windows. Alternatively, the energy input could force a chemical event or cascade, thereby stimulating natural events from an alternative starting point.

This overview of one aspect of electrical stimulation is probably just the visible part of a substantial iceberg. Other chapters have considered the effects of different energy forms (mechanical, electrical and electromagnetic), and the resultant picture should be one of excitement rather than despair. The key to progress is research both in the laboratory and in the clinical field, providing the key(s) that will enable utilisation of the endogenous bioelectric systems associated with healing and repair.

REFERENCES

Akai, M, Oda, H, Shirasaki, Y, Tateishi, T (1988) Electrical stimulation of ligament healing; An experimental study of the patellar ligament of rabbits. *Clinical Orthopaedics* **235**: 296–301.

Akers, TK, Gabrielson, AL (1984) The effect of high voltage galvanic stimulation on the rate of healing of decubitus ulcers. *Biomedical and Scientific Instrumentation* **20**: 99–100.

Albert, SF, Wong, E (1991) Electrical stimulation of bone repair. *Clinics in Pediatric Medicine and Surgery* **8**(4): 923–935.

Alvarez, OM, Mertz, PM, Smerbeck, RV, Eaglstein, WH (1983) The healing of superficial skin wounds is stimulated by external electrical current. *Journal of Investigations in Dermatology* **81**: 144–148.

Assimacopoulos, D (1968) Wound healing promotion by the use of negative electric current. *American Surgery* **34**: 423–431.

Bach, S, Bilgrav, K, Gottrup, F, Jorgensen, TE (1991) The effect of electrical current on skin incision. *European Journal of Surgery* **157**: 171–174.

Baker, LL, Chambers, R, DeMuth, SK, Villar, F (1997) Effects of electrical stimulation on wound healing in patients with diabetic ulcers. *Diabetes Care* **20**(3): 405–412.

Barker, AT, Jaffe, LF, Vanable, JW (1982) The glabrous epidermis of cavies contains a powerful battery. *American Journal of Physiology* **242**: R358–R366.

Barnes, TC (1945) Healing rate of human skin determined by measurement of the electrical potential of experimental abrasions. *American Journal of Surgery* **69**: 82–88.

Bassett, C, Land, A, Herrmann, I (1968) The effect of electrostatic fields on macromolecular synthesis by fibroblasts *in vitro. Journal of Cell Biology* **39**: 9A.

Becker, RO (1961) The bioelectric factors in amphibian limb regeneration. *Journal of Bone and Joint Surgery* **43A**: 643–656.

Becker, RO (1962) Some observations indicating the possibility of longitudinal charge-carrier flow in the peripheral nerves. *Biological Prototypes Synthetic Systems* **1**: 31–37.

Becker, RO (1967) The electrical control of growth processes. *Medical Times* **95**: 657–669.

Becker, RO (1974a) The basic biological data transmission and control system influenced by electrical forces. *Annals of the New York Academy of Sciences* **238**: 236–241.

Becker, RO (1974b) The significance of bioelectric potentials. *Bioelectrochemistry and Bioenergetics* **1**: 187–199.

Becker, RO (1982) Electrical control systems and regenerative growth. *Journal of Bioelectricity* **1**(2): 239–264.

Becker, RO, Bachman, CG, Friedman, H (1962) The direct current control system: A link between environment and organism. *New York State Journal of Medicine* **62**: 1169–1176.

Becker, RO, Bachman, CH, Slaughter, WH (1962) Longitudinal direct current gradients of spinal nerves. *Nature* **196**: 675–676.

Becker, RO, Murray, DG (1967) A method for producing cellular dedifferentiation by means of very small electrical currents. *Transactions of the New York Academy of Sciences* **29**: 606–615.

Becker, RO, Spadaro, JA (1972) Electrical stimulation of partial limb regeneration in mammals. *Bulletin of the New York Academy of Medicine* **48**(4): 627–641.

Becker, RO, Spadaro, JA, Marino, AA (1977) Clinical experiences with low intensity direct current stimulation of bone growth. *Clinical Orthopedics and Related Research* **124**: 75–83.

Biedebach, MC (1989) Accelerated healing of skin ulcers by electric stimulation and the intracellular physiological mechanisms involved. *Acupuncture and Electrotherapeutics* **14**: 43–60.

Black, J (1987) *Electrical Stimulation: Its Role in Growth, Repair and Remodelling of the Musculoskeletal System.* Praeger, New York.

Borgens, RB (1981) *Injury, Ionic Currents and Regeneration. Mechanisms of Growth Control.* Charles C Thomas, Springfield, IL, pp 107–136.

Borgens, RB (1982) What is the role of naturally produced electric current in vertebrate regeneration and healing? *International Review of Cytology* **76**: 245–298.

Borgens, RB (1984) Endogenous ionic currents traverse intact and damaged bone. *Science* **225**: 478–482.

Borgens, RB (1988a) Stimulation of neuronal regeneration and development by steady electrical fields. *Advances in Neurology* **47**: 547–564.

Borgens, RB (1988b) Voltage gradients and ionic currents in injured and regenerating axons. *Advances in Neurology* **47**: 51–66.

Borgens, RB, McCaig, CD (1989) *Endogenous Currents in Nerve Repair, Regeneration and Development. Electric Fields in Vertebrate Repair.* Alan R Liss, New York, pp 77–116.

Borgens, RB, Robinson, K, Vanable, JW, McGinnis, M (1989) *Electric Fields in Vertebrate Repair: Natural and Applied Voltages in Vertebrate Regeneration and Healing.* Alan R Liss, New York.

Borgens, RB, Vanable, JW, Jaffe, LF (1977) Bioelectricity and regeneration: Large currents leave the stumps of regenerating new limbs. *Proceeedings of the National Academy of Sciences, USA* **74**(10): 4528–4532.

Bourguignon, GJ, Bourguignon, LY (1987) Electric stimulation of protein and DNA synthesis in human fibroblasts. *FASEB Journal* **1**(8): 398–402.

Burr, HS, Harvey, SC, Taffel, M (1938) Bio-electric correlates of wound healing. *Yale Journal of Biology and Medicine* **11**: 103–107.

Carey, LC, Lepley, D (1962) Effect of continuous direct electrical current on healing wounds. *Surgical Forum* **13**: 33–35.

Carley, PJ, Wainapel, SF (1985) Electrotherapy for acceleration of wound healing: Low intensity direct current. *Archives of Physical Medicine in Rehabilitation* **66**: 443–446.

Chakkalakal, DA, Wilson, RF, Connolly, JF (1988a) Epidermal and endosteal sources of endogenous electricity in injured canine limbs. *IEEE Transactions in Biomedical Engineering* **35**: 19–29.

Chakkalakal, DA, Wilson, RF, Connolly, JF (1988b) Electrophysiologic basis for prognosis in fracture healing. *Medical Instrumentation* **22**(6): 312–322.

Chang, KS, Snellen, JW (1982) Bioelectric activity in the rabbit ear regeneration. *Journal of Experimental Zoology* **221**: 193–203.

Charman, RA (1990a) Bioelectricity and electrotherapy—towards a new paradigm: introduction. *Physiotherapy* **76**(9): 502–503.

Charman, RA (1990b) Bioelectricity and electrotherapy—towards a new paradigm: Part 1, The electric cell. *Physiotherapy* **76**(9): 503–508.

Charman, RA (1990c) Bioelectricity and electrotherapy—towards a new paradigm: Part 2, Cellular reception and emission of electromagnetic signals. *Physiotherapy* **76**(9): 509–516.

Charman, RA (1990d) Bioelectricity and electrotherapy—towards a new paradigm: Part 4, Strain generated potentials in bone and connective tissue. *Physiotherapy* **7**(11): 725–730.

Charman, RA (1990e) Bioelectricity and electrotherapy—towards a new paradigm: Part 5, Exogenous currents and fields—experimental and clinical applications. *Physiotherapy* **76**(12): 743–750.

Charman, RA (1991) Bioelectricity and electrotherapy—towards a new paradigm: Part 6, Environmental currents and fields—the natural background. *Physiotherapy* **77**(1): 8–14.

Cho, MR, Thatte, HS, Lee, RC, Golan, DE (2000) Integrin-dependent human macrophage migration induced by oscillatory electrical stimulation. *Annals of Biomedical Engineering* **28**(3): 234–243.

Chu, CS, Matylevich, NP, McManus, AT, Mason, AD, Pruitt, BA (1996) Direct current reduces wound edema after full-thickness burn injury in rats. *Journal of Trauma* **40**(5): 738–742.

Cooper, MS, Schliwa, M (1985) Electrical and ionic controls of tissue cell locomotion in DC electric fields. *Journal of Neuroscience Research* **13**: 223–244.

Dayton, PD, Palladino, SJ (1989) Electrical stimulation of cutaneous ulcerations. *Journal of the American Podiatric Medical Association* **79**(7): 318–321.

Dunn, MG (1988) Wound healing using collagen matrix: Effect of DC electrical stimulation. *Journal of Biomedical and Material Research* **22**(A2 Suppl): 191–206.

Eaglstein, WH, Mertz, PM (1978) New method for assessing epidermal wound healing: The effects of triamcinolone acetonide and polyethylene film occlusion. *Journal of Investigations in Dermatology* **71**: 382–384.

Erickson, C, Nuccitelli, R (1984) Embryonic fibroblast motility and orientation can be influenced by physiological electric fields. *Journal of Cell Biology* **98**(1): 296–307.

Feedar, JA, Kloth, LC, Gentzkow, GD (1991) Chronic dermal ulcer healing enhanced with monophasic pulsed electrical stimulation. *Physical Therapy* **71**(9): 639–649.

Forrest, L (1983) Current concepts in soft connective tissue wound healing. *British Journal of Surgery* **70**: 133–140.

Foulds, IS, Barker, AT (1983) Human skin battery potentials and their possible role in wound healing. *British Journal of Dermatology* **109**: 515–522.

Frank, CB, Szeto, AY (1983) A review of electromagnetically enhanced soft tissue healing. *IEEE Engineering in Medicine and Biology* **2**: 27–32.

Friedenberg, Z, Brighton, CT (1966) Bioelectric potentials in bone. *Journal of Bone and Joint Surgery* **48**(A): 915–923.

Gardner, SE, Frantz, RA, Schmidt, FL (1999) Effect of electrical stimulation on chronic wound healing: a meta-analysis. *Wound Repair and Regeneration* **7**(6): 495–503.

Gault, WR, Gatens, PF (1976) Use of low intensity direct current in management of ischaemic skin ulcers. *Physical Therapy* **56**: 265–269.

Gentzkow, GD, Miller, KH (1991) Electrical stimulation for dermal wound healing. *Clinics in Podiatric Medicine and Surgery* **8**(4): 827–841.

Goldman, R, Pollack, S (1996) Electric fields and proliferation in a chronic wound model. *Bioelectromagnetics* **17**(6): 450–457.

Griffin, JW, Tooms, RE, Mendius, RA, Clifft, JK, Vander Zwaag, R, Elzeky, F (1991) Efficacy of high voltage pulsed current for healing of pressure ulcers in patients with spinal cord injury. *Physical Therapy* **71**(6): 433–442.

Hinkle, L, McCaig, CD, Robinson, KR (1981) The direction of growth of differentiating neurones and myoblasts from frog embryos in an applied electric field. *Journal of Physiology* **314**: 121–135.

Illingworth, CM, Barker, AT (1980) Measurement of electrical currents emerging during the regeneration of amputated finger tips in children. *Clinical Physics and Physiological Measurement* **1**(1): 87–89.

Im, MJ, Lee, WPA, Hoopes, JE (1990) Effect of electrical stimulation on survival of skin flaps in pigs. *Physical Therapy* **70**(1): 37–40.

Jaffe, LF, Vanable, JW (1984) Electric fields and wound healing. *Clinics in Dermatology* **2**(3): 34–44.

Kincaid, CB (1989) Inhibition of bacterial growth in vitro following stimulation with high voltage, monophasic, pulsed current. *Physical Therapy* **69**: 651–655.

Kloth, LC, Feedar, JA (1988) Acceleration of wound healing with high voltage, monophasic pulsed current. *Physical Therapy* **68**: 503–508.

Kloth, LC, McCulloch, JM (1996) Promotion of wound healing with electrical stimulation. *Advances in Wound Care* **9**(5): 42–45.

Konikoff, JJ (1976) Electrical promotion of soft tissue repairs. *Annals of Biomedical Engineering* **4**: 1–5.

Lundberg, T, Kiartansson, J, Samuelsson, U (1988) Effect of electrical nerve stimulation on healing of ischaemic skin flaps. *Lancet* **2**(8613): 712–714.

Mulder, GD (1991) Treatment of open skin wounds with electric stimulation. *Archives of Physical Medicine in Rehabilitation* **72**: 375–377.

Okihana, H, Uchida, A, Shimorura, Y (1985) Effects of direct current on the cultured growth of cartilage cells. In: Fukada, E, Inoue, S, Sakou, T, Takahashi, H, Tsuyama, N (eds) *Bioelectrical Repair and Growth*. 4th Annual Meeting of Biological Repair and Growth Society, Nishimura, Japan, pp 103–108.

Patel, NB (1986) Reversible inhibition of neurite growth by focal electric currents. *Progress in Clinical and Biological Research* **210**: 271–278.

Patel, NB, Poo, M-M (1982) Orientation of neurite growth by extracellular electric fields. *Journal of Neuroscience* **2**(4): 483–496.

Politis, MJ, Zanakis, MF, Miller, JE (1989) Enhanced survival of full thickness skin grafts following the application of DC electrical fields. *Plastic Reconstructive Surgery* **84**(2): 267–272.

Pomeranz, B (1986) Effects of applied DC fields on sensory nerve sprouting and motor nerve regeneration in adult rats. *Progress in Clinical and Biological Research* **210**: 251–260.

Reed, BV (1988) Effect of high voltage pulsed electrical stimulation on microvascular permeability to plasma proteins—A possible mechanism in minimising edema. *Physical Therapy* **68**: 491–495.

Reger, SI, Hyodo, A, Negami, S, Kambic, HE, Sahgal, V (1999) Experimental wound healing with electrical stimulation. *Artificial Organs* **23**(5): 460–462.

Reich, JD, Cazzaniga, AL, Mertz, PM, Kerdel, FA, Eaglstein, WH (1991) The effect of electrical stimulation on the number of mast cells in healing wounds. *Journal of the American Academy of Dermatology* **25**(1): 40–46.

Ross, SM, Ferrier, JM, Aubin, JE (1989) Studies on the alignment of fibroblasts in uniform applied electric fields. *Bioelectromagnetics* **10**: 371–384.

Rowley, BA (1985) Electrical enhancement of healing. *Proceedings of the IEEE National Aerospace and Electronics Conference (NAECON)*. IEEE, Dayton, OH.

Rowley, BA, McKenna, JM, Wolcott, LE (1974) The use of low level electrical current for enhancement of tissue healing. *Biomedical Scientific Instrumentation* **10**: 111–114.

Rubinacci, A, Black, J, Brighton, C, Friedenberg, Z (1988) Changes in bioelectric potentials on bone associated with direct current stimulation of osteogenesis. *Journal of Orthopaedic Research* **6**: 335–345.

Sheffet, AA, Cytryn, S, Louria, DB (2000) Applying electric and electromagnetic energy as adjuvant treatment for pressure ulcers: a critical review. *Ostomy Wound Management* **46**(2): 28–33, 36–40, 42–44.

Sisken, BF (1983) Nerve and limb regeneration. *IEEE Engineering in Medicine and Biology* **2**: 32–39.

Stanish, W, MacGillvary, G, Rubinovich, M, Kozey, J (1985) The effects of electrical stimulation on tendon healing. In: Fukada, E, Inoue, S, Sakou, T, Takahashi, H, Tsuyama, N (eds) *Bioelectrical Repair and Growth*. 4th Annual Meeting of Bioelectrical Repair and Growth Society, Nishimura, Japan, pp 311–318.

Stefanovska, A, Vodovnik, L, Benko, H, Turk, R (1993) Treatment of chronic wounds by means of electric and electromagnetic fields: Part 2: Value of FES parameters for pressure sore treatment. *Medical and Biological Engineering and Computing* **31**: 213–220.

Stromberg, BV (1988) Effects of electrical currents on wound contraction. *Annals of Plastic Surgery* **21**(2): 121–123.

Taskan, I, Ozyazgan, I, Tercan, M, *et al.* (1997) A comparative study of the effect of ultrasound and electrostimulation on wound healing in rats. *Plastic Reconstructive Surgery* **100**(4): 966–972.

Vanable, JW (1989) *Integumentary Potentials and Wound Healing. Electric Fields in Vertebrate Repair*. Alan R Liss, New York, pp 171–224.

Vodovnik, L, Karba, R (1992) Treatment of chronic wounds by means of electric and electromagnetic fields. *Medical and Biological Engineering and Computing* **30**: 257–266.

Vodovnik, L, Miklavcic, D, Sersa, G (1992) Modified cell proliferation due to electrical currents. *Medical and Biological Engineering and Computing* **30**: CE21–CE28.

Watson, T (1995) *The Bioelectric Correlates of Musculoskeletal Injury and Repair*. PhD thesis, University of Surrey.

Watson, T (2000) The role of electrotherapy in contemporary physiotherapy practice. *Manual Therapy* **5**(3): 132–141.

Weiss, DS, Eaglstein, WH, Falanga, V (1989) Exogenous electric current can reduce the formation of hypertrophic scars. *Journal of Dermatology, Surgery and Oncology* **15**: 1272–1275.

Weiss, DS, Kirsner, R, Eaglstein, WH (1990) Electrical stimulation and wound healing. *Archives of Dermatology* **126**: 222–225.

Wilber, MC (1978) Surface direct current bioelectric potentials in the normal and injured human thigh. *Texas Reports on Biology and Medicine* **36**: 197–204.

Winter, GD (1964) Epidermal regeneration studies in the domestic pig. In: Montagna, W, Billingham, RE (eds) *Advances in the Biology of Skin*. Pergamon Press, Oxford, pp 113–127.

Wolcott, LE, Wheeler, PC, Hardwicke, HM, Rowley, BA (1969) Accelerated healing of skin ulcers by electrotherapy. *Southern Medical Journal* **62**: 795–801.

Wu, KT, Go, N, Dennis, C, Enquist, I, Sawyer, PN (1967) Effects of electric currents and interfacial potentials on wound healing. *Journal of Surgical Research* **7**: 122–128.

CONTENTS

Appendix: Safety in practice

Sarah Bazin

Safety including regular maintenance is of paramount importance in the application of all electrophysical agents, and the general aspects are covered in this Appendix. (Particular contraindications are addressed in the relevant chapters.) Recently there has been a greater emphasis on risk management and a tightening of health and safety regulation.

SAFE APPLICATION

Irrespective of the mode of treatment used, physiotherapists have a duty of care to the patient and should confine themselves to their scope of practice in the use of electrophysical modalities, taking into account physiological and therapeutic effects, safe application, precautions and contraindications. There should be access to relevant literature, equipment evaluation reports, safety bulletins, hazard notices and clinical research papers.

It is important that all treatment interactions are documented and signed. These should include assessment, indications for use, results of skin sensation tests, modality and machine used, time setting and treatment parameters and effects—beneficial or adverse—and outcome. As part of the assessment process, any drugs being taken by the patient must be identified as these could sensitise them or mask their condition and therefore alter their response to the intervention. Note that electrotherapy must *never* be used in the treatment programme for patients who are unable to understand warnings and instructions.

Before treatment, a visual check is made of the equipment in relation to plugs, cables, leads, electrodes, controls, dials and indicator lights, and the output should have been tested prior to use. The patient is then made comfortable and the area to be treated is exposed and inspected, both before and after treatment.

The patient must be able to contact the physiotherapist at all times during the treatment session. Patients should be advised not to move during treatment or touch the machine or controls, unless the equipment is fitted with a patient switch-off device, in which case they should be instructed in its use. It is important to ensure that the leads do not touch the patient or trail on the floor and/or that the machine is not within the field of another modality that could distort the field and alter the effectiveness of treatment. Electrodes and cables should not be adjusted whilst the apparatus is in operation.

MAINTENANCE OF EQUIPMENT

Correct maintenance ensures that electrotherapy equipment is in the optimal condition for use. Faults should be reported immediately and the machine or part must be removed from use until repaired.

Advice on the safe management of electro-medical equipment is laid down in *Health Equipment Information HEI 98* produced by the UK Department of Health.

Regular maintenance minimises breakdown. When purchasing electrotherapy equipment for use in the UK National Health Service, MLQ request forms are sent out by supplies departments to suppliers to reduce the risk of buying equipment which does not comply with BS 5724 and its supplements, which are synonymous with the International Electrotechnical Commission Standard IEC 601. The aim is to prevent faulty equipment being put into use and to ensure that correct equipment records are maintained.

Maintenance contracts

Procedures for the testing of new machinery are outlined in *Health Equipment Information HEI* 95 and should be undertaken by the supplier before use. In the UK National Health Service the machine will also be checked for safety and function by the electromedical engineer.

Maintaining equipment in good working order is important, and a check should be made once a year as a minimum, though if there is heavy usage twice a year is desirable. This should be undertaken by a reputable company on a maintenance contract. The credentials of the company should be checked to ensure that it is appropriately licensed to maintain different manufacturers' equipment and to obtain and fit specialised spare parts. Maintenance contracts can be set up with individual suppliers to service their own equipment. The practitioner should check that the full maintenance contract includes planned preventative maintenance, all breakdown callouts and the cost of labour, travel and spares. The cost of maintenance options varies widely, but the most comprehensive contract should cost less than 10% per annum of the capital cost of the equipment.

It is important to monitor the service contract, to check that visits are made, that all equipment is checked as agreed, and a report on its condition and the work done is received and kept. In the UK no one other than the agreed contractor should repair equipment, as this may remove liability under the Product Liability Act and the Consumer Protection Act. Maintenance service specifications should meet the needs of the service.

THE ENVIRONMENT

It is important that there are facilities for the safe storage of equipment. The area should be kept clean and dry, and care should be taken over trailing leads.

EQUIPMENT LOAN

Equipment is often loaned to patients on a trial basis. It is most important that the equipment is checked to be electrically safe. Patients must be well instructed in its use, effects and maintenance, backed up by written instructions. These must include information about a contact point in case of problems. Regular contact must be kept with the patient during the loan period to ensure adherence. Records must be kept of each item loaned.

Indemnity

Where machinery is loaned by a company on a trial basis, an indemnity form must be completed by both the supplier and a representative of the NHS Trust or practice. This protects the practitioner/hospital from litigation or damage as a result of any failure of the loaned equipment.

STAFF EXPOSURE

Operators must minimise their exposure to the effects of the treatment being applied.

PLANNED REPLACEMENT

It is recommended that there should be a policy to ensure that equipment is replaced in a planned manner; new equipment is likely to have a manufacturer's specified life expectancy.

Index

Multimedia CD-ROM
Single User License Agreement

1. NOTICE. WE ARE WILLING TO LICENSE THE MULTI-MEDIA PROGRAM PRODUCT TITLED "CD-ROM TO ACCOMPANY ELECTROTHERAPY: EVIDENCE-BASED PRACTICE ELEVENTH EDITION" ("MULTIMEDIA PROGRAM") TO YOU ONLY ON THE CONDITION THAT YOU ACCEPT ALL OF THE TERMS CONTAINED IN THIS LICENSE AGREEMENT. PLEASE READ THIS LICENSE AGREEMENT CAREFULLY BEFORE OPENING THE SEALED DISK PACKAGE. BY OPENING THAT PACKAGE YOU AGREE TO BE BOUND BY THE TERMS OF THIS AGREEMENT. IF YOU DO NOT AGREE TO THESE TERMS WE ARE UNWILLING TO LICENSE THE MULTIMEDIA PROGRAME TO YOU, AND YOU SHOULD NOT OPEN THE DISK PACKAGE. IN SUCH CASE, PROMPTLY RETURN THE UNOPENED DISK PACKAGE AND ALL OTHER MATERIAL IN THIS PACKAGE, ALONG WITH PROOF OF PAYMENT, TO THE AUTHORISED DEALER FROM WHOM YOU OBTAINED IT FOR A FULL REFUND OF THE PRICE YOU PAID.

2. **Ownership and License.** This is a license agreement and NOT an agreement for sale. It permits you to use one copy of the MULTIMEDIA PROGRAM on a single computer. The MULTIMEDIA PROGRAM and its contents are owned by us or our licensors, and are protected by U.S. and international copyright laws. Your rights to use the MULTIMEDIA PROGRAM are specified in this Agreement, and we retain all rights not expressly granted to you in this Agreement.

- You may use one copy of the MULTIMEDIA PROGRAM on a single computer.
- After you have installed the MULTIMEDIA PROGRAM on your computer, you may use the MULTIMEDIA PROGRAM on a different computer only if you first delete the files installed by the installation program from the first computer.
- You may not copy any portion of the MULTIMEDIA PROGRAM to your computer hard disk or any other media other than printing out or downloading non-substantial portions of the text and images in the MULITMEDIA PROGRAM for your own internal informational use.
- Your may not copy any of the documentation or other printed materials accompanying the MULTIMEDIA PROGRAM.

Neither concurrent use on two or more computers nor use in a local area network or other network is permitted without separate authorisation and the payment of additional license fees.

3. **Transfer and Other Restrictions.** You may not rent, lend, or lease this MULTIMEDIA PROGRAM. Save as permitted by law, you may not and you may not permit others to (a) disassemble, decompile, or otherwise derive source code from the software included in the MULTIMEDIA PROGRAM (the "Software"), (b) reverse engineer the Software, (c) modify or prepare derivative works of the MULTIMEDIA PROGRAM (d) use the Software in an on-line system, or (e) use the MULITMEDIA PROGRAM in any manner that infringes on the intellectual property or other rights of another party.

However, you may transfer this license to use the MULTIMEDIA PROGRAM to another party on a permanent basis by transferring this copy of the License Agreement, the MULTIMEDIA PROGRAM, and all documentation. Such transfer of possession terminates your license from us. Such other party shall be licensed under the terms of this Agreement upon its acceptance of this Agreement by its initial use of the MULTI-MEDIA PROGRAM. If you transfer the MULTIMEDIA PROGRAM, you must remove the installation files from your hard disk and you may not retain any copies of those files for your own use.

4. **Limited Warranty and Limitation of Liability.** For a period of sixty (60) days from the date you acquired the MULTIMEDIA PROGRAM from us or our authorised dealer, we warrant that the media containing the MULTIMEDIA PROGRAM will be free from defects that prevent you from installing the MULTIMEDIA PROGRAM on your computer. If the disk fails to conform to this warranty you may as your sole and exclusive remedy, obtain a replacement free of charge if you return the defective disk to us with a dated proof of purchase. Otherwise the MULTIMEDIA PROGRAM is licensed to you on an "AS IS" basis without any warranty of any nature.

WE DO NOT WARRANT THAT THE MULTIMEDIA PROGRAM WILL MEET YOUR REQUIREMENTS OR THAT ITS OPERATION WILL BE UNINTERRUPTED OR ERROR-FREE. THE EXPRESS TERMS OF THIS AGREEMENT ARE IN LIEU OF ALL WARRANTIES, CONDITIONS, UNDERTAKINGS, TERMS AND OBLIGATIONS IMPLIED BY STATUTE, COMMON LAW, TRADE USAGE, COURSE OF DEALING OR OTHERWISE ALL OF WHICH ARE HEREBY EXCLUDED TO THE FULLEST EXTENT PERMITTED BY LAW, INCLUDING THE IMPLIED WARRANTIES OF SATISFACTORY QUALITY AND FITNESS FOR A PARTICULAR PURPOSE.

WE SHALL NOT BE LIABLE FOR ANY DAMAGE OR LOSS OF ANY KIND (EXCEPT PERSONAL INJURY OR DEATH RESULTING FROM OUR NEGLIGENCE) ARISING OUT OF OR RESULTING FROM YOUR POSSESSION OR USE OF THE MULTIMEDIA PROGRAM (INCLUDING DATA LOSS OR CORRUPTION), REGARDLESS OF WHETHER SUCH LIABILITY IS BASED IN TORT, CONTRACT OR OTHERWISE AND INCLUDING, BUT NOT LIMITED TO, ACTUAL, SPECIAL, INDIRECT, INCIDENTAL OR CONSEQUENTIAL DAMAGES. IF THE FOREGOING LIMITATION IS HELD TO BE UNENFORCEABLE OUR MAXIMUM LIABILITY TO YOU SHALL NOT EXCEED THE AMOUNT OF THE LICENSE FEE PAID BY YOU FOR THE MULTIMEDIA PROGRAM. THE REMEDIES AVAILABLE TO YOU AGAINST US AND THE LICENSORS OF MATERIALS INCLUDED IN THE MULTIMEDIA PROGRAM ARE EXCLUSIVE.

5. **Termination.** This license and your right to use this MULTIMEDIA PROGRAM automatically terminate if you fail to comply with any provisions of this Agreement, destroy the copy of the MULTIMEDIA PROGRAM in your possession, or voluntarily return the MULTIMEDIA PROGRAM to us. Upon termination you will destroy all copies of the MULTIMEDIA PROGRAM and documentation.

6. **Miscellaneous Provisions.** This Agreement will be governed by and construed in accordance with English law and you hereby submit to the non-exclusive jurisdiction of the English Courts. This is the entire agreement between us relating to the MULTMEDIA PROGRAM, and supersedes any prior purchase order, communications, advertising or representations concerning the contents of this package, No change or modification of this Agreement will be valid unless it is in writing and is signed by us.